HEALTH PLANNING
AND REGULATION
THE DECISION-MAKING PROCESS

HEALTH PLANNING
AND REGULATION
THE DECISION-MAKING PROCESS

Drew Altman

Richard Greene

Harvey M. Sapolsky

AUPHA Press
Washington, D.C.   Ann Arbor, Michigan

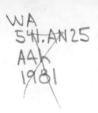

Library of Congress Cataloging in Publication Data

Altman, Drew.
    Health planning and regulation.

    Bibliography: p.
    Includes index.
    1. Health planning—New England. 2. Medical
policy—New England. 3. Health facilities—New
England—Planning. I. Greene, Richard, 1938–
joint author. II. Sapolsky, Harvey M., joint author.
III. Title. [DNLM: 1. Health planning—New England.
2. Facility regulation and control—New England.
WA541 AN25 A4h]
RA395.N44A47   362.1′068   80-23231
ISBN 0-914904-57-4
ISBN 0-914904-58-2 (pbk.)

AUPHA Press is an imprint of Health Administration Press

Health Administration Press
School of Public Health
The University of Michigan
Ann Arbor, Michigan 48109
313-764-1380

Association of University Programs
in Health Administration
One DuPont Circle
Washington, D.C. 20036
202-659-4354

To Pam, Olga, and Karen

Contents

Acknowledgments

This volume is one of the products of a study of health planning and regulation in New England supported by the Department of Health, Education and Welfare. The work was done under contract from the Health Resources Administration to The Codman Research Group, Inc., Contract No. 291-76-0003.

The authors are indebted to a large number of individuals who assisted them throughout the course of this three-year study. In particular it is a pleasure to acknowledge the excellent staff work of Malcolm Curtis, Helen Darling, Cheryl Lurye, Alan Pardini, Jessica Townsend, Sanford Weiner, and Nancy Worthington. We thank Wentworth Boynton III for his technical assistance in the area of nursing home financing. The encouragement and support of our colleagues John Wennberg and Alan Gittelsohn is gratefully acknowledged.

The information developed for this book was derived from many individual interviews with health planners, regulators, and providers of health care. To all those persons who so generously participated in these interviews we wish to extend our most sincere thanks. We also are appreciative of the assistance of HEW staff. In particular we wish to thank Richard Phillips, Anabel Crane, and Daniel Zwick for their guidance and help in this effort.

We benefited from the assistance of staff members of the Maine Health Data Service and the Rhode Island Health Services Research Inc. (SEARCH), organizations which provided us with data on hospital and nursing home utilization and costs in their states. In particular we are indebted to John Putnam and David Soule of the Maine Health Data Service for their invaluable help. The reader should be aware that certain hospital-use data are confidential and, for this reason, we have disguised the names of some hospitals discussed in this book.

Finally we wish to thank Judy Spitzer for her untiring, if somewhat cantankerous, efforts in preparing the final manuscript. It was enjoyable to work with someone who could place health planning and regulation in proper perspective.

Preface

Detailed governmental planning and regulation of medical services are new phenomena in the United States. They are consequences primarily of budgetary problems experienced by federal and state governments since the implementation of Medicaid and Medicare programs in the late 1960s. Whereas government once sought to expand the access to health care services, it now seeks to limit the expenditures incurred in financing health services. Restricting health care facility and equipment expansion is thought to be an effective way to reduce future health benefit expenditures. In this book we describe health planning and regulatory processes in New England as they have evolved under the National Health Planning and Resources Development Act of 1974 (PL 93–641), the most recent in a series of federally created control measures for health care facilities.

The analysis focuses on the decision-making process in health planning and regulation and, more specifically, on how decisions were made in health plan development, Certificate of Need (CON) and Section 1122 reviews and, where present, rate-setting programs. Our findings are based on extensive field work conducted between 1976 and 1979. Most of the observations were made in Maine, Massachusetts, New Hampshire, and Rhode Island. Vermont and Connecticut were studied in less detail. We have conducted more than 700 interviews with individuals active in health delivery, planning and regulation activities in New England. In order to increase our confidence in the accuracy of the information gathered, we sought an interview sample that encompassed the full range of possible perspectives on health facility control and planning. Those interviewed included federal, state, and local health planners, rate setters, politicians, consumers, providers, and staff members of state hospital associations, representatives of community organizations, health insurers, and officials of Professional Standards Review Organizations. To gauge the generalizability of our findings, we have supplemented our observations in New England with interviews in non-New England states (California, Georgia, Florida,

Michigan, Minnesota, and New York among others), with interviews with federal officials and others monitoring national developments, and with analysis of published materials describing health planning and regulation activities throughout the country.

We chose not to be limited by a formal interview questionnaire, but instead to structure our interviews through the use of a topic guide which identified issues to be covered but not the specific questions or their sequence. In order to test what was learned in the interview process, we also conducted a series of case studies in each state. The case studies were developed through reviews of planning files and interviews with knowledgeable participants. Not surprisingly, the case studies raised further questions to pursue in our general study of health planning and regulation in New England. Follow-up interviews were conducted in each state at regular intervals throughout the three-year period in order to monitor changes in the process.

We recognize that the interview/case study methodology has major limitations. We believe, however, that it provides the best (indeed perhaps the only) mechanism for learning how the planning process actually works and how it might be improved. Policies, of course, continue to evolve as circumstances, administrations, and officials change. We feel confident though that the descriptions we present reflect accurately the planning system as it existed through 1979 and the bounds of its likely evolution.

Our work is organized in two parts. The first provides a description and analysis of the key issues in health planning and regulation. In this part we present a synthesis of findings rather than a state-by-state account. The second part consists of a set of complementing case studies that illustrate the range or problems facing planners and regulators and the variety of approaches they employ in solving them.

PART ONE

Health Care
Planning and Regulation:
Opportunities and Constraints

Chapter 1

Introduction

The health planning system established by the National Health Planning and Resource Development Act of 1974 (PL 93-641) has become an integral element in the federal government's regulatory strategy for containing health care costs. To be sure, the planning system also "plans" by involving local health care consumers and providers in a structured dialogue designed to map the road to a more desirable local arrangement of health services, but this is a subsidiary activity to the system's regulatory orientation and one greatly influenced by it. Given federal policies that bound its actions, the prime objective of the planning system has had to be to constrain the growth of local hospitals and nursing homes so as to limit the future cost of health care services. Thus, health planning as it is now practiced is a form of regulation, at times coercive, more often cajolative, but almost always directed toward implementing the new federal health policy doctrine, shared by at least some states, that "less is best" when applied to the capacity to deliver health care services.

This was not always the case. Much of the history of government-sponsored health planning involved attempts to improve the public's access to health services. For example, the first federally supported health planning program, established in 1946 by the Hospital Survey and Construction Act and best known as the Hill-Burton program, was concerned with setting priorities among hospital expansion projects in order to distribute construction subsidies.[1] The belief at the time of the enactment of the Hill-Burton program—and one that persisted through the 1960s—was that the nation faced a shortage in the availability of health services that limited the public's access to these services. Other subsidies to enhance the supply of health services followed, each with its own planning objective and administrative structure. Thus, by the mid-1960s the federal government was subsidizing not only the construction of hospital beds, but also the expansion of medical schools, the training of physicians, nurses, and allied health workers, the establishment of neighborhood health centers, and the diffusion of specialized medical services.

The policy turning point came in the late 1960s, after the passage of the Medicare and Medicaid programs which involved the federal government in the direct financing of health services for the first time and which significantly improved the access to health services of the elderly and the poor, the most medically underserviced groups in the population. A rapid increase in the cost of health services resulted. Soon the government's attention began to focus on cost containment activities.

Table 1.1 shows the increase in per capita expenditures for personal health care services and changes in the contribution of third-party payers that occurred between 1965 and 1977. Because of Medicare and Medicaid, government has become the major financier of health care services in the United States. Although this burden is primarily a federal one, certain state governments have also experienced considerable increases in their health care expenditures during this period.

The 1977 distribution of governmental expenditures for the Medicare and Medicaid programs is listed in Table 1.2. Of the federal expenditures for these programs, overall hospital services accounted for 60.3 percent, physician services 17.5 percent, nursing home services 12.7 percent, and drug and dental services 2.5 percent of the combined expenditures. Medicare, however, is primarily a program for hospital services, while the Medicaid program, for which the federal and state

Table 1.1

Personal Health Care Expenditures Per Capita by Year
with Percent by Payment Source

		Percent Contribution by Payment Source				
					GOVERNMENT	
Year	Per Capita Expenditures	Direct Payment	Private Health Insurance	Philanthropy	Federal	State and Local
1965	$170.32	52.5	24.7	2.0	8.5	12.3
1970	289.76	40.4	24.0	1.5	22.3	11.9
1975	495.80	31.2	26.2	2.2	27.7	12.8
1977	646.11	30.3	27.6	2.0	27.9	12.2

Source: R. M. Gibson and C. R. Fisher, National Health Expenditures, Fiscal Year 1977, *Social Security Bulletin* 41(7):3–20, July, 1978.

Table 1.2

Estimated Expenditures for Medicare and Medicaid,
Fiscal Year 1977,
and Percent of Expenditures by Payment Category

	Total Expenditures X 1,000,000	PERCENT OF EXPENDITURES PAID FOR:				
		Hospital Care	Physician Services	Dentist Services	Drugs	Nursing Homes
Medicare	$21,591	71.9%	20.5	—	—	1.7
Medicaid	17,103	34.9	10.7	2.3	5.9	37.3
State Share	7,389					
Federal Share	9,713					
Federal Expenditures for Medicare and Medicaid (combined)	31,304	60.3	17.5	0.7	1.8	12.7

Source: R. M. Gibson and C. R. Fisher, National Health Expenditures, Fiscal Year 1977, *Social Security Bulletin* 41(6):3–20, July, 1978.

governments share the costs, is significantly oriented toward nursing home services. Thus, federal interest tends to focus on hospital costs while the states have a greater incentive to contain nursing home expenditures.

The rate of increase in total governmental (state and federal) health care expenditures since the passage of the Medicare and Medicaid program has been enormous. Between 1965 and 1970 the annual rate of increase was 21.6 percent. In absolute terms, governmental outlays for health increased from $9.5 billion to $25.4 billion during this period. By 1974, the year in which PL 93–641 was enacted, the total had reached $41.5 billion. It is not surprising then that governments would seek to impose constraints on health care expenditures, especially those which they must absorb. For the federal government this has meant abandoning the Hill-Burton subsidies for hospital construction and adopting ever more antagonistic stances toward the expansion of hospital capacity and costs. The health facility planning system created by PL 93–641 provides a convenient vehicle for expressing at least some of this concern.

The Development of Capital Expenditure Controls

Public policies are rarely consistent or well coordinated. Certainly in the health area government has worked against itself by pursuing conflicting policy objectives. Thus, despite an announced desire to restrain capital growth in the health sector, and despite the termination of Hill-Burton construction grants, the federal government still provides incentives for hospital expansion. One way it does this is by offering several types of subsidized loans for hospital renovations and construction. Among the agencies sponsoring such loans are the Federal Housing Administration (FHA), the Small Business Administration (SBA), the Economic Development Administration (EDA), and the Farmers Home Administration (FHA), all of which hold authority independent of the former Department of Health, Education and Welfare (HEW). Another is by reimbursing Medicare and Medicaid hospital service providers on the basis of their incurred costs rather than their standard charges. With cost-based reimbursements, hospitals have an incentive to expand their capital base for they are essentially assured payment for invested capital irrespective of its source or productivity. (Blue Cross is also a cost-based payer so that in 1974 nearly 60 percent of hospital reimbursements in the United States were cost-based).[2]

Hospitals clearly have responded to these incentives. Table 1.3 lists the increases in hospital plant assets that occurred after the start of the Medicare and Medicaid programs. It should be noted that the level of hospital capital formation accelerated after 1970 when the ratio of acute hospital beds per 1,000 population in the United States passed 4/1000, the ratio now believed appropriate.

State governments were the first to counteract the rapid increase in health sector capital investments. The budgetary pressures of rising Medicaid utilization and expense were soon felt by the state governments. Beginning in the 1960s, the most hard pressed among them began enacting Certificate of Need (CON) laws that required governmental approval of major capital investments by hospitals and nursing homes.

The initial federal effort to control the growth in health sector capacity as a means of containing its own health care costs was the "1122" program which was included among the 1972 amendments to the Social Security Act. Similar to CON, the 1122 program requires hospitals and nursing homes to submit major capital project proposals for state review and approval. But state participation in the program is voluntary, necessitating a formal contractual arrangement between HEW and state agencies for the performance of the reviews before the controls take effect. Moreover, the 1122 penalties are weaker than those of CON laws. Projects denied approval under 1122 procedures are

Table 1.3

Change in Hospital Plant Assets
1964–1977

Year	Plant Assets ($ millions)	Increase In Actual Dollars ($ millions)	Increase In Constant 1972 Dollars* ($ millions)
1964	8,217		
1965	9,078	861	1,333
1966	9,752	674	1,000
1967	10,457	705	1,001
1968	11,490	1,033	1,402
1969	12,523	1,033	1,283
1970	13,783	1,260	1,433
1971	15,529	1,746	1,844
1972	17,007	1,478	1,478
1973	18,945	1,938	1,796
1974	20,963	2,018	1,590
1975	24,005	3,042	2,198
1976	26,827	2,822	2,045
1977	30,455	3,628	2,485

*Implicit price deflator—nonresidential building construction—Department of Commerce—Bureau of Economic Analysis.

Source: American Hospital Association, *Hospital Statistics 1978*.

ineligible for Medicare and Medicaid interest and depreciation reimbursements, usually a less severe sanction than the legal barriers to construction that occur upon CON denial.[3]

In 1974, when the future structure of the national health planning system was being considered, half of the states were still without stringent capital controls. Twenty-one states relied solely on the 1122 program while another five lacked even that level of restraint on health sector capital expansion. Recognizing the weakness of the 1122 sanctions, HEW pressed the inclusion in PL 93–641 of a requirement that all states adopt a CON program by 1980. The HEW proposal became part of the new planning law, thus making CON the preferred national instrument for limiting health sector expansion.[4]

The 93-641 Planning System

PL 93-641 mandated the delineation of health service areas in each state and the creation of a Health Systems Agency (HSA)*, generally a nonprofit entity whose governing board must have a consumer majority and a membership economically and socially representative of its area.†[5] Approximately 205 health service areas have been delineated, a dozen being statewide in coverage and another dozen convened by interstate compacts. Under the CON provisions of the planning law, the HSAs review applications for permission to make capital investments filed by health care institutions, passing their recommendations on to a state-level CON decision making body. States are required to designate State Health Planning and Development Agencies (SHPDAs) with the responsibility of coordinating health planning at the state level. Most often the SHPDAs are also the CON decision-making bodies or serve as staff to a gubernatorily appointed council which makes the final CON decisions. Each HSA prepares a health plan which is combined into a draft state health plan by the SHPDA. The final approval of the State Health Plan resides in a gubernatorially appointed State Health Coordinating Council (SHCC), 60 percent of whose members are selected on nomination of the state's HSAs. Unlike previous planning efforts, which permitted health care providers to absorb a substantial share of the expenses, nearly the entire cost of the planning system is borne by taxpayers and the private contributions allowed are carefully specified.[6]

The law appears to have broad goals and to give much responsibility to the HSAs. Their mandate lists the following ambitious tasks:

(1) improving the health of residents of a health service area.
(2) increasing the accessibility (including overcoming geographic, architectural, and transportation barriers), acceptability, continuity, and quality of the health services provided them.
(3) restraining increases in the cost of providing them health services, and
(4) preventing unnecessary duplication of health resources. . . .[7]

In reality, though, the power the law confers is narrowly focused, confined primarily to the state agencies, and directed almost entirely

*Rhode Island and Hawaii are not required to have HSAs.

†Local governments are eligible to be designated HSAs, as are public regional planning bodies. Of the 205 HSAs, 180 are nonprofit, nongovernmental organizations.

toward the regulation of health sector capital investments. It is the exercise of this regulatory function that is of most interest to health care providers who, after all is said, are the ultimate planners of the nation's health care system.

Health Planning in the Context of the New Regulatory Strategy

The health planning agencies do not operate as isolated regulatory bodies, but rather are a part of government-created entities engaging in containing the cost of health (primarily hospital) care. In addition to capital controls applied through the planning structure, regulation of two other aspects of hospital operations emerged in the early 1970s: the control of inappropriate use of hospital beds by Medicare and Medicaid patients and the control of the rate of increase of hospital (and also nursing home) budgets. If fully implemented and coordinated, these programs, in combination with capital investment controls, could result in an effective regulatory strategy to contain certain, but not all, increases in health care costs.

Regulation of inappropriate hospital use by federally financed patients is mandated through a section of PL 92–603, the 1972 act which authorized the development of 200 local physician corporations termed Professional Standards Review Organizations (PSROs). PSROs are to review all admissions and hospital stays of Medicare and Medicaid patients and certify the appropriateness of bed use as a precondition of payment for service,[8] such review to take place at the time of admission (concurrent review) to avoid retroactive denial of payments to the hospitals and other health care providers. Although PSROs have the additional charge of improving the quality of hospital services provided to federal patients, to date the great bulk of their resources have been expended on the cost control aspect of the program.

Hospital budget controls have existed in some states since the 1960s. Nine states currently operate programs that regulate the rate of increase in hospital budgets, generally termed rate setting.[9] Although the Carter Administration failed to obtain enactment of a national hospital budget control program in both the Ninety-fifth and Ninety-sixth Congresses, it continues to place high priority on the passage of such a bill.

It should be emphasized that all current health regulatory programs focus on institutional medical services. Local and state regulatory agencies have little influence over physician manpower production and distribution. Given current doctrines in health economics which hold that physicians have a high degree of control over the demand for medical and hospital services, it is becoming clear that a regulatory strategy aimed solely at institutions will have limited effect on overall health care costs as long as the physician manpower pool continues to expand.[10]

Only the most naive among us can expect that government will soon implement the integrated and comprehensive policies needed to control health care costs. Policy makers must be content with simpler aspirations: seeking to discover, before great damage is done, the extent to which current programs make things worse and hoping to achieve the legislative corrections needed to keep policies headed in the correct direction.

In this book we describe our observations of the effectiveness of the health facilities planning system established by PL 93-641. In doing so we have tried to keep in mind the political environment in which programs must operate so as not to be utopian in our expectations. Not surprisingly, we were driven to make an analysis of that environment a central feature of our work.

Our observations took place in the six New England states, and primarily within Maine, Massachusetts, New Hampshire, and Rhode Island. Within Massachusetts, a state with six HSAs, we have concentrated on the Metropolitan Boston and Central Massachusetts (Worcester) HSAs. It is to a description of these areas that we turn next.

Notes

[1] Judith R. Lave and Lester B. Lave, *The Hospital Construction Act: An Evaluation of the Hill-Burton Program, 1948-1973* (Washington, D.C.: American Enterprise Institute for Public Policy Research, 1974).

[2] The precise figures for 1972 are as follows: Blue Cross, $6,501 million; Medicare, $5,835 million; Medicaid, $2,557 million; Total Hospital Expenditures for non-Federal Short Term Hospital Care, $25,549 million.

[3] Lewin and Associates, Inc., *Evaluation of the Efficiency and Effectiveness of the Section 1122 Review Process* (Washington, D.C.: Lewin, 1975).

[4] Section 1521 9(d), PL 93-641. The planning law does not mandate a CON program; it only threatens noncomplying states with the loss of all federal funds for planning, and public health activities, alcohol rehabilitation, and mental health services.

[5] A detailed description of the mechanics of the 1974 planning system is available in Steven Sieverts, *Health Planning Issues and Public Law 93-641* (Chicago:

American Hospital Association, 1977). See also Stanley H. Werlin, Alexandra Walcott, and Michael Joroff, "Implementing Formative Health Planning Under PL 93-641," *New England Journal of Medicine* (September 23, 1976), pp. 698–702, and Herbert H. Hyman, editor, *Health Regulation: Certificate of Need and 1122* (Germantown, MD: Aspen Systems, 1977).

6 The financing of HSAs is discussed in Elsa R. Kelberg, *et al., An Analysis and Assessment of Non-Federal Funding of HSAs,* Final Report HRP-0900002, JRB Associates, McLean, VA, 1977.

7 Section 1513, PL 93-641.

8 PSROs are required also to review the appropriateness of admission and length of stay of Title V (Maternal and Child Health Program) patients, but payment for service to these patients is not tied to PSRO certification.

9 In a number of other states Blue Cross performs a similar rate review on its member hospitals.

10 *The Supply of Health Manpower; 1970 Profiles and Projections to 1990* (Washington, D.C.: BHRD/HRA, 1974).

Chapter 2

The New England Setting

The variety of approaches to health planning and regulation adopted by New England states range from near abstinence to some of the most stringent CON and rate-setting programs in the nation. In describing the implementation of PL 93-641 in New England three factors are of particular importance: the state of development of the health care industry, the per capita costs for health care (and specifically, the Medicaid burden carried by the state government) and, perhaps most important, the political attitude of the state government toward regulation of industry in general and the health care industry in particular.

Based on these factors, there appear to be two clusters among the New England states. The three northern states (Maine, New Hampshire, and Vermont), more rural in character, generally have less sophisticated health care facilities, carry a smaller per capita Medicaid burden, and demonstrate a greater reluctance to regulate. In contrast, the three southern states (Massachusetts, Connecticut, and Rhode Island) generally have more sophisticated facilities, higher medical costs, larger Medicaid expenses per capita, and governments more inclined to intervene in the operations of private sector institutions be they in the health sector or not.

Table 2.1 lists selected health resources statistics for New England. Massachusetts provides the most costly care and New Hampshire the least costly. Massachusetts has the largest number of physicians per capita and Maine the least. Vermont and Maine have the largest hospital-bed-to-population ratios while Connecticut and Rhode Island have the smallest. But the table cannot convey well the variations in service availability and quality that exist among the states. The three southern New England states, with their larger cities, tend to possess extremely sophisticated medical facilities. Massachusetts and Connecticut, in particular, have institutions with worldwide reputations, such as

Table 2.1

Selected Health Resource Statistics
For New England States

	CT	ME	MA	NH	RI	VT
Number of hospitals*	40	40	127	29	14	16
Bed/1,000 population	3.5	4.8	4.5	4.3	3.7	4.8
Admissions/1,000	134	163	152	157	137	156
Patient days/1,000	1,010	1,227	1,293	1,110	1,114	1,312
Hospital expenditures/capita	$247	$229	$350	$189	$262	$207
Nursing care beds/1,000 residents over 65 years old†	60	51	57	62	51	56
Physicians per 100,000‡	178	113	186	135	162	162

*Acute hospital statistics are taken from *Hospital Statistics*, American Hospital Association, from their 1977 survey. All figures are for short-term nonfederal hospitals. Utilization and expenditure rates are not true rates, since the numerator includes hospitalizations of out-of-state residents and lacks data on out-of-state hospitalizations for state residents. These figures are, however, useful approximations for comparative purposes.

†*Health Resources Statistics*, Health Manpower and Health Facilities 1976–1977, National Center for Health Statistics.

‡All ratios are for patient care physicians. From HRA staff-personal communication; based on 1976 AMA Survey. Total U.S. rate = 174 patient care/physicians/100,000 population.

the Massachusetts General Hospital, the Peter Bent Brigham Hospital, the Lahey Clinic, Massachusetts Eye and Ear Infirmary, Children's Hospital, and Yale-New Haven Hospital. Boston alone has three of the region's ten medical schools, with two others less than 50 miles away in Worcester and Providence.

Medicaid expenditure variations are reported in Table 2.2 Massachusetts offers the most expensive coverage, more than double the per capita cost of New Hampshire's program. Rhode Island lags behind Massachusetts by only five dollars on a per capita basis. Because the federal contribution in Connecticut is the lowest in New England, that state's quite modest program costs its taxpayers an amount nearly comparable to that borne by the taxpayers of Massachusetts and Rhode Island. New Hampshire's program is both the most heavily weighted toward nursing home care and the least expensive.

The governments of the New England states also have differed sharply in their propensity to regulate the cost and distribution of health care services. Again the contrast is basically between the northern tier and southern tier states.

Until recently, at least, it was clear that the Massachusetts state

Table 2.2

Selected Medicaid Statistics, New England

	CT	ME	MA	NH	RI	VT
Total Medicaid Expenditures per capita	$71	$80	$122	$54	$117	$86
State share per capita	$36	$24	$ 58	$20	$ 50	$28
Percent expenditure for:						
Acute hospitals	26%	25%	36%	20%	37%	21%
Long-term care	49%	45%	38%	56%	40%	40%
Physician service	6%	14%	6%	9%	4%	13%

Source: Medicaid Statistics Fiscal Year 1977; HCFA, April, 1978. Per capita expenditure rates are based on total state population figures for 1975, Bureau of the Census.

government offered hospital and nursing home providers one of the toughest regulatory environments in the nation in which to operate. State regulation of provider costs and charges began in 1968 and was made progressively more stringent. A CON program (known in Massachusetts as the Determination of Need Program) was put in place in 1971, three years before Congress passed the law encouraging the diffusion of this type of health sector regulation and a year before the weaker 1122 controls became part of the Social Security Act. The persons appointed to regulatory posts by Governors Francis Sargent (R 1970-1975) and Michael Dukakis (D 1975-1979) were never considered friendly toward the industry, and some cultivated just the opposite image. The election of Governor Edward King (D), an avowed opponent of governmental intervention in the economy, has, however, raised expectations that major changes in the administration of state regulatory programs, including those affecting health care providers, are possible.

Rhode Island's regulation of health facility investments began harmoniously enough in 1966 as an industry-initiated effort supported by state government and conducted through a voluntary, nonprofit Health Planning Council composed of the representatives of the state's major health provider groups. The Council's work was buttressed in 1970 with the enactment of a certificate of need program that formally involved state government in the industry's planning activities. Two years later, following the denial of a Blue Cross rate increase request by the state, all of Rhode Island's hospitals agreed to participate with the state government's budget office in an experimental prospective reimbursement program. So as not to disturb this apparently cooperative environment, Rhode Island, with provider support, requested and gained an exemption from the basic organizational requirements of the federal health planning act passed in 1974. All authority and responsibilities of PL 93-641 were, as a result, vested in the State Department of Health. (There is no HSA in Rhode Island.) The Department strengthened its already considerable role in health planning and facilities review while the voluntary Health Planning Council lost much of its previous importance. Providers are now beginning to demonstrate concern over the increased power state government has in Rhode Island.

Connecticut also has imposed tough controls on health care providers, but only since Governor Ella Grasso (D) took office in 1976. Three years earlier the legislature had enacted rate-setting and CON programs, placing administrative responsibility for both in a single agency, the Commission on Hospitals and Health Care. Governor Grasso appointed an experienced health care regulator from Rhode Island to head the Commission. His emphasis on rate regulation has precipitated conflict with the state's health care providers and the State Department of Health which, independent of the Commission, holds responsibility for the coordination of health planning activities and whose constituency is Connecticut's five HSAs.

The three northern New England states are all states with a single HSA, and many of their health planning efforts to date have been absorbed in sorting out the relevant organizational jurisdictions.[1] In Vermont, for example, the governor delayed full implementation of PL 93–641 for several years in the hope of obtaining a waiver from HEW of the requirement for establishing an HSA. Failing that, Vermont has commingled the staffs of the HSA and SHPDA and utilized a single board of directors for both the HSA and SHCC, clear reflections of the persistent desires of state officials to avoid the creation of a health planning unit operationally independent of state government. It is only within the last year that attention has begun to focus on the application of investment controls.

Maine has been the scene of an acrimonious dispute between the HSA and state officials managing the SHPDA over the relative roles of the agencies and the appropriate philosophy for health sector regulation. While state officials initially concentrated on strengthening the 1122 review process for acute care hospitals, the HSA staff sought both co-equal status in directing health planning activities and more rigorous review procedures for nursing home and ambulatory care projects. Personality conflicts further complicated the relations between the agencies. At one point in the dispute the state even considered opposing the renewal of the HSA's charter. Pressed apparently by rising health

benefit costs, state officials did, however, begin to seek an accommodation. Both a CON program and a voluntary rate-setting arrangement were instituted in 1978. The election that year of a new governor
seems to have resolved the dispute, as he has placed the former director
of the HSA in charge of the SHPDA.

New Hampshire's state government has lagged behind those of
Maine and Vermont in its willingness to control health sector
expansion. The administration of Governor Meldrin Thomson (R
1975–1979), in particular, was especially unsympathetic to the notions
of federal guidance, consumer participation, and formal planning embodied in PL 93–641. As a result, it maintained an openly antagonistic
attitude toward the HSA and failed to utilize fully the regulatory
powers vested in the designated state agency by the law. Personality
conflicts, as in Maine, exacerbated the strained relations between the
HSA and the SHPDA. It is uncertain, though, whether or not the new
governor will move to alter the situation, given the apparent popularity
of laissez-faire doctrines in New Hampshire.

Table 2.3 records the year of enactment of CON and rate-setting
programs in New England. The question is how effectively have they
been implemented? We begin this analysis by describing the stances
various participants have assumed toward these programs and health
regulation in general.

Table 2.3

Regulatory Programs of the New England States,
Year of Enactment or Establishment

	1122 Agreement	Certificate of Need	Rate Setting
Connecticut	—	1973	1973
Maine	1973	1978	1978 (Voluntary Program)
Massachusetts	—	1971	1968
New Hampshire	1973	1979	—
Rhode Island	—	1970	1972
Vermont	1975	1979	—

Note

[1] For a discussion of the problems that have developed in one HSA state see U.S. General Accounting Office, *Status of the Implementation of the National Health Planning and Resource Development Act of 1974*, HRD-77-157, November 2, 1978, and *Study of Single HSA States and Section 1536 States*, Arthur D. Little, Inc., Cambridge, MA, Contract No. HRP-0900117, 1978.

Chapter 3

Providers

Assessments of the health planning system are contradictory. On the one hand, there are those who believe that the planning system serves only the interests of health care providers—primarily hospitals, nursing homes, and physicians.[1] On the other hand, there are those who believe that the planning system has been a useful mechanism for controlling health care costs and thus for serving the public interest.[2] These assessments parallel the contending evaluations of the efficacy of government regulation of industry in general, evaluations in which regulation is portrayed as either being invariably captured by the regulated industry or as providing necessary and effective protection for the public against the economic consequences of imperfect markets.[3]

Advocates of the capture theory argue that regulation protects the regulated, not the public, from the rigors of competition, creating market imperfections where none existed. The regulated industry uses instruments of governmental authority to limit competition within the industry and to blockade entry of potential competitors in order to increase profits. Whether or not industry is the instigator of the initial regulatory effort matters not at all, for invariably it is the beneficiary of regulation. Thus comes the cynic's advice that no industry should pass by the opportunity to be regulated.[4] The costs of regulation, though potentially quite large, are not noticed by consumers since each consumer bears only a small part of the burden.[5]

Applied to the health care industry, the capture theory holds that providers use the powers of the planning law for their own ends. Certificate of need regulation gives hospitals and nursing homes an essentially protected franchise. Limits on expansion are used to block the entry of potential competitors, yet existing providers can gain approval for most, if not all, of the new equipment and service changes they desire by using arguments about enhancing quality. Health insurance and government health care subsidies absorb the cost of the local inefficiencies such a regulatory system produces while hiding their ultimate cause from the public.[6]

Adherents of a public interest theory of regulation argue that regulation can be effective in protecting consumers from firms seeking to exercise their overwhelming power when markets fail. Without regulation certain (usually poor) consumers would not be served, prices would be higher, and the quality of goods and services would deteriorate. Regulation redistributes power, strengthening consumers in their dealings with firms unconstrained by market forces.[7]

According to the proponents of the health care planning system, PL 93–641 does effectively compensate for the nonexistent and largely unobtainable market in health care services. Certificate of need regulation in particular prevents some, though of course not all, wasteful duplication of facilities that is fostered by the subsidies that insurance and government provide to health care consumers. Billions of dollars in needless construction costs, equipment purchases, and operating expenses have been avoided, they claim, because of the regulatory constraints placed on the expansion plans of health care providers, billions which ultimately would have been paid by consumers through higher taxes or lower purchasing power. And, they argue, all this has been achieved with no noticeable diminution in the access to services and with some enhancement of quality.[8]

We take a different position. We believe the planning system as legislated is an evolving charter between two conflicting forces, both of which stand to realize important gains or losses through its particular configuration and both of which have major internal divisions.[9] The contending forces are the institutional providers of health care services, especially hospitals but also nursing homes, and the government, especially the federal government, which carries an increasing share of national health care costs. On the provider side there are divisions among hospitals with different types of ownership and different types of services and among different types of physicians and other health care specialists. On the government side there are divisions between the advocates of markets and increased regulation, and among the various levels and branches of government.

The legislative framework for planning, the charter which records what level of government will hold what amount of regulatory authority and who will or will not be regulated, is the product of bargaining within and between the contending forces. Providers seek to have rivals restricted and their own freedom of action protected. The federal government seeks to limit its own health benefit costs while not doing too much violence to other cherished objectives. Each side knows that the particular bargain struck is subject both to adjustments in practice and to subsequent legislation. No one among the participants can expect to capture the resulting system totally or believes that the public interest will be harmed if their side gets the best of the bargain.

In this chapter we describe briefly the evolution of the planning system and its current balance. We examine in detail the cleavages among providers that enhance the government's opportunities to extract benefits from the planning system and the strategies providers use to protect themselves individually from the exercise of regulatory controls over their plans for expansion and, at times, their very survival.

The Evolution of Health Planning

The conflict between the institutional providers of health care services and certain financiers of health care is clearly evident in the history of American health planning efforts.[10] The initial impetuses for planning came both from hospitals and from philanthropic and business donors who supported local efforts to acquire major health facilities and who helped pay for the care of the poor before these tasks became largely governmental. The hospitals sought the benefits of cartelization while donors sought to protect themselves from the insatiable demands of medical care providers.

The Great Depression sharpened these interests as it stripped many Americans of the resources to pay for their own care. Private nonprofit hospitals organized both to create insurance mechanisms for spreading the financial risks of illness and to encourage government to absorb the burdens of caring for the destitute, either through the direct provision of services in public hospitals (as happened in some cities) or by means of welfare grants available more broadly. In communities such as Pittsburgh and Rochester where civic leadership was strong and wealthy donors organized to rationalize the system for providing care and particularly for requesting support to renew or expand the investment in health care capital.[11]

The economic strains of the Great Depression followed by the Second World War caused most communities to postpone the replacement of aging hospital plants and equipment. The geographic spread of population and its urbanization also created a need for the construction of new hospitals by the end of the war, as did the belief that public works projects were the only way to employ a demobilized army. Thus it was easy to conceive of the Hill-Burton Program, the federal government's first major venture into the financing of privately provided health care and a precursor of much more. The happy task was the expansion of hospital facilities and it was endorsed both by provider groups and civic leaders.[12]

Within two decades government came to supplant private charity as the prime source for health care capital. The supremacy of government as the benefactor for hospitals was marked by the passage of the Medicare and Medicaid programs in 1965. Soon government, like private charity before it, was seeking ways to constrain the appeals of health care providers for new facilities. The conflict between hospitals and their financial guardians was now largely one between hospitals and the federal government.

Health care providers, hospitals among them, had benefited greatly from the government programs that followed the Hill-Burton Program even though they at times offered stout resistance to their enactment. Government moved from subsidizing the supply of health services to direct subsidization of the purchase of health services. The public resources made available for use by the private sector were without parallel in domestic affairs. The role of private charity and civic benefactors in controlling the local distribution of health services declined rapidly as the federal government became the major financier of health care services.

Subsequent federal interest in planning was to ensure that services were quickly and evenly distributed to meet the growth in demand which its service and supply subsidies generated. The Regional Medical Program was established in 1965 to diffuse advances in diagnosis and treatment for major diseases achieved in research. Through this program, assistance was provided to aid the growth of voluntary agreements among medical schools, hospitals, and research institutions for the dissemination of medical knowledge.[13] The next year saw the passage of the Comprehensive Health Planning Program which offered grants for state and local planning efforts and the training of health planning professionals.[14] By the early 1970s, however, both of these programs had been converted to efforts intended to control by resource rationalization the growth of health care facilities in line with emerging federal priorities.[15]

The Comprehensive Health Planning Program, in particular, marks the beginning of the contest between the providers and the federal government over the design of the regulatory system for the allocation of health care capital. The program in essence federalized the pre-existing local planning agencies, though new ones were created where none had existed before and a new layer of state planning agencies known as "a" agencies (after a section in the enabling legislation) was established. With it the federal government had acquired a framework for involving itself in the decisions guiding the development of local health care facilities.

Federal legislation followed, with the purpose of using the regulatory framework to limit the duplication of medical facilities. A 1967 amendment to the Public Health Service Act required state "a" agencies to assist hospitals in developing plans for capital expenditures. Another amendment in 1970 mandated that grant applications for health services development assistance be reviewed by local planning agencies. And in the 1972 amendments to the Social Security Act, a voluntary, state-administered program was created which would deny Medicare, Medicaid, and Maternal and Child Health reimbursements for depreciation, interest or return on equity for capital expenditures in excess of $100,000 made by health facilities that were not approved by state health planners.[16]

The ability of the federal government to use the planning system effectively for regulatory purposes, however, was frustrated by the fact that health care providers tended to dominate the system. Hospital associations and insurers financed most of the cost of the local planning agencies. Hospital administrators and physicians usually constituted a majority of the local board members. State politics often permitted provider associations to control the policies of the state agencies. Despite the federal government's growing interest in regulating capital finances, little regulation actually occurred.[17] Thus, when the legislative authority for the Comprehensive Health Planning Program, the Hill-Burton Program, and the Regional Medical Program expired in 1974, the administration sought their consolidation into a more easily manipulated arrangement.

Health planning was not a priority concern for national provider associations in 1974. The implementing regulations for the Professional Standards Review Organizations were being debated then, as were major changes in the federal financing of health manpower training and the outlines of the program to promote health maintenance organizations as a mechanism for restructuring delivery of health services in the United States. At the same time there was the threat of renewal of the rate control which had been established under the Economic Stabilization Program and which had been continued for health care providers a year longer than for other industries. In addition, everyone in Washington was diverted by the culmination of the Watergate crisis.

Hospital and physician lobbyists made certain that the planning legislation did not contain any new powers, blocking attempts to include proposed provisions for rate setting and recertification of health care facilities.[18] Once these goals were achieved they tended to ignore the bills. A restructuring of the planning system held little interest for their associations since the resulting arrangements would still remain locally based and be limited in scope and authority. Their view of legislation was apparently confirmed by a Senate staff member who was quoted as saying that without a recertification provision the legislation would be "an industry protection bill."[19]

Yet important changes in the planning system were achieved with the enactment of PL 93–641. The federal government, not providers, would finance the planning system. Local boards were required to have consumer majorities. The definition of provider representation was broadened to include other health care professionals beyond hospital representatives, physicians, and nursing home administrators. The federal government was authorized to establish guidelines for health plans which the local agencies and the states were mandated to produce. And states were required to implement CON programs to strengthen the regulation of capital expenditures for health care facilities and equipment. Because of these changes the regulation of health care capital has evolved into a competition for allies among consumers and state governments between the federal government and providers. What was once a system dominated by providers is now a more indeterminate and conflictual arrangement. It is not surprising that provider associations have had second thoughts about the value of the system.[20]

Provider Cleavages

If health care providers were united they could easily fend off federal attempts to regulate their capital expenditures. Certificate of need reviews are case-by-case analyses of the medical need for health care capital projects, both renovations and additions. Providers are perceived by the public to be the experts in determining medical need. They are, after all, medical professionals. Their unified opposition to any standard of need the federal government might seek to impose on project review decisions would likely be decisive. Certainly state and local agencies would have great difficulty sustaining actions that sought to limit the acquisition of medical facilities and equipment in the face of unamimous professional judgments to the contrary. The deference afforded to medical authorities by society is too great to expect otherwise.

Health care providers are united in the belief that capital regulation, if it is to take place, is best done on the local level and is best when locally directed. This is the often-stated preference for "bottom up" planning. The decentralized structure of national provider organizations requires such a stance as does the general perception that providers, though of great influence in Washington, will fare better in the hands of state and local, rather than national, regulators. The more locally based the regulation, the more likely that the regulators will have the choice of saying yes or no to their own doctor or hospital administrator.

But at the local level providers are sharply divided. This is due in part to the franchising nature of the regulation that is being attempted. Existing providers seek to protect the growth opportunities for themselves. Market shares are at stake when certificates of need are being decided. Thus the hospitals serving growing populations in the suburbs to the west of Boston opposed vigorously the application made by the Lahey Clinic to relocate its facilities in Burlington and the decision of the Harvard Community Health Plan to open a HMO unit in Wellesley. If there are opportunities for new services the existing franchise holders seek to claim them. Certainly they do not wish their territories invaded by aggressive new competitors.

There are, however, other reasons for divisions among providers. The definition of provider was broadened when PL 93–641 was enacted to include allied health professional and noninstitutional health care providers. The HSAs not only must allocate board and committee seats to physicians, hospital and nursing home representatives, but also to nurses, dentists, optometrists, home health care specialists, and HMO representatives who either compete with the more established professions and institutions for clients and/or who are disdainful of their authority and prestige. In Rhode Island, for example, osteopathic physicians have demanded that a separate category of "osteopathic need" be established for capital expenditure review. In Maine, the state health plan was attacked as not devoting sufficient attention to the service skills of chiropractors and alcoholic rehabilitation specialists. Gone is the time when provider interests could be judged as being coterminous with the interests of allopathic physicians and the hospitals in which they held affiliations. Providers in general may hold up to 49 percent representation on HSA boards and committees, but physicians and hospital administrators do not.

Provider associations are beset by internal cleavages and are challenged by competing organizations. The state hospital association must contend with its rural hospital members as well as its major tertiary care center members. Physicians affiliated with medical schools or neighborhood clinics may not be happy with the pronouncements of the medical society. Nursing home representation is often divided between a proprietary association and a nonprofit association. Optometrists oppose the dominance of ophthalmologists, and both are well-organized.

In Maine, for example, the three largest hospitals—The Maine Medical Center, Eastern Maine Medical Center, and Mid-Maine Medical Center—have formed an alliance that is viewed with great suspicion by other hospitals, especially by Central Maine Medical Center in Lewiston, the next largest hospital in the state. The fear is that these hospitals have agreed to divide major medical opportunities among themselves, excluding others from early access to approval for advanced services and equipment.

A final important division among local providers is the split between public and private care delivery. City and state hospitals worry about the competition for patients in an era when most of their traditional clients are eligible for government subsidies to obtain private care. Private providers in turn are concerned about the exemptions from certificate of need given Veterans Administration (VA) and other federal hospitals, and the political protection available to city- and state-supported institutions. The University Hospital in Worcester, part of the University of Massachusetts for example, successfully evaded CON review by the local HSA for over a year while private hospitals could not. VA representatives sit in judgment over the applications of private providers while their own expansion or modernization plans are not subject to local or state approvals.

These cleavages among providers make them more vulnerable to regulation than would otherwise be the case. At the national level providers usually can agree to oppose attempts to extend federal regulatory jurisdiction. Thus the American Medical Association, the Council of Community Hospitals, the American Federation of Hospitals and several other groups oppose federal proposals for mandatory revenue controls and a capital cap. But at the local level the conflicts among and within provider groups permit the exercise of regulatory authority already gained and even the implementation of federal standards so apparently distasteful to providers.

Regulation is like every other environmental factor affecting competition among institutions; it provides opportunities for individual gains as well as losses.[21] Although philosophical opposition to regulation is frequently expressed, local competitors can see advantages in its exercise against current or potential rivals. Division among providers prevents their unified action against regulation, especially when specific awards or denials are at issue. Individual providers face the threat of regulation on their own, knowing that others may rejoice in any misfortune which may befall them and that none will risk their future opportunities by coming to their aid.

Provider Strategies

Although local provider associations will be forced into neutrality when specific regulatory actions are being considered, providers need not meet their regulators naked. Available to them are a wide range of specialists—accountants, lawyers, construction managers, equipment salesmen, and consultants—who count among their expertise the ability to foil regulators. Moreover hospitals and nursing homes are increasingly being absorbed by chains or are contracting for management services, where the specific advantages of group affiliation are the skills gained in dealing with regulators.[22] Regulation encourages consolidation among the regulated and the growth of counter expertise.[23]

Regulation also strengthens the position of administrators within health care institutions. Even if outside assistance is sought to help keep regulators at bay, there is a need for inside knowledge of potential regulatory threats and the methods for dealing with them. Administrators have the time to become knowledgeable about regulation and can use their knowledge to assert their importance within the organization. Although physicians may still dominate within hospitals and boards of directors hold legal responsibility for major decisions, their power is eroded by regulation and the need for specialized knowledge to cope with it. Administrators, not surprisingly, may be advocates for increased regulation or find it useful to emphasize its increasing threat.[24]

Whether or not the threat of regulation is exaggerated, strategies have been devised to cope with it. Below we describe coping strategies we know to have been utilized.

The Data Overload Strategy

An important advantage a health care institution most often has over its regulators is its medical expertise and ability to assemble and manipulate complicated data. Thus when challenged by a regulatory agency a health facility may opt to flood the agency with technical data apparently justifying its position. The need for expansion, for example, may be supported with elaborate analyses of utilization experience which may or may not be relevant, but which can easily impress the uninitiated. One hospital administrator we interviewed arrived fresh from an encounter with a HSA and was still chuckling over the mound of data he had presented their project review committee. He was particularly amused by a consumer representative on the committee who had asked to take home a copy of the computerized report he had presented so that she could check its calculations at her leisure.[25]

The Litigation Strategy

Another advantage a health care institution has is the opportunity to litigate. The courts are available for the appeal of most regulatory decisions and are extremely sensitive to procedural errors which infringe upon due process rights. Regulators, eager for quick and significant changes in the health care industry, can easily stumble over requirements for proper notice, public hearings and the opportunity for a full consideration of the issues. Often regulators lack the resources for proper legal representation or must rely on state legal staffs inexpert in health affairs. The standards regulators adopt are rarely scientifically based and thus are vulnerable to judicial scrutiny.

The Connecticut rate-setting commission achieved quick success in controlling hospital costs only to fall victim to suits brought by nearly all of the state's 36 hospitals. The court found the commission's actions in the lead case to be "illegal, unconstitutional, and arbitrary" and required that they be done over. In its desire to control hospital costs, the commission had, in the court's view, ignored the necessity for fair regulatory rulemaking imposed by the state's administrative practices statute including the holding of hearings, publication of standards, collection of evidence, and the preparation of an adequate record.[26] Other jurisdictions such as Massachusetts have been kinder to regulators than Connecticut, but the threat of legal challenge remains an effective strategy for providers as it forces regulators to be cautious or face the likelihood that their decisions will not survive judicial review.

The frustrations the legal process holds for regulators are seen clearly in the Castine (Maine) Community Hospital case. The hospital had closed its obstetrical unit in 1973 when the only physician in town who delivered babies retired, but sought its reestablishment in 1976 when a replacement physician arrived. Overall occupancy at the hospital was about 50 percent and there was no expectation births would total much beyond 40 per year, both figures well below state and national standards. In turn the HSA, the state Department of Human Services (the 1122 agency), and the state's PSRO had rejected Castine's application to reopen the unit, arguing that its likely low utilization among other factors made the service undesirable and potentially dangerous. Castine sought binding arbitration and won the right to reopen an obstetrical unit when the arbitrator ruled that application of established criteria and standards to a specific case was arbitrary and discriminatory as the state had not demonstrated that Castine's care was certain to be poor quality. Maine was forced to certify the unit and pay all legal fees.[27]

The Political Intervention Strategy

A third strategy providers pursue is political intervention. The national administration had sought to prevent local politicians from having a role in the health planning process when PL 93–641 was being drafted because it feared that they would be unable to resist provider pressures for expansion, a position confirmed by our observations.[28] Friendly relations with the state legislature or the governor can, we discovered, be effective protection for providers against enthusiastic or even dutiful regulators. In Massachusetts the state legislature has willingly overturned certificate of need decisions unfavorable to well connected constituents through the enactment of special exemptive legislation.[29] Because Governor Thomson and major providers shared an ideology, virtually no regulation occurred in New Hampshire during his administration. It is not surprising that hospitals have increasingly placed prominent public officials on their boards and physicians are numbered among the best political campaign contributors.[30]

The Loaf and a Half Strategy

Another strategy is to ask for more than you expect to get. By enlarging a project providers give regulators the opportunity to look tough without jeopardizing anything really desired. A hospital might ask for a 120-bed addition when it only expects and wants 80. Or a nursing home might request permission for 100 Level III and 75 Level II beds when it is willing to settle for 50 of each. Providers know that regulators have to do some cutting if only to justify themselves to HEW.

A variation of this strategy is to apply for more CONs than you expect to win. One proprietary hospital chain we interviewed reported that it monitors closely CON approval rates. When they drop, the chain increases its applications in order to maintain preestablished investment goals.[31] Thus, the record of projects rejected or applications trimmed that planning agencies report may not accurately reflect their impact on health care capital expenditures. There is, after all, an element of provider anticipation to consider in these achievements.[32]

There is yet one more variation of this strategy. Providers may be tempted to offer regulators something they know the regulators want in order to protect a project the provider truly prefers. Regulators, of course, may seek to impose conditions on their CON approvals, but the wise provider is easily persuaded to accept such a deal. The University Hospital in Worcester, for example, would most likely be willing to open an outpatient facility on the site of Worcester City Hospital if only City Hospital's bed quota were transferred to University Hospital.

The Constituency Strategy

A fifth major strategy is building a constituency. Providers who gain the support of a constituency are obviously less vulnerable to adverse regulatory decisions than those who do not.[33] The constituency may be religious, ethnic, or geographic. It can be traditional or newly acquired. But whatever its basis it must be cultivated. Increasingly, hospitals have begun to advertise. For example, there is hardly a hospital in Boston that does not circulate a flier within its service area, some quite expensively done, that extols hospital facilities. In Lewiston, Maine, St. Mary's Hospital stresses it ties to the French Canadian community while Central Maine Medical Center seeks feeder relationships with neighboring rural hospitals and towns. When buses full of Leonard Morse Hospital supporters roll up to meetings, the HSA staffs and the consumer board members cannot fail to notice the power of constituency (see Leonard Morse Case, Part Two). And as officials in New York City are now discovering, the racial and religious ties of hospitals, as well as their unionized work forces, will make it extremely difficult to achieve the bed closure objectives that have been set.[34]

Hospitals are sometimes each other's constituents. That is, they arrange to support one another in dividing the market. They may agree to trade services or regulatory approval opportunities. Regulators at times encourage these arrangements, but the providers are the prime beneficiaries as they are in essence cartelizing hospital services. The actions of the three major hospitals in Maine are along these lines; they gain the tacit support of regulators as they appear to be limiting the acquisition of major equipment and new services. The nonprofit community hospitals in Worcester seem willing to trade services such as consolidating obstetrics and allowing one hospital to specialize in cancer treatments while another holds the lead in heart surgery. Their opposition to regulatory limitations imposed on proprietary, public, and rural hospitals in their area is almost nonexistent.[35]

The Open Job Offer Strategy

An old but still potentially effective strategy is to try to buy off the regulators. Patent Office examiners often become patent attorneys. A year or two with the Federal Communications Commission provides excellent training for lawyers seeking positions with Washington law firms specializing in communications law. Health care providers too know this strategy. Providers pay larger salaries than government and often offer better long-term career opportunities. The turnover is high on HSA staffs and in state agencies with the forwarding addresses often being state hospital associations, PSROs or major hospitals. The first head of certificate of need review in Massachusetts left to join a Boston teaching hospital. Her successor recently quit also, taking a post at a major suburban community hospital. Their former colleague responsible for the preparation of planning standards is now with the hospital association in an adjoining state. Several HSA staff members also now work for hospital councils or local providers. No one can say judgments of regulators are compromised by the prospects of future employment with the industry, but no one can say they are not.

The Code Requirements Strategy

Code compliance is another strategy used to thwart regulators. Arguments that vital services will lose accreditation and qualification for reimbusement unless permission is granted for renovation and modernization to meet code requirements are difficult to resist. The fact that those standards are largely industry-generated and are often somewhat arbitrary in their origins is not always made clear. Intervention by courts to enforce standards can prevent normal regulatory review as has occurred in the case of state-operated facilities for the care of the retarded in Massachusetts. Millions of dollars in reconstruction expenses have been mandated by the courts. Even when regulators are free to reject applications for code improvements they are reluctant to do so as rejection would drastically alter the competitive balance among providers. Unions, patient groups, and physicians in training have all been articulate advocates for projects that are justified in terms of the need to comply with quality and safety codes.[36]
Code conformance can also be used as an opportunity to justify a modernization project that is more expansive than simple compliance would entail. Often it is difficult for planners to locate the line between mere compliance and compliance "plus". Even when this can be determined, the logic of a total renovation now rather than a piecemeal and

gradual fix-up is hard to resist. This is especially true when the financing required flows mainly from the federal government. In one example of this, the Boston HSA declined to question a major renovation project at Boston City Hospital which had been expanded to take advantage of federal subsidies to upgrade public hospitals. The HSA allowed the project to go forward without challenge despite the fact that the agency staff and Executive Director harbored serious doubts about the need for the project.

The Deception Strategy

A final strategy is deception. The cost and scope of projects can easily be understated. The regulators have insufficient staff to monitor projects, especially once a certificate of need is issued. Providers pressure for quick decisions and then pursue projects leisurely, adding and subtracting elements without much fear of detection. One provider, for example, failed to mention a research building that was to be constructed jointly with an approved outpatient clinic. Others are thought to have altered plans while construction was in progress. The complexity of projects, their long lead times, the turnover of regulatory staff, and the difficulty government agencies have in coordinating their programs all prevent close scrutiny of providers and encourage cheating.

The first nationwide planning system for health care capital expenditures was established in 1966 by legislation ironically titled The Partnership for Health Act. There is no partnership for the planning of health care capital expenditures. Rather there is continuing conflict between the federal government and health care providers over the design of the system for regulating capital. The federal government wishes to have a system that will limit capital expenditures. Providers prefer a system that guarantees their autonomy in determining the location and type of health services which they will offer.

As the system has evolved since 1966, it has provoked a competition between the federal government and providers for the support of consumers and state governments who have been made participants. The relevant consumers are not only those who serve on the boards of local planning agencies, but also those who are the clients of local providers. State governments are best seen as variable coalitions composed of regulators, providers, health care payers, and politicians. Neither contestant can be certain of the allies they gain among consumers and state government nor the permanency of the bargain struck. The chapters that follow discuss why this is the case.

Notes

[1]Roger G. Noll, "The Consequences of Public Utility Regulation of Hospitals," in R. Hanft and P. Rettig, editors, *Controls on Health Care* (Washington: National Academy of Sciences, 1975), pp. 25–48; Joel May, "The Planning and Licensing Agencies," in C. Havighurst, editor, *Regulating Health Facilities Construction* (Washington: American Enterprise Institute, 1974).

[2]H. E. Klarman, "National Policies and Social Planning in Health Services," *Health and Society*, Vol. 54, No. 1 (Winter 1976), pp. 1–28. See also Stuart Altman and Sanford Weiner, "Regulation as a Second Best," in W. Greenberg, editor, *Competition in the Health Care Sector* (Germantown, MD: Aspen, 1978), pp. 339–358.

[3]For a discussion of alternative perspectives on government regulation see Bruce M. Owen and Ronald Braeutigan, *The Regulation Game* (Cambridge: Ballinger, 1978).

[4]Ibid.

[5]Ibid.

[6]Clark Havighurst, "Controlling Health Care Costs: Strengthening the Private Sector's Hand," *Journal of Health Politics, Policy and Law* (Winter 1977), pp. 471–98.

[7]The advocates of regulation are strangely inarticulate as a set and without credible academic supporters. As a result, most of the literature tends to be highly critical of regulation. For the best available balanced view of health regulation see P. Feldman and R. J. Zeckhauser, "Sober Thoughts on Health Care Regulation," in C. Argyris, editor, *Regulating Business: The Search for an Optimum* (San Francisco: Institute for Contemporary Studies, 1978), pp. 93–124.

[8]American Health Planning Association Survey of Health Planning Agencies, September, 1978.

[9]See James Q. Wilson, "The Politics of Regulation" in J. W. McKie, editor, *Social Responsibility and the Business Predicament* (Washington: Brookings, 1974), pp. 135–168.

[10]Eli Ginzberg, editor, *Regionalization and Health Policy* (Washington: HEW-HRA, 1977) discusses the history of health planning in the U.S. Another important source is David A. Pearson, "The Concept of Regionalized Personal Health Services in the United States, 1920-1955," in E. W. Saward, editor, *The Regionalization of Personal Health Services* (New York: Prodist, 1976), pp. 3–51.

[11]Ginzberg, op. cit.

[12]For an evaluative history of the program see J. R. Lave and L. B. Lave, *The Hospital Construction Act: An Evaluation of the Hill-Burton Program 1948-1973* (Washington: American Enterprise Institute, 1974). Note also M. DuBois, "Areawide Planning: Where It Came From, Where It's Going," *Hospitals*, Vol. 40, No. 23 (1966).

[13]Officially The Heart Disease, Cancer, and Stroke Amendments of 1965 (Public Law 89-239).

[14]The Comprehensive Health Planning and Public Health Services Amendments of 1966 (Public Law 89-749).

[15]U. S. General Accounting Office, *Status of the Implementation of the National Health Planning and Resources Development Act of 1974,* Washington, D.C., November 2, 1978, pp. 2 and 3.

[16]The Social Security Amendments of 1972 (Public Law 92-603) which added Section 1122 to the Social Security Act.

[17]The experience of the Comprehensive Health Planning Program is reviewed in John T. O'Connor, "Comprehensive Health Planning: Dreams and Realities," *Health and Society,* Vol. 54, No. 4 (Fall 1974), pp. 391-413. See also Harold S. Luft and Gary A. Frisvold, "Decisionmaking in Regional Health Planning Agencies," *Journal of Health Politics, Policy, and the Law,* Vol. 4, No. 2 (Summer 1979), pp. 250-72.

[18]*Congressional Quarterly Weekly Report,* November 23, 1974, p. 1770.

[19]Ibid., p. 1771.

[20]AMA units opposed and forced a suit against the implementation of the bill. For current opposition see Jerome Brazda, "Washington Report," *The Nation's Health,* June, 1979, p. 3; *National Journal,* January 25, 1975, p. 147. For historical analysis of the law see S. H. Werlin, A. Waliott, and M. Joroff, "Implementing Formative Health Planning Under PL 93-641," *New England Journal of Medicine* (September 23, 1976), pp. 698-702. Note also Jonathan P. West and Michael P. Stevens, "Comparative Analysis of Community Health Planning: Transition from CHPs to HSAs," *Journal of Health Politics, Policy, and the Law,* Vol. 1, No. 2 (Summer 1976).

[21]Owen and Braeutigan, *The Regulation Game.*

[22]Interviews. See also any recent issue of *Modern Healthcare,* an industry journal specializing in the activities of hospital management chains.

[23]Peter F. Drucker, *Management: Tasks, Responsibilities, Practices* (New York: Harper & Row, 1974).

[24]The bureaucratization of hospital administration, including the growth of specialists in regulation monitoring and manipulation, is rapidly occurring, but as yet largely unrecognized in the sociological literature on the hospital.

[25]Interview.

[26]New Britain General Hospital v. Commission on Hospitals and Health Care, Court of Common Pleas, Hartford, Connecticut, June 21, 1977.

[27]In the Matter of Arbitration between Castine Community Hospital and the Designated Planning Agency, State of Maine, August 5, 1977, American Arbitration Association, Case Number 110-0021-77.

[28]*Congressional Quarterly Weekly Report,* November 22, 1974, p. 1769.

[29]See St. Joseph Nursing Home case, Case 2, Part Two.

[30]Senator Edward Kennedy, for example, sits on the board of Lahey Clinic. Former Governor James Longley of Maine was a trustee of Central Maine Medical Center in Lewiston before he took office. The list could easily be expanded.

[31]Interview.

[32]The claims of vast savings stemming from the planners must therefore be viewed with some skepticism. See also David S. Salkever and Tom W. Bice, "The Impact of Certificate of Need Controls on Hospital Investment," *Health and Society,* Vol. 54 (1976).

[33]Paul Danaceau, *The Health Planning Guidelines Controversy: Report from Iowa and Texas* (Hyattsville, MD: HRA, 1979).

[34]"Closing Hospitals With Care," *New York Times,* June 29, 1979, p. A26.

[35]See Worcester City Hospital case, Case 3, Part Two.

[36]Codman Research Group, Progress Report No. 5, Contract 291-76-0003, April, 1978.

Chapter 4

Citizen Participation

Since the early 1960s citizen participation has been a feature of the policymaking process in the United States. The citizen's role in policymaking has taken a variety of forms ranging from spontaneous grass roots protest to highly structured participation in local organizations. In health planning citizen participation is mandated by the federal government and institutionalized through the board structure of Health Systems Agencies. Thus, it is an integral part of an organized and highly complicated regulatory effort.

In this chapter we will assess its role, dividing our analysis into four parts: the roots of citizen participation in health planning; the mechanics of citizen participation; the underlying theory and assumptions; and the impact of citizen participation in health planning in practice. Our overall conclusion is that citizen participation on HSA boards in New England has proven to be more supportive of health planning goals than had generally been predicted, but that this support can be offset when health planning issues reach the community arena and local citizens (nonboard members) become involved.

The Roots of Citizen Participation in Health Planning

In part, citizens are involved in health planning because citizen participation became a public program norm in the 1960s and has been insisted upon ever since. The presence of consumers on the boards of the regional "b" agencies established under the Comprehensive Health Planning Program in 1966 set a clear precedent for a consumer role in health planning. Similarly, the Neighborhood Health Center and Community Mental Health Center Programs also set a precedent for citizen involvement in health planning. Other health programs contributed to the institutionalization of citizen participation as well, but to a lesser degree. These include the Regional Medical Program established under the Heart Disease, Cancer and Stroke Amendments of 1965, the Experimental Health Services Delivery Program initiated by HEW in 1971, and the Emergency Medical Systems Program established in 1973.

Of course, impetus for citizen participation also came from some very important nonhealth programs. In the late 1950s and early 1960s, the Ford Foundation developed its "gray areas" programs, providing financial support for direct community action organizations in a number of cities. A New York City effort called Mobilization for Youth (MFY) established community boards to deal with problems of juvenile delinquency and became a model for action elsewhere. Most important of all was the Community Action Program established under the Economic Opportunity Act of 1964. Consistent with the program's initial goal of "maximum feasible participation" Community Action Agencies were established in over 1,000 locations around the country. Citizen participation was also an integral part of the Model Cities Program, established in part as a response to the 1964 act. Taken together, these programs created a constituency which would demand that citizen participation be included in all future domestic policy initiatives.

In addition to being based in historical precedent, citizen participation in health planning receives support because it fits the agenda of the two most prominent groups currently committed to changing the health system in the United States. The first and currently more prominent is the agenda of the Cost Controllers, those who are alarmed by the steady rise in health care costs. The cost control agenda is embraced most fully, but not exclusively, by officials in state and federal governments, by Blue Cross and private insurers, and by some large unions and employers.

A second agenda for change is that of the Institutional Reformers, those who criticize professionalism and bureaucracy in medicine. The medical profession, in their view, is oriented towards the rewards of institutionally based acute care medicine and unresponsive to the primary and preventive care needs of the poor and the elderly. It is also thought to be overly impersonal and bureaucratic.[1] Among those who hold this perspective are the Nader-affiliated Health Research Group, the National Consumer Alliance, and the National Health Law Project.

In the context of health planning, Cost Controllers and Institutional Reformers are natural allies. Although the former emphasize runaway costs and the latter focus on professional dominance and autonomy, the two groups point to the same set of structural characteristics as the causes of these problems. They believe that the current mixture of specialized, high-technology, hospital-oriented care, fueled by a distorted reimbursement system, is responsible for the respective evils they highlight. But most importantly, citizen participation fits the strategic purposes of both groups.

For Cost Controllers, citizen participation is a means to an end. They recognize it is difficult politically to impose soon the tough, federally directed, regulatory system needed to halt spiraling health care costs. Citizen participation structured within a federal health planning program offers an imperfect, but practical, mechanism for pursuing and legitimizing cost control objectives and, in the process, for drawing public attention to health costs as an important national issue. For Institutional Reformers, citizen participation is both a means and an end in itself.

For the Bureau of Health Planning in HEW, consumer representation on HSA boards serves the added function of providing a simple measure for evaluating agency performance. Given the difficulties of evaluating the performance of the HSAs, all of which operate in very different local environments, this is particularly important to HEW. Compliance with governing body regulations is a leading criterion in HEW's ongoing monitoring and evaluation of the HSAs. The Bureau of Health Planning has developed a formula for measuring compliance with the representational requirements of the law.

The Mechanics of Citizen Participation in Health Planning

Under the National Health Planning and Resources Development Act of 1974, more than two hundred HSAs were established across the United States. These local health planning organizations constitute the lower tier of a three-tiered planning structure that also involves both state and federal government. The HSAs and the communities they serve provide the primary forum for citizen participation in health planning.

Citizen participation in health planning is institutionalized through the board structure of the HSAs. The statute requires that a majority, up to 60 percent, of the members of the HSA governing boards must be "consumers." Since virtually everyone in one sense or another is a consumer of health care, the statute further specifies the characteristics of bona fide HSA consumers. Consumers are persons who have not been "direct providers" for 12 months preceding their appointment to the HSA board; providers being defined as those whose "primary activity is in the provision of health care . . . or the administration of facilities." In addition, consumers may not be "indirect providers"—those who have a fiduciary interest in a provider or are married to a provider. The son or daughter of a drug company executive, for example, could not serve as a consumer member of an HSA board. A retired person receiving income from dividends of a hospital supply company would also be disqualified.

More important than the simple fact that consumers are in the majority on HSA boards are two other requirements. First, consumers must be residents of the geographical area covered by the HSA. Second, and most significantly, they must "be *broadly representative* of the social, economic, linguistic, and racial populations, and geographic areas of the health service area."[2]

In practice, the structure for representation is even more complicated than this quick recitation of the law indicates. Many HSAs, particularly in metropolitan areas and in the states with only a single HSA, operate a system of sub-area councils. Where they exist, these sub-area councils serve as the initial decision point for all planning activities performed by the HSA. Thus, in New Hampshire, a single-HSA state, a series of sub-area councils that conform to the geographical coverage of the old Comprehensive Health Planning ("b" or local level) agencies has been established. In Boston, there is a sub-system of five "metro-councils." Typically, the composition of these bodies conforms to the representational requirements of HSA boards. As of February 15, 1978, there were 474 sub-area councils reported in operation in 88 of 205 HSA areas in the country. These 474 sub-area councils included 15,466 members, with a range by HSA area of 15 to 1,802 sub-area council members.

HSAs also establish numerous internal sub-committees (e.g., plan development, project review, nominations, etc.) and generally make similar efforts at representational coverage in these sub-committees. And there are sometimes structures that stand between the sub-area councils and the HSA. For example, in Boston there is a "multi-metro working committee," an intermediary body that stands between the Boston HSA and its five Metro Councils. Nationally, approximately 52 percent of HSA board members are "consumers" and 48 percent are "providers." A more precise breakdown based on a sample of 136 HSA boards is provided in Table 4.1.

Implicit in the structure of the boards are the assumptions that a few categorizations such as race, occupation, place of residence and income are the appropriate characteristics for consumer representatives and that individuals who have these characteristics, no matter how identified, can in fact represent others with the same attributes more effectively than anyone else. Challenges have come from groups not initially included in the categories selected and from those wishing to represent specific interests, even though they themselves lack the distinguishing characteristics. The necessity of applying some limit on the size of the boards and committees means that many plausible interests are not represented and that others are represented poorly. It also means that there is potential for doing harm to the very objectives sought by those who advocated the inclusion of citizen participation provisions in the law.

Not surprisingly, there were predictions that such a structure would fail to produce reform, that interest representation on the boards would dissolve into conventional pork barrel politics where small groups collude to divide up available resources. As Bruce Vladeck put it:

> There are no majorities in such a system, only a series of fragmented and largely autonomous minorities. Under these conditions, the only way in which an institution can function at all is to develop very strong norms of reciprocity and log rolling. I get mine if you get yours; that is and must be the general rule.[3]

The belief was that the logic of local interests would prevail over the planners' efforts to restrain health sector growth. The situation would be aggravated where HSAs include a network of sub-area councils. Here the game would begin earlier and last longer; staff resources would be especially thin, but providers would always be well-represented. Providers and consumers, it was thought, would find easy agreement on serving themselves rather than any broader conception of the public interest.[4]

It is worth noting that behavior based on rigid definitions of self-interest (e.g., economic interest maximization) is not universally regarded as dysfunctional. Anthony Downs, for example, has written about the positive effects of rational self-interest applied to political behavior.[5] Indeed, most arguments in favor of market policies are based on the same claims. Nevertheless, the predictions concerning the negative effects of HSA group bargaining and health consumer parochialism were plausible. They were sufficiently compelling that, as one observer put it, "the behavior that needs to be explained is the effort anyone [labeled a consumer] would make to control health costs."[6]

HSA Consumer Behavior in Practice

In New England, at least, there is considerable variation in consumer motivations and in the results of HSA interest-group bargaining. To be

Table 4.1

Selected Breakdowns of HSA Governing Board Membership
for 136 HSA Boards

		Number	Percentages
A.	Consumer-Provider		
	Consumer members	3,105	52
	Provider members	2,835	48
	TOTAL	5,940	100
B.	Consumer Minority Members		
	Blacks	581	77
	Hispanics	121	16
	Native Americans	44	6
	Orientals	13	2
	TOTAL	759	100
C.	Sex		
	Male	4,399	74
	Female	1,541	26
	TOTAL	5,940	100
D.	Providers		
	Direct	1,785	64
	Indirect	574	20
	Not classifiable	476	17
	TOTAL	2,835	100
E.	Providers by Representative Category		
	Physicians (incl. DOs)	673	24
	Dentists	136	5
	Nurses	165	6
	Health care institutions	869	31
	Health care insurers	144	5
	Health professional schools	159	6
	Allied health professionals	235	8
	Not classifiable	454	16
	TOTAL	2,835	100
F.	Public Officials		
	Consumer members	594	68
	Provider members	277	32
	TOTAL	871	100

Table 4.1, continued

G.	Elected/Appointed		
	Elected officials	472	54
	Appointed officials	294	34
	Not classifiable	105	12
	TOTAL	871	100
H.	State/Local/Other		
	State officials	72	8
	Local officials	669	77
	Other officials	25	3
	Not classifiable	105	12
	TOTAL	871	100

Source: Bureau of Health Planning and Resources Development Memorandum, R.L. Petersen, September 22, 1976.

sure, there are instances where the HSA consumers support technological expansion and capital investment (e.g., a CAT scanner, a new building, more beds, etc.) based on perceived local interests. Parochial HSA consumer behavior is seen in its purest form in rural areas where consumers often fall in line behind the goal of making their town "medically self-sufficient." But there are also a surprising number of cases where HSA consumers support staff efforts to contain health sector growth. All the New England HSA boards have recommended disapproval of hospital requests for new acute beds and medical technology. HSA boards in Massachusetts and New Hampshire, for example, participated in establishing periodic moratoria on the acquisition of CAT brain and body scanners. Some HSA boards have also worked to limit growth in the long-term care sector and (a much more difficult task politically) to discourage renovation and replacement of existing facilities.

We see five major reasons for this. One of the most important relates to the size of the geographic areas covered by health systems agencies. HSA areas are sufficiently large that board consumers only rarely would be required to sacrifice any perceived local and personal interest in voting against a particular certificate of need application. The Boston HSA area, for example, contains 65 of the 351 towns and cities in Massachusetts, and a population of 2,225,000. It, in turn, is divided into five "Metro" sub-areas, displayed in Figure 4.1. The Metros range in population from 500,000 to 800,000. The Central (Boston) Metro

Figure 4.1

Health Service Area IV

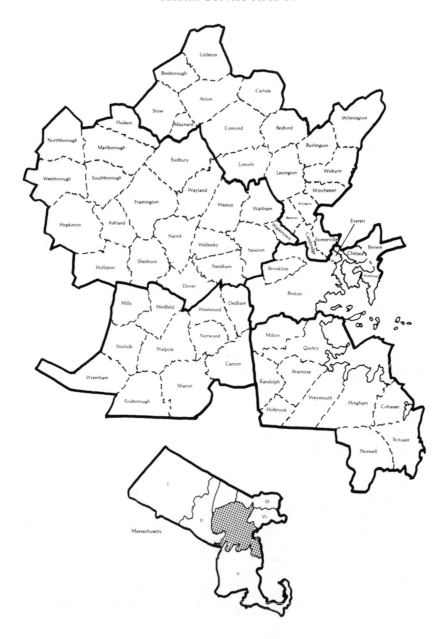

contains 5 towns and cities, and the West Metro as many as 20 different towns and cities. A consumer representative of the Boston HSA board from the Northwest Metro may have little or no "interest" in a CON application from, say, the South Metro area. Often, of course, this will hold within Metro areas as well as between them.[7] Public opinion surveys give some clue as to why the size of HSA areas lends itself to regulation. They show that most Americans subscribe to the notion that there is a "crisis" in United States health care, but that most are satisfied with the care they personally receive. Thus, the size and fragmentation of the HSA areas offer board consumers the opportunity to support regulation in order to address the "crisis," but at someone else's expense. This tendency will be reinforced as planning is more successful at placing overall limits on medical resources. Under such circumstances, board consumers may be reluctant to approve expansion in another community if they believe that to do so would threaten future changes for their own.

Although the size of the HSA areas is important, it does not give a full explanation of consumer behavior on HSA boards. This is because where board consumers do have a tangible interest in a particular CON project, they still are often supportive of staff recommendations for disapproval. One reason for this is that consumer members of HSA Boards are often committed to planning goals as a matter of ideology and past experience. Many are community activists with a history of participation in voluntary organizations who come to the HSA already in support of planning goals.[8] As the experience of the neighborhood health centers indicates, the people most likely to seek positions in such organizations are community activists and professional advocates.[9] Thus, consumer members of HSA boards are often community activists who see cost control and citizen participation in health as not unlike other "public interest" issues they have supported in the past. These people, who providers often derisively label "professional consumers," are often willing to sacrifice a measure of localism in behalf of a perceived greater good.

Consumers on HSA boards, by virtue of the fact that they are joiners and are participating, are at least in some sense unlike the broader population they are meant to mirror. Studies of neighborhood health centers tend to confirm this. In one study, board members of a New York health center were described as having "more explicitly political attitudes towards problems" than the average person in the community.[10] Trainees in a California Consumer Health Training Project (for members of community health boards) were described as "willing to speak out" and as "suspicious of professionals."[11] The behavior of consumers on HSA boards calls into question the assumption that consumer representatives will think and act like the groups they purportedly represent simply because both share certain ascriptive social characteristics. In urban areas, at least, health planning agencies enjoy the relative luxury of a pool of available consumer representatives who fit the representational requirements of the law while also being committed to planning goals and ideology.

There are other reasons for consumer support of planning on HSA boards. In many of their earlier organizational roles, consumer representatives on HSA boards have had previous encounters with health care institutions. Often these have involved consumer/provider conflicts over such issues as hospital land holdings in the community, hospital hiring practices, the environmental impact of hospital facilities, the racial and ethnic composition of the hospital staff, the perceived quality and comfort of the outpatient department, the extent and quality of community services, and community representation on governing boards. Even where HSA consumers have not had antagonistic experiences with a particular health care institution, a general history of community/institutional conflict will influence, indeed sometimes oblige, consumer representatives to be supportive of planning. A history of community/institutional conflict, then, even where board members are not personally involved, is a third reason for consumer support of planning on HSA boards. This kind of consumer support motivated by general political conflict is most likely to occur in urban areas where community organizations are both more numerous and more active, the population more heterogeneous and hospital expansion more likely to have an immediate and very visible impact.

Hospitals have traditionally prepared their plans for modernization or expansion in private and exclusively in terms of institutional priorities. Consumers on HSA boards have been particularly concerned when community groups are not included in developing hospital plans. Sometimes this is because the members themselves are from the community in question. More often, however, it is because HSA consumers regard such practices as a violation of the spirit of the planning process. This was an issue when Harvard University attempted to combine three of its teaching hospitals in the Affiliated Hospital Center. Harvard's plans were blocked for almost three years pending resolution of a number of community objections, including the claim that Harvard had not adequately involved the community and its various health planning agencies in its planning process. HSA consumers voiced similar criticism when the New England Baptist Hospital, less than a mile away, attempted to replace its 250-bed facility. HSA consumers argued that the Baptist, oriented towards specialty care, had never been responsive to community needs and, in any event, "had just not played ball with the planning process in developing its plans."[12] Not surprisingly, the hospital turned this argument on its head, claiming that it is a unique worldwide health resource and, therefore, should be exempt from normal processes for determining community need.

There is a fourth reason for HSA consumer support of planning: HSA consumers gradually develop support for planning through on-the-job learning. Faced for the first time with a host of expansion requests of varying validity, consumers may learn to discriminate among them. In some cases this merely reinforces already supportive attitudes. In other cases (even among providers) board members interviewed indicated that they had been "converted" as a result of their experience on the HSA board.

A fifth and very important factor is that HSA consumers come to share the interests and goals of the organization as a whole, and behave in ways that serve the needs of organizational maintenance and enhancement. In order to win initial designation and funding, and continued funding and redesignation, HSAs must meet the standards for performance set by HEW. Some of these standards are exceedingly vague, others quite specific and easily monitored. Generally, they demand that HSAs meet a number of procedural requirements (including the "broadly representative" standard for consumer representation) while displaying a commitment to HEW's agenda for regulation and cost control. However, at the same time as they must meet these requirements, HSAs must establish organizational independence and identity. They cannot alienate providers by appearing to be agents of federal or state government, nor can they alienate community groups by violating the ethos of "bottom up" planning by automatically accepting the government's agenda for change. Since HSAs have limited formal authority, such independence is crucial to developing the credibility necessary to operate effectively in the health planning arena.

In the last analysis, however, HSAs cannot stray too far in establishing their independence. They know that they will be evaluated, both by HEW and Congress, on the basis of their ability to make hard cost control decisions. Their future role in health, particularly under a national health insurance system, will depend upon their cost control performance. In order to insure that they are participating in a meaningful endeavor as members of an organization that will grow in importance and responsibility, HSA consumers must accept this system of organizational rules and rewards. Few want to behave in ways that will diminish the viability of the organization in which they are participating and to which they give long hours. The need to establish a strong cost control record, albeit one with an independent flair, is recognized by both staff and consumer representatives as the key to organizational maintenance and success.

From the HSA to the Community Arena

Health systems agencies operate in a potentially turbulent local environment. When health planning conflicts move beyond the confines of the HSA board, a new set of actors and interests are engaged. Providers who cannot find the necessary support on HSA boards to carry the data often pursue strategies that destroy the resolve of HSA consumers to adhere to planning objectives.

Expanding the scope of conflict in any particular instance is a relatively simple matter.[13] The issues involved in CON review often touch upon important aspects of community members' lives; their own health and the health of their relatives and neighbors may be regarded as being at stake. Since health facilities are invariably a major source of employment, providing jobs for over five million people nationally, the livelihood of many individuals and the health of the local economy can be made an issue. Tradition of community service, ethnic or religious ties, and civic pride may also spark community interest.

Where health planning attempts to reduce the availability of local health services, it threatens a community with the loss of services that is only partially offset by widely dispersed benefits. This situation, concentrated costs and dispersed benefits, lends itself to local mobilization and increased participation.[14] When it occurs, conflict also often escalates quickly. The controversy surrounding the addition of a few nursing home beds may soon be transformed into a conflict over local control, the proper role of government, and economic freedom.

Community interests typically line up on different sides of a CON dispute. Some providers are for the applicant, some against, and others conspicuous in their disinterest. But neighborhood consumers, often recruited and organized by the applicant, are usually outspoken in the support of the CON project. Most politicians will support local projects, identifying themselves as being pro-employment, pro-health care, pro-local applicant. Only a few may be sufficiently entrepreneurial as to want to carve an image as cost controllers. Sometimes, local and statewide public interest organizations provide a countervailing influence to the aggrieved applicant and assorted local allies. This is particularly true in urban areas where entrenched and experienced community groups with access to the political system and the media are more likely to be found. But, in general, when conflict escalates to the community arena, the forces for expansion have an edge. This is particularly true where HSAs attempt to deny applications for renovation and replacement. Communities may sometimes be mobilized when they cannot get something new, but it is predictable that they will be mobilized when health planning threatens to rob them of what they already have or leave them with "second-rate" facilities by attempting to let obsolescence run its course. Politically, it is always difficult for planning to effect reductions below existing resource levels, whatever they may be. A recent experience, one that has been replicated throughout the country, illustrates this point nicely.

On September 23, 1977, in accordance with the health planning law, the Department of Health, Education, and Welfare published a set of Proposed National Guidelines for Health Planning in the *Federal Register*. The Guidelines established quantitative standards for services in a variety of areas. For example, they set a goal of 4.0 acute beds per 1,000 population for the country. For maternity services, they proposed that hospitals in SMSAs with a population of 100,000 or more operate at a minimum level of 2,000 deliveries per year, an exceedingly tough standard that only a few hospitals can meet. The implicit purpose of the Guidelines, it could be argued, was to constrain local flexibility and to commit local agencies to something approximating the numerical goals set in the Guidelines. However, the Guidelines would at the same time assist those HSAs already interested in aggressive regulation. Like the union negotiator arguing that his hands are tied, the standards could be used by such HSAs to gain bargaining leverage. In Massachusetts, however, two HSAs encountered considerable difficulty in attempting to apply these standards on a communitywide basis.

The Draft Health Systems Plan for the Boston HSA called for quantitative targets in a number of areas. The target for maternity services generated the most controversy. According to the Draft Plan, "Hospital Maternity Services, that are performing fewer than 1,000 deliveries should be required to immediately close or consolidate with other maternity services, subject to geographic restraints." The HSA standard fell below the state's 1,500 delivery minimum, and well below the 2,000 minimum contained in the proposed National Guidelines. Nevertheless, the more lenient HSA standard generated local opposition sufficient to force the HSA to abandon the effort to apply the standard to particular local communities.

Suburban community hospitals in particular mobilized to protest the HSA standard. The Leonard Morse hospital southwest of Boston

mounted an especially aggressive protest.[15] Although the hospital performed about 700 deliveries per year, it argued (with considerable
documentation) that both its quality of care and efficiency were
relatively good. By busing employees and local consumers to public
hearings and effectively utilizing local and citywide media, the hospital
brought the HSA standard under close scrutiny. Meeting in committee,
HSA staff conceded that the targets were essentially arbitrary; they
could not document the efficacy of the goals advanced in the Draft Plan.
In December, the HSA board voted a number of changes in the Draft
Plan, among them the decision to abandon the effort to push ahead with
the maternity standards.

In Worcester County the draft of the maternal and newborn component of the Health System Plan experienced a similar fate. It called for
consolidation of maternity services, including the elimination of one-
half the currently available obstetric beds in the HSA North County
sub-area. Protest from supporters of the three North County hospitals
affected came quickly. It was sufficiently strong to force the HSA
virtually to abandon the plan.[16]

What was occurring in Boston and Worcester was also occurring
throughout much of the country. HEW received some 55,000 letters of
protest and criticism regarding the Draft Guidelines. Indeed, Congress
soon passed a resolution assuring community hospitals that HEW had
no authority to use the Guidelines to force consolidation or closure.
HEW has since amended the Guidelines, promulgating the now revised
and diluted goals reserving a lowered annual delivery frequency of
1,500 for "hospitals providing care for complicated obstetrical problems. . . ."[17]

In the foregoing examples providers mobilized consumer support in
the community in response to specific planning policies and decisions.
Sometimes, however, community consumers may be involved before
rather than after the fact. This is what happened in Rhode Island in one
of the most controversial certificate of need cases to date.

During the mid-1970s Suburban Memorial Hospital[18] in Rhode
Island, experiencing high occupancy rates, moved to develop a strategy
for expanding the hospital's capacity. To accomplish this, Suburban
Memorial formed a Citizens Advisory Committee composed of a cross
section of citizens from the hospital's service area. After a year of
intensive study, the committee submitted its recommendations. They
included the addition of 50 acute medical and surgical beds to the
hospital's 309-bed supply. When the state's certificate of need decision-
making body, the Health Services Council, sought to block the new
beds, Suburban Memorial already had at its disposal an organized and

effective citizens' group equipped with its own set of statistics and its own leadership. Members of the Citizens Advisory Committee testified before the Health Services Council, the first time members of the public had been allowed to present their views before the Council. Local hearings at the hospital were well-attended, attracting considerable media attention. Although the Council stood firm, its denial was eventually overturned on a procedural technicality in an administrative hearing in March, 1978. The Director of the State Health Department decided to accept the hearing officer's ruling rather than appeal to the Superior Court, risking a defeat and further public controversy. The fact that Suburban Memorial had community consumers organized and on board prior to submitting a CON request and prior to any ruling appears to have contributed to the hospital's success in winning one of the very few new acute bed additions in Rhode Island in recent years.[19]

Although some counter examples are available, interest group bargaining in the community arena is almost always less supportive of planning goals than is interest group bargaining confined to the HSA board room. The potential for communitywide conflict is real. Roughly 20 percent of the HSA areas currently fall below the federally mandated goal of 4.0 beds per 1,000 population. They are fertile ground for equity arguments to expand up to the 4.0 level. More interestingly, even where states or HSA areas exceed 4.0 in the aggregate, a number of smaller geographic divisions currently fall below the 4.0 target. Planners in these areas will be particularly hard pressed to prevent expansion or to push for reductions should conflict reach the community arena.

Both providers and health planners attempt to manage the planning process in order to enhance their chances for success. Planners attempt to limit the scope of conflict, processing decisions as a matter of routine within the confines of the HSA structure, where consumer representatives are supportive and provider interests are generally fragmented.[20]

Providers are able to operate much more effectively in the community and political arenas, and disaffected providers often work to expand the scope of conflict to the community arena where support is more readily available. Not all planning issues, however, reach the community agenda. Many times planners would rather compromise than commit the resources necessary for a protracted political dispute in an arena where their chances for success are reduced. For their part providers will seek to expand the scope of conflict only as a last recourse. This is because mobilizing consumer support and placing a case on the community agenda requires a major organizational effort. It is also because providers are wary of earning a reputation for circumventing the planning process. Like the shepherd in the fable, they can cry wolf only so often. The potential for causing community conflict is a valuable resource in the bargaining that occurs between providers and planners at the local level and, as such, must be husbanded.

Notes

[1] For the clearest discussion of the Institutional Reformers perspective see Eliot Freidson's well-known book, *Professional Dominance* (Aldine Co., 1970).

[2] Public Law 93-641, Section 1512 (b) (3) (c).

[3] Bruce Vladeck, "Interest Group Representation and the HSAs: Health Planning and Political Theory," *American Journal of Public Health* (January, 1977), p. 25.

[4] Aaron Wildavsky, "Can Health Be Planned?" Michael Davis Lecture, Graduate School of Public Policy, University of California at Berkeley, 1976.

[5] Anthony Downs, *An Economic Theory of Action in a Democracy* (Columbus: Bobbs-Merrill, 1967).

[6] Harvey M. Sapolsky, "The Political Sociology of Health Regulation," unpublished paper, January, 1977.

[7] The picture across the country is similar. Five HSA areas contain 3 million people. Although the population of 47 HSAs is less than 500,000, none fall below 200,000.

[8] Previous participatory experience for HSA consumers was reported in a study by KOBA Associates. Of 70 Board consumers surveyed in the KOBA study, only 3 did not record an affiliation in addition to their HSA membership. At least 30 reported affiliation with at least 2 other specific groups, including educational, religious, and civic organizations in addition to health organizations. The KOBA study concluded: "representatives of target groups are not people 'off the streets', but have a history of participation." (KOBA Associates, Inc., Washington, D.C., "An Analysis of Representation of Minority and Other Target Groups in Health Systems Agencies and State Health Planning and Development Agencies," July, 1978).

[9] George Golbert, Fredrick Trowbridge, and Robert Bucksbaum, "Issues in the Development of Neighborhood Health Centers," *Inquiry*, Vol. 16, No. 1 (March, 1969), pp. 34-47. On professional advocates see the role played by Urban Planning Aid in Allan Lupo, et al., *Rights of Way*.

[10] Ana Dumais, "Organizing the Community Around Health," *Social Policy* (January/February, 1971).

[11] Alberta Parker, "The Consumer as Policymaker—Issues of Training," *American Journal of Public Health* (November, 1970).

[12] Interview.

[13] See James Coleman, *Community Conflict* (New York: The Free Press, 1957).

[14] James Q. Wilson, "The Politics of Regulation" in James McKie, editor, *Social Responsibility and the Business Predicament* (Washington: Brookings, 1974).

[15] See the Leonard Morse case, Case 7, Part Two.

[16] Codman Research Group, "The Plan Development Process," January, 1978.

[17] *Federal Register,* March 28, 1978, p. 13046.

[18] The name at this hospital has been disguised in keeping with Codman's agreement with SEARCH on data confidentiality.

[19] See the Suburban Memorial case, Case 5, Part Two.

[20] This is unnecessary in Rhode Island where, as a result of a waiver, there is no Health Systems Agency. Thus the task facing health planners in Rhode Island is simplified. Although the Rhode Island Hospital Association frequently raises the issue, the relative lack of citizen participation in the state has not been a major public concern. This, in part, is due to the fact that the presence of an independent consumer-oriented agency, the Health Planning Council, serves to diffuse the citizen participation issue in the state.

Chapter 5

Planners

In the preceding chapters we have examined the roles of health care providers and consumers in the health planning process. Here we will examine the role played by health planners, focusing on the different strategies that have been developed by health planners in the New England states. We are most concerned with describing and explaining the policies developed by HSAs and SHPDAs under PL 93–641 in New England. Thus, we will discuss the policies developed by the staff of other agencies such as PSROs, rate-setting commissions, and hospital associations mainly as they bear on the actions of HSAs and SHPDAs. As we have done elsewhere, we will use the terms "planners" and "regulators" interchangeably, reflecting our belief that the primary purpose of PL 93–641 is cost control. In fact, the distinction commonly made between agencies with a long-range planning orientation and a regulatory orientation does not accurately describe differences between agencies in practice, except as "planning" orientation is merely intended as a euphemism for a weak regulatory effort. Most health planning agencies in New England accept regulation as their first priority, but differ across a broad spectrum in terms of regulatory philosophy and policy and with regard to their reading of what can realistically be accomplished in their respective areas.

Expectations of Planners' Behavior

The dominant perspective on the behavior of planning/regulatory agencies is the "capture theory," a loose collection of writings that picture regulatory agencies as controlled by industry, more passive than aggressive, and lacking in expertise and political skill; a picture not unlike that generally associated, in health, with the performance of planning agencies under the Comprehensive Health Planning Program. Over time, this loose collection of studies has been lumped together and afforded the status of a "theory." In fact, there are a number of variations of the capture theory. Three are most relevant to the behavior of planning agencies under PL 93–641.[1]

One of the most prominent capture theories is the notion that there is a natural "life cycle" for a regulatory agency, popularized by Marver Bernstein in his book, *Regulating Business by Independent Commission*. A typical "life cycle" for a regulatory agency works like this: the agency is first established under circumstances of public concern and political consensus; in order to pull together the coalition necessary to support regulation, the agency is given a very broad mandate, often with vague, conflicting, or unobtainable goals. Over time, however, the public loses interest in the increasingly technical affairs of everyday regulation. With public apathy comes a withdrawal of legislative and executive support. Isolated, the agency gradually strikes a bargain with the industry it was designed to regulate. Over time, as key original staff depart, the process of surrender is completed.

A second version of the capture theory can be called the "regulator as job hunter" view. Regulators rarely make regulation a career; terms are short, reappointment can be difficult, newly elected politicians typically bring in their own people. Command of the technical details and skills of regulation are not highly marketable qualities, except in the regulated industry. Thus, in order to ensure future positions, regulators engage in what some have called "minimal squawk" behavior.

Still a third version of the capture theory, and by far the most sophisticated, is the notion of protectionism. According to this view, entrenched industry takes advantage of the state's power in order to protect its market position. Typically, the regulated industry plays a major role in the creation of regulatory agencies. In the words of George Stigler, one proponent of this view, "regulation is acquired by industry and is designed and operated primarily for its benefit."[2] Protection via regulation is not regarded as costless. Rather, the costs of regulation to industry are seen as worth the price of market protection. This version of the capture theory focuses on the motivation of the industry rather than the regulators, a perspective we discussed in Chapter 3.

Taken together, these three versions of the capture theory—the life cycle view, the regulator as job hunter, and regulation as protectionism —help frame a set of expectations about the behavior of planners and planning agencies under PL 93–641. Simply put, planners would be much less than aggressive in pursuing the regulatory mandate under the planning law. However, the behavior we have observed in New England forces one to recognize the complexities of the regulators' motivations and behavior. Thus, the notion of protectionism which sees regulatory agencies as black boxes appears to be too simplistic. It does not fully recognize that regulatory agencies are organizations with all the incentives for maintenance and growth of other organizations and that regulation can provide opportunities to grow. Further, it misses the significance of the commitment made by many planners to a set of beliefs regarding inequities in the existing system and the importance of redressing these through regulation. In short, it misses the fact that regulatory agencies can have an organizational mission of their own and are not simply available for capture. The life cycle view does recognize the importance of organizational interests in regulatory agency behavior, but sees these interests as uniformly consistent with surrender rather than with the equally feasible tough regulatory stand. The life cycle view predicts gradual weakening and surrender, but increased regulatory toughness over time may be as likely.

The capture theory was developed to explain the behavior of federal-, or in some cases, state-level independent regulatory commissions. It did not envision a highly decentralized three-tiered regulatory system involving federal, state, and local agencies such as exists under PL 93–641, where interaction between regulatory agencies becomes a major determinant of policy and where varying degrees of capture or regulatory toughness are possible at different levels and in different parts of the country. Developing as it did around experiences with federal- and state-level commissions, the capture literature also does not address the role of citizen participation in a decentralized regulatory system. As this ex post facto revision of the capture theory implies, it is reasonable to expect variation in the behavior of regulatory agencies under PL 93–641, with at least some state agencies and HSAs taking a tough regulatory stand. This is exactly what we have observed in New England.

The Spectrum of Regulation in New England

As noted in Chapter 2, New England encompasses a broad range of regulatory effort. Generally, the southern New England states (Rhode Island, Connecticut, and Massachusetts), have adopted a tough regulatory posture, while the northern New England states have been less inclined towards intervention. Among the northern New England states, Maine has been by far the most active in health planning and regulation. New Hampshire has been the least committed of the New England States to regulation in health.

In the southern New England states regulation in health predated the passage of PL 93–641 in 1974. Certificate of need was first passed in Rhode Island in 1970, in Massachusetts in 1971, and in Connecticut in 1973. In addition, each of these states operates its own hospital rate regulation programs, generally regarded among the toughest in the nation. Prior to the passage of PL 93–641, none of the northern New England states had passed certificate of need legislation. CON legislation was enacted in Maine in 1978 and in Vermont in 1979; New Hampshire did not pass a CON law until 1979.

The specific intervention strategies adopted by planners in New England states are different, even among states occupying roughly similar positions on the regulatory spectrum. The strategies employed by state-level planners in New England can be characterized in the following manner.

Capital and Revenue Containmment Through Regulation

This category includes those states that have moved aggressively through certificate of need and rate regulation to prevent capital expansion and to limit increases in hospital budgets. The first priority of the containment strategy is to hold the line at existing levels and to limit increases in service intensity by controlling the modernization of existing capital stock through certificate of need actions. A secondary goal, one that given present authority cannot be readily effected, is to achieve reductions below existing levels. A common denominator of the containment strategy is a focus on hospital beds. Typically, the analytical component of the containment strategy focuses on bed-to-population ratios and hospital occupancy rates. For New England, the containment strategy is characteristic of Connecticut, Rhode Island, and Massachusetts. For each of these states a different approach to containment can be discerned.

Centralized and formalized is the approach taken in Connecticut, where both certificate of need and rate setting are integrated within a single agency, the Commission on Hospitals and Health Care. The Commission operates independently of the SHPDA, SHCC, and the HSAs established under PL 93–641. CON and rate setting in Connecticut are linked in more than an organizational sense. In most cases, CON and rate reviews occur simultaneously. Review panels (3 of 17 commissioners per panel), assisted by staff analysts from both the finance and planning divisions, review CON applications and hospital rate requests for any services involved in or affected by the CON application. The aggressive containment policy in Connecticut (in 1977 the Commission denied more than half of the $802 million hospital budget requests) is formalized in a series of rate-setting formulas and CON decision standards.

Decentralized and formalized is the approach to cost containment practiced in Massachusetts. As in Connecticut, Massachusetts has taken an aggressive stand towards capital expansion and hospital budgets. Massachusetts has been particularly strict in the area of acute hospital expansion and in controlling hospital revenues. As in Connecticut, the overall regulatory policy is formalized in quantitative rate-setting formulas and in a series of decision methodologies for acute and long-term care. Both have been and continue to be a focus of controversy and debate. Unlike Connecticut, however, the regulatory structure in Massachusetts is highly decentralized. Rate setting and planning in Massachusetts are separate, the former falling under the jurisdiction of the Massachusetts Rate Setting Commission and the latter the Department of Public Health. On the planning side, authority is also fragmented; the state health plan is prepared by the Office of State Health Planning, CON reviews are performed by the Determination of Need Office, and CON decisions are made by the Public Health Council.

Decentralized and adaptive is the approach taken in Rhode Island. As in Massachusetts, the regulatory apparatus in Rhode Island is fragmented, although it is much less fragmented. Planning and rate setting in Rhode Island are separate, with certificate of need falling within the jurisdiction of the Department of Health (DPH) and budget review conducted through a unique negotiating process involving the State Budget Office, Blue Cross, and individual hospitals. Thus, planning and rate setting are organizationally separate, although in practice there is considerable interaction between DPH planners and rate setters. For its part, planning in Rhode Island is centrally directed. As a result of a waiver under Section 1536 of PL 93–641, Rhode Island has no HSAs and all of the powers of HSAs and SHPDAs are integrated within the DPH. However, planning in Rhode Island is somewhat less centralized than the casual observer would suspect. This is because a voluntary non-profit planning agency first created in 1966, the Health Planning Council, still operates and has input into the planning process. The HPC conducts its own advisory reviews of many CON proposals and, in addition, provides reviews and priority rankings of major hospital program changes for use by rate setters in the budget review decision process. Unlike both Connecticut and Massachusetts, the aggressive regulatory strategy in Rhode Island has not been formalized in a set of quantitative formulas or decision rules. Hospital budget increases are negotiated with individual hospitals. And planners in Rhode Island have operated without developing complex quantitative CON decision standards. Instead, they prefer to base decisions on general policy and situation-specific analyses. Obviously, the size of the state and of the hospital industry (there are only 14 acute care hospitals in Rhode Island) facilitates this approach.

In 1979, the Rhode Island Department of Health published a "Preliminary (Draft) State Health Plan" containing quantitative resource targets in a number of areas and spelling out strategic priorities for the Department's regulatory policy. The Draft Plan, required by PL 93–641, marks a departure from previous regulatory tactics, and may signal a shift towards the more formalized approach, and perhaps, a more contentious program similar to those found in Massachusetts and Connecticut. Not surprisingly, the Draft Plan has generated considerable controversy and debate.[3]

The Analytical Approach

In contrast to the policy of cost containment practiced in Connecticut, Massachusetts, and Rhode Island, the overall regulatory strategy in Maine has been both more moderate and more mixed. Although the SHPDA in Maine has been increasingly aggressive in regulating hospital facilities, it has been less stringent in other areas. This has been especially true in long-term care, where official state policy has encouraged the addition of new nursing homes in order to trigger competition between the new homes and the many older, lower-quality homes.

Whatever its record in the area of regulation, one important distinguishing feature of the health planning program in Maine has been its analytical orientation. State-level planners in Maine have utilized state-of-the-art, population-based analytical techniques available through the Maine Health Data Service file covering all hospitalizations in the state. In contrast to the planners' focus on bed-to-population ratios and hospital occupancy rates in the three southern New England states, planners in Maine have focused on small area per capita variations in hospital use and, in some instances, have included variations in hospital use and surgical procedures between areas, and within an area over time, in the facilities review decision process. Although data-sharing relationships between SHPDA planners and the Maine Health Data Service have not resulted in a full integration of population-based data into the review process, it is important to recognize that when planners assess the medical delivery system in Maine they do so through an analytical lens that differs in important respects from the planning perspective in most other states. (The use of population-based analytical techniques in facilities review in Maine is described in the "A" General Hospital case in Part Two).

In important respects, the regulatory philosophy of Vermont parallels that of Maine. Planners in Vermont share with those in Maine an analytical focus that emphasizes population-based data and small area variations in hospital use. Planners in Vermont are also beginning to utilize analyses of population-based data in facilities review. Regulation in Vermont, however, has been much more moderate than in Maine. Facilities review has not been a hot issue in Vermont; in the past, the limited number of applications submitted have been approved after only minimal reviews. This is, in part, a consequence of delay in the implementation of PL 93-641 in Vermont resulting from an unsuccessful effort to obtain a Section 1536 waiver that would have allowed Vermont to function without an HSA. Vermont is moving towards a more aggressive regulatory program grounded in an analytical perspective that emphasizes population-based data and small area variations in hospital use (see Chapter 6).

Pre-Regulation

New Hampshire is a state where planners have yet to develop a clear regulatory strategy. This is a result of New Hampshire having had an administration unalterably opposed as a matter of record and political philosophy to government intervention in the economy. Much of the first four years of PL 93-641 in New Hampshire have been characterized by intramural conflict, with New Hampshire's HSA attempting to prod an inattentive and understaffed SHPDA into action. Even after five years of PL 93-641, very little facility regulation has occurred in New Hampshire. With the change in the state administration in 1978 and recent changes in leadership at both the HSA and the SHPDA, the preconditions for the development of an identifiable regulatory strategy may have at last been met.

Thus, planners in New England states embrace a broad spectrum of regulatory philosophy—from aggressive cost control and capital containment in the southern states, to a focus on analysis with moderate regulation in Maine and more recently in Vermont, to the situation in New Hampshire, where planners operating in a political vacuum have yet to articulate a clear operating philosophy. What remains is to consider the causes of these variations. We will focus our analysis at two levels in order to attempt to identify the key determinants of overall state support for regulation, as well as the factors that influence the specific policies developed by SHPDA and HSA planners operating within different political contexts.

State Policy Towards Health Planning

Most of the New England states regarded the passage of PL 93-641 in 1974 with some apprehension. The majority of states apparently held the same view. Working through the National Governors Association, state governments lobbied for changes that would give them greater control of the planning program. They allied themselves with similar interests in representing county government, specifically the National Association of Counties, an organization which had taken an even earlier interest in the planning law. Some lobbying occurred during the development of the legislation. Perhaps the best-known outcome of these efforts was a modification of the eligibility criteria for HSAs. The law was changed so that, in addition to private nonprofit corporations, units of county or regional government could become HSAs as well. The important state and county lobbying, however, occurred during the early stages of regulation development for PL 93-641. Most of the issues raised then involved further efforts to expand the state and county role in the planning program. In some cases the states and counties were successful; in others, issues were deferred and surfaced in 1978 and 1979 as proposed amendments to the planning law.

The early state attitude towards PL 93-641 was somewhat surprising. For all the talk of "planning with teeth" that surrounded the passage of the law, almost all of the teeth were state teeth. Final authority for certificate of need and appropriateness review, the key regulatory activities under PL 93-641, rests with the states. Indeed, a state-directed certificate of need program is made mandatory under the law. The most important health plan developed under the law is the State Health Plan; in theory it integrates the HSA's Health System Plans into an overall planning document consistent with the needs of the state as a whole. PL 93-641 also encouraged state rate-setting experiments, subsequently administered and funded by the Social Security Administration, significantly strengthening the hands of the states receiving rate-setting experiment funds.

In contrast, virtually all HSA powers are advisory. HSAs serve as the initial points of review for CON and appropriateness review and develop regional health systems plans. The only exception to this is the

HSA power to "review and approve or disapprove" proposals from their areas for certain federal funds. And here the HSA's review authority is not binding; the Secretary of HEW can fund projects despite unfavorable HSA reviews. Although the balance of authority was tipped towards the states from the start, as a group they voiced strong objections to the planning program. In part, the states were concerned that HSA-conducted appropriateness, CON, and federal funds reviews, and HSA-prepared health plans would impinge upon the states' ability to set priorities for spending and development. This, in turn, would impinge upon important political prerogatives, including the power to broker federal dollars and to cultivate political support and discourage political opponents. More fundamental to the states' early reaction to the planning law, however, was a general feeling that it represented an unfavorable balance of federalism, one that states and counties had resisted in the past and would not welcome in the future. PL 93–641, with its consumer-majority Health Systems Agencies, reminded governors, mayors, and county officials of the OEO community action programs of the 1960s. In their view, it contradicted recent efforts— revenue sharing being the most important—to shore up traditional units of government and disarm local "para governments" which the states, counties, and cities had regarded as troublesome in the past. Most especially, the balance of federalism under PL 93–641 appeared to be establishing a precedent for a reduced role for the states in future health regulation and perhaps even under a national health insurance plan.

Despite this early reaction from the states, it became clear as PL 93–641 was implemented that HSA powers were in fact limited and that federal legislation in health regulation and national health insurance would proceed slowly. As the planning program became a reality, some states reacted to it as an opportunity to effect cost control in health while others remained opposed or disinterested. These differences in response to PL 93–641 set the context for health planning in particular states. Indeed, the state posture with regard to health regulation is perhaps the key factor explaining the considerable variation in program performance that has occurred in New England as well as around the country.

One obvious factor that might discriminate between states that utilized PL 93–641 as a regulatory opportunity and states that are more passive is health care costs, particularly the burden placed on state budgets by expenditures for Medicaid. If we look at Medicaid as a percentage of state budget in New England (Table 5.1) at around the time of the passage of PL 93–641, we see some differences that

Table 5.1

State Expenditures for Medicaid
as Percent of State Budget,
1974, 1975

State	1974	1975
Connecticut	4.5%	4.4%
Maine	3.2	3.1
Massachusetts	6.5	6.4
New Hampshire	2.3	2.5
Rhode Island	5.5	5.3
Vermont	2.9	3.1

Table 5.2

Dollar Expenditures for Medicaid
in New England States,
1974, 1975 (x 1000)

State	1974	1975
Connecticut	$ 66,936	$ 80,970
Maine	14,734	19,540
Massachusetts	217,604	253,522
New Hampshire	8,132	10,554
Rhode Island	26,722	31,365
Vermont	8,615	10,287

correspond to the differences in support for regulation described earlier in southern and northern tier states.

Tables 5.3 and 5.4 show a similar difference between the southern and northern New England states during the same period. Table 5.3 provides a measure of the level of benefits provided by each state. Table 5.4 provides a measure that can be used in comparing the total Medicaid burden for the different states.

Finally, we can consider two measures of the visibility and political significance of Medicaid expenditures in the New England states (Tables 5.5 and 5.6).

Table 5.3

State Expenditures for Medicaid per Low Income Resident, 1974

State	1974
Connecticut	$302
Maine	109
Massachusetts	495
New Hampshire	127
Rhode Island	263
Vermont	182

Table 5.4

State Expenditures for Medicaid Per Capita, 1974, 1975

State	1974	1975
Connecticut	$22	$26
Maine	14	18
Massachusetts	37	43
New Hampshire	10	13
Rhode Island	28	34
Vermont	18	22

Table 5.5

State Expenditures for Medicaid as Percentage of *Increases* in State Budgets Over Time

	1975		1976		1977	
	State Medicaid Expendit.	State Budget	State Medicaid Expendit.	State Budget	State Medicaid Expendit.	State Budget
Connecticut	+21.0%	+27.3%	+19.5%	+19.3%	+10.8%	−2.6%
Maine	+32.6	+36.9	+32.4	+24.0	+ 1.2	−9.4
Massachusetts	+16.5	+17.7	+15.8	+ 8.2	+17.2	−2.1
New Hampshire	+29.8	+18.0	+22.4	+16.2	+25.6	−2.7
Rhode Island	+17.4	+21.5	+24.8	+25.8	+20.4	−4.6
Vermont	+19.4	+26.5	+18.9	+ 8.8	+ 8.2	−1.4

Table 5.6

State Expenditures for Medicaid as Percentage of
State Budget Over Time

State	1974	1976	1977
Connecticut	4.5%	4.4%	5.1%
Maine	3.2	3.3	3.7
Massachusetts	6.5	6.8	8.2
New Hampshire	2.3	2.6	3.4
Rhode Island	5.5	5.2	6.6
Vermont	2.9	3.4	3.7

Sources for Tables 5.1–5.6

State Budget = total state expenditures minus revenue from the federal government.

State Medicaid expenditures = total amount of medical payments under Title XIX minus federal Medicaid Assistance Percentage. Sources: *Medicaid Statistics* – HEW.

Population from the Annual Abstract of Statistics – Census Bureau.

All this suggests differences in the burden of Medicaid expenditures that correspond to differences in support for regulation. Nevertheless, the data should be interpreted very cautiously. For one thing, it is not at all clear that a cause-and-effect relationship between Medicaid costs and willingness to regulate can be established. Both may independently be the products of other factors, including the political tradition of the state—a record of providing comprehensive benefits and services and a willingness to intervene in the private sector. Moreover, the burden of Medicaid expenditures does not explain why the southern New England states have launched broad regulatory programs. Presumably, a state concerned primarily with Medicaid expenditures could focus its regulatory efforts on Medicaid alone. It could also focus even more narrowly on the long-term care sector, which consumes the largest share of Medicaid expenditures. Certainly, states respond to health-related financial pressures above and beyond their Medicaid costs. For example, in Rhode Island repeated Blue Cross requests for premium increases provided the immediate stimulus for the state's Department of Business Regulation to initiate the development of Rhode Island's innovative rate-setting program. In Massachusetts, the Dukakis administration supported the development of tough rate-setting and CON programs, in part because they believed that rising health care costs would exacerbate the "fiscal crisis" in the state, increasing the burden on consumers and further discouraging business from entering the state.

Figure 5.1 shows a sharp rise in per capita hospital revenues in Maine between 1974 and 1977. Perhaps not entirely coincidentally, both the previous and the current administrations in Maine have shown increasing support for regulation in health. Maine has moved from a nonregulatory posture to a regulatory stance that much more closely resembles its southern neighbors, embarking on a voluntary hospital budget review program and passing CON legislation in 1978. However, Figure 5.1 also shows a sharp increase in hospital revenues per capita in New Hampshire, a state which is just now beginning to address health planning and facilities review under PL 93-641. Thus, even when we include not just Medicaid, but other health-related costs and the condition of the state economy as well, differences in the burden of health care costs do not adequately or reliably explain state policy toward regulation.

What is undoubtedly the most important factor is clearly the most difficult to measure—the political ideology and culture in a state, including in particular the willingness of the state to intervene in the private sector. New Hampshire clearly has a tradition of nonintervention, one which it advertises widely to attract industry to the state. And obviously the Thomson administration was not reluctant to assert its philosophical opposition to government intervention in general and to federal intervention in state affairs in particular whenever the opportunity arose. Just as obviously, Massachusetts has traditionally been regarded as an interventionist state. However, beyond these and similar general observations it is difficult to discriminate among states on the basis of political culture.

One might, however, take as a proxy for political culture, as it is expressed in the health area, the level of regulation already in place at the time of the passage of PL 93-641. Here one can clearly see a close fit between the state behavior prior to PL 93-641 and the state response to the law and record since. And that, of course, should not be surprising. PL 93-641 offered existing health planning agencies in the southern New England states an opportunity to expand their authority and importance. Often these agencies and the officials in them, rather than the governors or state legislatures, were the key advocates of cost control and regulation in their respective states. And it is for that reason that PL 93-641 implementation was immediate in pro-regulatory states, while political opposition and start-up time have been major problems in others. We will turn next to the factors that influence the specific policies developed by health planners in the HSAs and SHPDAs in New England, operating within the context of obviously different state attitudes towards regulation in health.

Figure 5.1

Per Capita Hospital Revenue Trends

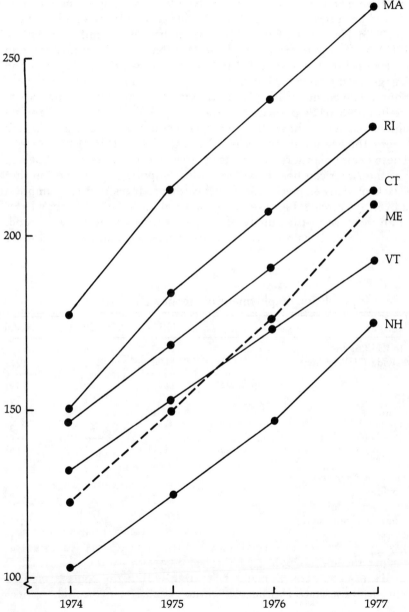

The Policymaking Process in the HSAs and SHPDAs

Taken together, the HSAs and SHPDAs have an aggregate staff of more than three thousand nationally, Of these, approximately two thousand are professional staff. HSA staffs range from a high of more than 75 in New York City to just a handful in a number of HSAs. SHPDA staffs range from a high of 74 in New Jersey to just three in New Hampshire.[4] As Table 5.7 indicates, the majority of SHPDA and HSA agency directors have previous experience in a variety of organizations involved in health planning, with the majority having experience in PL 93–641's predecessor, the Comprehensive Health Planning Program. Table 5.8 shows that in terms of education, the largest degree category for agency directors is a Master of Public Health.

These health planners, to one degree or another, share a set of beliefs about the American health system.[5] Most important is the notion that the lack of market mechanisms in health produces overconsumption and overinvestment. Because of a widely held belief in "Roemer's Law" that an increase in the supply of hospital beds induces more demand, planners regard it as essential to restrict hospital-induced demand by

Table 5.7

Prior Employment of Agency Directors

		HSAs	SHPDA	Total
State CHP agency		3	24	27
Areawide CHP agency		120	2	122
	Subtotals	(123)	(26)	(149)
RMP		13	1	14
Hill–Burton		1	—	1
EHSDS		3	—	3
	Subtotals	(17)	(1)	(18)
Hospital		4	2	6
Other direct service provider		2	6	8
Local government		5	—	5
Regional planning body		7	—	7
University		2	1	3
Other		7	1	8
	TOTALS	167	37	204

Source: Bureau of Health Planning and Resources Development Program Information Note 77-2, February 25, 1977.

Table 5.8

Degrees of Agency Directors (8)

	HSAs	SHPDA	Total
None	6	1	7
Associate	2	—	2
Bachelors	30	7	37
MBA	12	—	12
MHA	14	—	14
MPA	4	1	5
MPH	37	11	48
MSW	8	3	11
MUP	2	1	3
Other Masters	39	6	45
Ph.D.	6	4	10
M.D.	3	3	6
Other	4	—	4
TOTALS	167	37	204

Source: Bureau of Health Planning and Resources Development Program Information Note 77-2, February 25, 1977.

controlling the supply of hospital beds.[6] Generally, planners believe that by controlling the supply of resources they can bring some order to a haphazard system. Their goal is to develop regional delivery systems with predetermined sets of arrangements linking together the major components of the health care system, including acute care, ambulatory care, long-term care, and so forth. In theory, each regional system would be built around a core of more sophisticated tertiary care centers. Sophisticated and expensive technology too would be rationed in an economically efficient manner. The planners' view of the health system stands in sharp contrast to the notion, currently experiencing resurgence of its own in Congress, and generally, that market mechanisms can effectively be introduced into the health care system.

Despite this common set of beliefs, HSA and SHPDA planners operate in rather different organizational contexts. State agencies can act directly through certificate of need, rate setting, or licensing. HSAs, in contrast, must bargain and cajole, always cognizant of the need to accommodate their various component groups. When they emerge from this bargaining and negotiating process, HSAs still cannot act authoritatively; instead they make recommendations in an attempt to influence state policy. As a consequence, key state agency officials view themselves as agents of state government. They are governmental decisionmakers operating within the bounds of departmental and gubernatorial policy. Key HSA staff, in contrast, view themselves as professional planners. They are advocates for a set of beliefs and skills, who bargain for their policy positions within a more pluralistic and participatory structure. Whatever the analytical method used in need determination or in plan development,[7] the availability of different organizational resources (including both technical and political resources), perceptions of organizational interests, and the interaction between agencies are consistently important determinants of planning policy and key elements of the health planning policymaking process.

One of the most graphic examples of the recognition by health planners of the importance of organizational position and resources in health planning comes from Vermont. Implementation of PL 93–641 in Vermont was delayed considerably while state officials, including the Governor, the Secretary of Human Services, and the Commissioner of Health, engaged in a prolonged effort to win approval for HEW for a Section 1536 waiver. The waiver would have enabled Vermont to function under PL 93–641 as Rhode Island does, without a health system agency, and with HSA and SHPDA powers integrated within a single unit. Vermont officials were opposed in these efforts by three groups, including one representing providers and another representing the existing CHP "b" agencies, each interested in becoming Vermont's single HSA. One two occasions, HEW Secretary Mathews rejected the waiver request. As a next step, the state legislature, acting on the request of the Governor's Commission on Health, created the Health Policy Council, with the ultimate goal of having the Council serve as HSA, SHPDA, and SHCC. In effect, this move represented an attempt to accomplish a Section 1536 waiver through state legislation. As a first step towards accomplishing this plan, the Council applied for and received designation as the SHPDA in Vermont. However, it was to be an incomplete SHPDA. Section 1122 review (Vermont did not then have a CON program) and appropriateness review were to be vested in the state's Department of Human Services.

When the Council applied for designation as Vermont's HSA, however, HEW denied the application, reasoning that the Council, technically a unit of state government, could not serve as both SHPDA and HSA. Thus rebuffed, the Council opted to establish itself as an HSA rather than a SHPDA, severing itself from state government, leaving its SHPDA functions to the Department of Human Services, and establishing itself as the Vermont Health Policy Corporation Inc. In order to strengthen its chances, VHPC also managed to coopt its two remaining rivals for the HSA slot, People for a Healthy Vermont, and a group representing the medical society known as Vermont Health Systems Agency Inc.

Apparently not satisfied with its status as an HSA, the VHPC next sought to establish itself as Vermont's statewide Health Coordinating Council as well. This could be accomplished by allowing the Governor to appoint members of the HSA board and adding the twist that appointment to the board would automatically constitute a nomination for gubernatorial decision on appointment to the SHCC. In effect, appointments to the HSA and the SHCC would occur simultaneously. When HEW approved the three separate applications for HSA, SHCC, and SHPDA, Vermont had accomplished almost all at once an interesting and unusual feat of organizational gymnastics—the SHPDA had become the HSA, the Department of Human Services had become the SHPDA, and the HSA had become the SHCC. In the end, Vermont had also accomplished something very similar to the 1536 waiver it had originally sought. In practice, the SHPDA and the HSA/SHCC, although under separate leadership, share a common location, a common phone system, even a common photocopier, the ultimate test of organizational cooperation. Obviously, health officials in Vermont recognized the importance of husbanding organizational resources under PL 93–641 and the difficulties a more fragmented planning structure in a rural, single-HSA state would bring.

A similar degree of attention to organizational interests in health planning can be seen in Connecticut and Rhode Island. In Connecticut, both rate setting and certificate of need are integrated within the Commission on Hospitals and Health Care, thus delegating to the Commission and its leadership the key regulatory functions in the state. HSAs in Connecticut provide advisory CON reviews to the Commission rather than to Connecticut's SHPDA. For its part, the SHPDA is left to concentrate its efforts on plan development and to building up a constituency and a base of support among the HSAs. In Rhode Island, as discussed elsewhere, the Section 1536 waiver enabled the Department of Health and the Health Services Council (its CON decision body) to gain the upper hand in a long-standing rivalry with unofficial, but influential, Health Planning Council. That planners recognize organizational interests and that regulation provides opportunities for organizational enhancement should not be surprising. Perhaps more important is the way in which interaction between planning agencies based on those interests shapes the policies health planners develop.

This can be seen, for example, in New Hampshire, where protracted personal battles between HSA and SHPDA directors effectively blocked the implementation of PL 93–641 and the development of planning policy. HSA planners and board members were continually frustrated when their negative 1122 recommendations were overturned by a very permissive SHPDA. Single-HSA states represent, at best, a difficult organizational arrangement. In a situation where both the SHPDA and the HSA have statewide jurisdiction, whose 1122 or CON review is controlling? Whose health plan counts most, the HSA's or the SHPDA's? What is the role, in such cases, of the SHCC?

These are the questions that have dominated the health planning scene in Maine, another single-HSA state. During the Longley administration, the SHPDA staff in Maine seized upon the opportunity provided by PL 93-641 to assume a leadership position in health regulation, moving the state from a laissez-faire to a moderate regulatory posture. Governor Longley, a critic of the HSA, clearly favored a leadership position for the SHPDA. During this time the HSA sought to achieve organizational identity and recognition by developing policies that clearly distinguished it from the SHPDA. Thus, the HSA advocated tougher regulation in non-hospital areas, notably in long-term care (where the SHPDA advocated a laissez-faire approach), and physician practice (where the HSA advocated inclusion of physicians' offices under 1122 and CON). Over time, as the HSA's identity problems were partially resolved, tensions between the two agencies gradually diminished. With the election of Governor Brennan in 1978, the leadership roles in health planning appear to have changed hands. Key SHPDA staff have departed and the former HSA director has become Deputy Commissioner for Health.

Obstetrical services provide another example of how bargaining between planning agencies determined a specific planning policy. In the summer of 1977, the Secretary of HEW convened a high-level working group to develop a set of proposed National Guidelines for Health Planning. Working without benefit of any substantial new empirical evidence, the group produced a set of proposed guidelines in less than three weeks. On September 23, 1977, the standards developed by the group appeared in the *Federal Register* as a Notice of Proposed Rulemaking on National Guidelines for Health Planning. The proposed guidelines contained numerical standards in ten areas, the best known being the four per thousand standard for acute care hospital beds. One of the most controversial standards, as discussed briefly above, was in the area of obstetrical services.[8] The proposed national standard called for a minimum of 2,000 deliveries annually in obstetrical services located in SMSAs with a population of 100,000 or more.[9]

The 2,000 delivery standard was an exceedingly difficult one for most hospitals to meet. In Massachusetts, the SHPDA responded to the HEW standard by promulgating its own, more moderate 1,500 delivery target. Locally, the Boston HSA was hard pressed to deal with the situation it faced as a result of the federal and state OB standards. The guidelines were HEW's attempt to bind them to federal goals. In theory, the tough federal standard would appear to offer the HSA some bargaining leverage by partially removing responsibility for a strict regulatory policy. The staff and board members at the Boston HSA, however, believed that this advantage would come at an unacceptable organizational cost. The HSA staff and board saw as a higher priority the establishment of organizational credibility and recognition locally, both with their constituent groups, the providers and interested community residents, and with state health planning agencies. They believed that their effectiveness depended upon the establishment of an independent track record. For this reason, they thought that it was essential to maintain at least the semblance of "bottom up" planning and avoid appearing as pawns of HEW policy.

At the same time, however, the HSA recognized that it existed within an HEW-defined reward structure. Its license to operate, its funding, its recognition nationally would depend upon HEW's assessment of its performance. HEW's performance standards, although vague, were thought to rely heavily on HSA conformance with the national guidelines. The HSA recognized that it could stray from the HEW standards in order to serve its local organizational interests, but it also recognized that it could not stray too far. As a result, despite the fact that the HSA staff and plan development subcommittee members were unequivocal that they had no empirical evidence on which to base their own standard, the HSA opted for "the reasonable compromise." The draft of the HSA's Health Systems Plan issued in the fall of 1977 contained a standard of 1,000 deliveries per year—still a tough standard, one that few Boston area hospitals could meet, but obviously less rigid than either the state or the HEW targets. Subsequently, the Boston HSA encountered considerable opposition even to this "least onerous" standard, and eventually the 1,000 delivery target was modified in the final version of the HSA's first Health Systems Plan.[10] The development of numerical standards for OB services is a clear example of how bargaining among planning agencies at three levels based on differences in resources and organizational interests produced a very specific planning policy for OB services.

Conclusion

We began this chapter by examining various versions of the capture theory of regulation—a loose set of expectations regarding the behavior of planners and regulators predicting an ineffective and somewhat less than aggressive regulatory effort. We then highlighted some of the many inadequacies of the capture theory, pointing out a variety of reasons to expect considerable variation in regulatory behavior, with aggressive and effective regulation occurring in at least some cases. It was not our intention to set up a straw man. Certainly many of the weaknesses of the capture theory have been recognized in recent years, and the theory itself has undergone considerable refinement. Rather, our purpose was to provide a conceptual context for the analysis of our observations in New England. What we observed in New England is precisely what the amended theory would lead one to expect— considerable variation in regulatory effort, with aggressive regulation in a significant number of instances and less in others.

State interest in and support for health regulation is perhaps partly a result of the burden of Medicaid expenditures on the state budget, and the burden of rising health costs in general during periods of fiscal strain. But the data are at best suggestive in showing a cause-and-effect relationship between health costs and regulatory response. The fact that Maine has moved towards more aggressive regulation and New Hampshire has not, despite sharply rising costs in both states, may mean that political ideology and tradition is a more important discriminator of state behavior.

The policies developed by SHPDAs and HSAs reflect the differences in organizational character of the two agencies. The specific policies that are developed by planning agencies are influenced significantly by the pulling and hauling that develops among federal, state, and local agencies, producing variations in policies that are explained not so much by differences in analytical techniques—indeed the analytical techniques used by SHPDAs and HSAs are usually quite similar—as by obvious differences in organizational interests. The play of these different interests in New England since 1974 suggests that PL 93-641 provided an opportunity for states already committed to an intervention strategy in health to strengthen their regulatory hand. In Maine, it provided the resouces and a structure to support a swing towards regulation that, although in its infancy, was already in progress. But the record in New Hampshire suggests that PL 93-641 could do little more than place planning issues somewhere near the bottom of the political agenda—using the pressure of a federally created and guided HSA to accomplish the task—pending a change in administration that would produce a state government more receptive to the purposes of the planning law.

Notes

[1] Perhaps the best presentation of the capture theory can be found in Douglas Anderson's "The Politics of Regulation," unpublished, Harvard Business School, March, 1978. Portions of this summary of the capture theory follow Anderson fairly closely.

[2] George Stigler, "The Theory of Economic Regulation," *Bell Journal,* Vol. 2, pp. 3–27.

[3] "Public Scorns Rhode Island Cost-Cutting Health Plan," *Medical World News* (March 17, 1980), p. 26. See also "Rhode Island Plan Creates Stir," *Washington Report on Medicine and Health/Planning Letter,* February 18, 1980, p. 3.

[4] Program Information Note 77-2, Bureau of Health Planning and Resources Development, February 25, 1977.

[5] The ideology of health planning is discussed in greater detail in Chapter 4.

[6] Milton I. Roemer, "Bed Supply and Hospital Utilization: A Natural Experiment," *Hospitals,* 35 (November 1, 1961).

[7] The technical aspects of planning are discussed in Chapter 6.

[8] The policymaking process for obstetrical services at the federal, state, and local level is described in brief in the Leonard Morse Hospital case, Case 7, Part Two.

[9] *Federal Register,* Vol. 42, No. 188, September 23, 1977.

[10] The provider opposition to the HSA standard and the resulting modifications in the plan are described in detail in the Leonard Morse Hospital case, Case 7, Part Two.

Chapter 6

Methodologies

The process of health planning in the acute hospital sector includes an assessment of the appropriateness of the services provided by each hospital, the development of a master plan for allocating hospital resources, and the review and approval or disapproval of specific capital projects under the CON and 1122 programs. Common to, and at the heart of, these planning and regulatory endeavors is the task of determining the need of discrete populations for medical facilities and resources.

Because of several unique attributes of the medical care market, needs assessment for institutional resources is a highly complex and uncertain process. Two characteristics of medical care delivery that complicate the efforts of planners to determine need for health resources are the influence of supply factors on the demand for medical care services and the problem of physician uncertainty surrounding the efficacy of many common medical interventions.

That the supply of hospital beds can influence the demand for hospital services was first suggested by Roemer in 1961.[1] He reported an analysis of a natural experiment—the impact of a significant expansion of beds on the utilization pattern of a community hospital in New York State. The hospital operated at 78 percent capacity prior to expansion; after beds were increased by over 40 percent, the annual number of admissions and the average length of stay increased. Demand expanded to fill the beds. Subsequent work of Feldstein provided more systematic evidence of the supply-demand relationship of hospital services.[2] Figure 6.1, adapted from Stevenson, shows a high degree of correlation between bed supply and bed use at the state level.[3]

Local physician supply has also been shown to correlate with the amount and kinds of medical services received by community residents.[4] For example, the data from the American College of Surgeons' study of

Figure 6.1

Hospital Bed Supply and Utilization

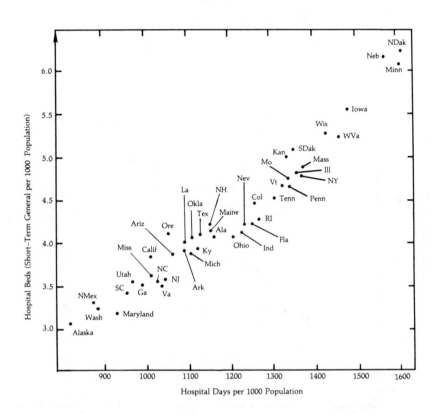

surgical services in the U.S. shows a direct relationship between the availability of surgeons in an area and the amount of surgery received by residents of that area (see Figure 6.2).[5]

The implications of supply-demand interaction in acute hospital services poses a serious dilemma for health planners engaged in determining need for, and appropriateness of, hospital services and resources. The demand for services, an easily measured statistic, cannot readily be related to the need for services.

The situation is further complicated by the observations that residents of similar, neighboring communities in New England receive widely different amounts and kinds of hospital services.[6] Among New England communities the rate of hospitalization per capita varies over

Figure 6.2

Relationship Between the Supply of Surgical Specialists
and Surgery Rate in
Four SMSA Areas in the United States

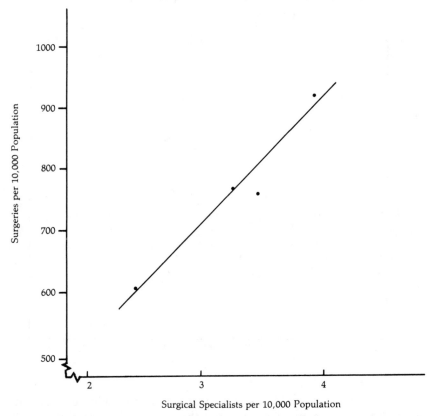

Surgical Specialists per 10,000 Population

Source: Data from *Surgery in The United States*, The American College of Surgeons
and The American Surgical Association, 1975.

threefold; the per capita surgery rate varies more than twofold and the
expenditure for acute hospital care varies over sevenfold.[7]

One interpretation of local variations in hospital use patterns and of
the supply-demand interaction is that medical science operates with
considerable uncertainty concerning the efficacy of many common
medical and surgical interventions. The variations in the rate of
consumption of specific medical and surgical services among similar

communities can be interpreted as reflecting the differences of opinion among local physicians and surgeons regarding the efficacy of specific treatments. Evidence to support this view comes from the fact that variations in use rates among communities are greatest for specific procedures.

For example, Figure 6–3 shows the variations in the rate of consumption of common surgical procedures in five Maine communities.[8] The variations in the rates of surgical consumption in these communities are demonstrated by comparing the specific local surgery rates to that of the state as a whole. It should be noted that while the total surgery rate varies 1.7-fold among these communities, the range for hemorrhoidectomy is fivefold (between Areas I and IV). Such differences in specific procedure rates are not uncommon and likely reflect the difference of opinion among local physicians as to the efficacy of these procedures. This interpretation is supported by the growing body of research which brings into question the efficacy of many common medical and surgical procedures.[9]

The evidence that local hospital bed and physician supply influence the demand for hospital services makes the process of analysis for CON review and plan development complex. Planners' assessments of need for hospital resources must be carried out with considerable uncertainty about the interpretation of data. Given this uncertainty it is instructive to review the approaches taken by health planning agency staffs in assessing the need for hospital beds. To date, the major forums for bed need assessments have been the facilities review (CON and 1122) and health plan development processes. We shall discuss each of these planning activities separately.

Assessment of Hospital Bed Need in Facilities Review

In New England, health planning agencies have expended considerable energy in assessing bed need when hospitals have attempted to expand their bed complement. Interestingly, little or no attention has been given to assessing the need for existing beds when hospitals applied for CON or 1122 approval of major renovation or replacement projects which do not include increases in bed complement.

The simplest arguments for hospital bed expansion have been based on institutional demand. When occupancy is high and elective admissions have to be postponed, hospitals have requested more beds. Such an example is the 1973 case of the Portsmouth Hospital (New Hampshire) application for 1122 approval of a renovation project

Figure 6.3

Ratio of Observed to Statistically Predicted Number of Selected Surgical Procedures, Five Largest Hospital Service Areas, Maine, 1975

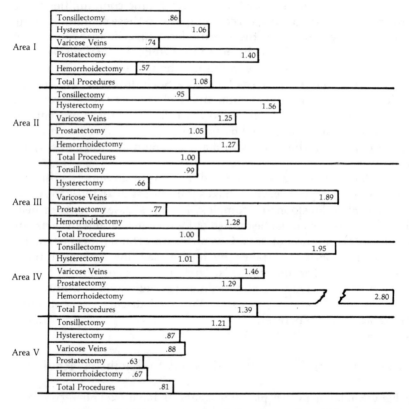

Source: J.E. Wennberg, "Using Localized, Population-based Data in Evaluating Planning Problems," in Papers on the National Health Guidelines, January, 1977, DHEW.

including a 10-bed expansion. The application cited the fact that up to 25 elective surgical procedures per week were postponed because of insufficient beds. The argument for more beds, based on overcrowding, was accepted without question by the state planning agency.

Similar arguments for expanding hospitals in Maine, Vermont, and Rhode Island have recently been challenged by planners using population-based data to compare the pattern of hospital use of local residents to that of the population of the entire state. In these states, independent hospital data services have maintained hospital data files containing information on virtually all discharges of state residents since 1969 in Vermont and since 1973 in Maine and Rhode Island. The files include the town of residence, diagnosis, and surgical procedures for each admitted patient. Thus, for any community in these states, the total number of hospital admissions per 1,000 residents can be compared to that of any other community or to the state as a whole. Moreover, the rate of use of specific hospital services, such as common surgical procedures, can be compared among communities. These data are beginning to play a major role in 1122 and CON reviews of hospital expansion proposals in Maine and Vermont.

Planners in Maine used population-based analysis of hospital use patterns to challenge a recent 1122 application for renovation and bed expansion. The "A" General Hospital ("A"GH), a rural 72-bed hospital, applied under Section 1122 for approval of a major renovation project including the addition of 11 new acute care beds plus shell space to accommodate future expansion.[10] The essential argument in support of additional beds was overcrowding. Between 1971 and 1975 the annual number of admissions had increased from 2,363 to 3,145; the occupancy rose from 60.5 percent to 75 percent. The SHPDA staff relied heavily on population-based analysis of the local hospital use pattern which showed that, on an age-adjusted basis, the residents of the area served by "A"GH were among the highest consumers of hospital services in Maine (248 discharges per 1,000 population compared to the state average of 164). Moreover, the rate at which "A"GH area residents underwent surgery was one-third higher than the state average, with the rates for appendectomy, hysterectomy, cholecystectomy, and hemorrhoidectomy over twice the average. These data were used by SHPDA staff to argue against the expansion portion of the project. The essential decision rule applied by planners in this case was that while bed need was difficult to assess, utilization rates dramatically exceeding the state average represented excessive use of hospital services.

The hospital staff maintained that the high use rates experienced by the community it served did not represent excessive hospital use. "A"GH staff argued that the community had special needs for hospital care. High rates of alcoholism, the presence of a small but poor American Indian population in the area, and the difficulty of travel to and from the hospital, especially in winter, were all presented as explanations for the high hospital use rates. To test their contention that the high use rates were justified, the hospital contracted with the

Maine PSRO to review the appropriateness of hospitalization of a sample of "A"GH patients. Based on process review of patient records, the PSRO reported that no inappropriate hospital admissions could be detected.

Thus the assessment of hospital bed need in the "A"GH case required weighing (1) institutional statistics showing increasing occupancy and admission frequency, (2) population-based data indicating residents of the area were extreme utilization outliers, and (3) the result of a process review of patient records offered as evidence of an appropriate admissions policy by the PSRO. It is important to stress that none of these sources of information provided an unequivocal argument for or against the need for additional beds. The hospital challenged the interpretation of the population-based analysis by arguing that the population served by "A"GH had more need than that of the average community in Maine. The SHPDA staff challenged the PSRO review on the grounds that the AMA process criteria used to assess appropriateness of admission were vague and permissive. In the end neither side was convinced of the other's argument, but the state did finally approve a revised application with eight, not eleven, new beds and no shell space.

The importance of the "A"GH case lies in the fact that in spite of the wealth of data and analysis available to the hospital and planners, no unequivocal technical solution to the bed need question was possible. The population-based analysis of hospital use patterns and the process review of patient records added analytic dimensions rarely available to planners attempting to assess bed need. But the results of both of these methods require considerable interpretation. The fact that a community uses 80 percent more hospital bed days than the average community in a state is not a priori evidence of unneeded hospitalization. The SHPDA staff applied a decision rule based on the assumption that the state average hospital use rate should be approximated in all communities. As will be seen in the recent Vermont case described below, other decision rules for interpreting population-based data can be used. Likewise, retroactive process review of patient records for appropriateness of admission is highly dependent on the stringency of criteria used and their application by the reviewers.[11] Thus, even in such circumstances where sophisticated, state-of-the-art analyses are available to planners, considerable uncertainty surrounds bed need assessments.

Another instructive example of the complexity of data interpretation for the purpose of determining bed need is provided by a recent 1122 application for renovation and bed expansion of "X" Memorial Hospital ("X"MH) in Vermont. The original application, submitted in December, 1978, included major renovations, the addition of both an ambulatory surgery center and an ambulatory obstetrics unit (a birthing room), an increase in bed complement from 175 to 200 beds, and shell space for an additional 25 beds. Again, the hospital's argument for bed need focused on increasing demand for services; occupancy and admission frequency were increasing in spite of a decreasing average length of stay.

The HSA planners used population-based analysis of local hospital use patterns to challenge the bed increase portion of the project. However, unlike the "A"GH case, the community residents served by "X"MH were not utilization outliers; their patient day rate per 1,000 residents was at the state average and the admission rate was only slightly higher than that of Vermont as a whole (see Figures 6.4 and 6.5). The Vermont HSA planners did not invoke a decision rule based on state average use rates. Their analysis included separating the "X"MH service area into two sub-areas—one rural, served primarily by young family physicians; the other more urban, served by older physicians. Table 6.1 compares the actual number of hospital admissions of residents of these two sub-areas to that predicted by extrapolating state average use rates (expected) to these populations.

HSA staff assumed that older physicians rely on hospitalization to a greater degree than younger physicians; the planners argued that Sub-area I would eventually experience lower use rates when the older physicians were replaced by younger colleagues. Moreover, the HSA staff applied a general decision rule which assumed that the communities with the lowest hospital use rates in the state received the correct amount of hospital service. The staff report on this application stated:

> It is important to restate that there is no evidence yet uncovered to suggest that the general health of the people of these low-use areas is different from the health of the high-use populations. This view leads straight to the policy issue. Should additional beds be authorized when the current supply is capable of delivering a reasonable number of patient days to serve the projected larger population of the service area?

The HSA further argued that the proposed ambulatory surgery center and the birthing room would reduce future admissions to "X"MH and thus would obviate the need for additional beds. While the hospital staff was unconvinced by the HSA arguments against bed expansion, a nego-tiated agreement was reached between the two parties; a revised application including only five additional beds was approved by both the HSA and SHPDA.

The "X"MH case example again demonstrates the fact that hospital

Figure 6.4

Average Number of Patients Discharged from
Hospitals per 1000 Population within each Hospital Service Area
(Age-adjusted, 1974–76)

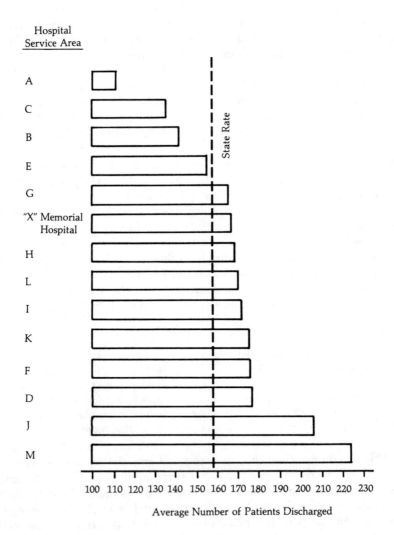

Source: The Vermont HSA staff review of "X"MH 1122 application.
Data from: "Dataset for Health Planning 1974–1976" CHIC-V.

Figure 6.5

Average Number of Days Spent in
Hospitals per 1000 Population within each Hospital Service Area
(Age-adjusted, 1974–76)

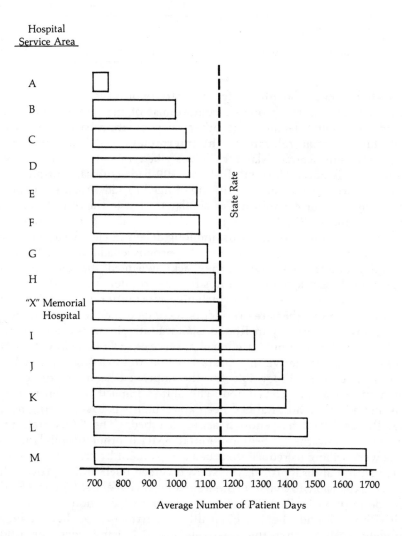

Source: The Vermont HSA staff review of "X"MH 1122 application.
Data from: "Dataset for Health Planning 1974–1976" CHIC-V.

Table 6.1

Actual/Expected Admissions and Physician Distribution

		Admissions (Number Per Year)			Number of Physicians by Age		
		Actual	Expected	Difference	Under 49	50–64	65+
I.	Relatively Urban Sub-area	5,804	4,533	+1,271	14	14	6
II.	Rural Sub-area	4,011	4,727	– 716	10	3	1

utilization data can be interpreted in a variety of ways. Bed need in this case was determined through a compromise of the two positions, one based on hospital demand, the other on population-based statistics.

A third example relevant to the interpretation of bed need comes from a recent Rhode Island case described in detail in Part Two. Suburban Memorial Hospital (SMH), a 309-bed acute care hospital in a suburban area, requested a certificate of need to add 50 acute care beds. The argument for expansion was similar to that in the other examples described above; SMH was experiencing increased overcrowding requiring the use of corridor beds and long delays in elective admissions.

The CON staff argued against the proposed addition of beds on several grounds. First, while they acknowledged the fact that the population-based hospital use rates for area residents were at the state average, data on health status, including mortality rates and disability day rates, showed that area residents were healthier than residents of the average community in Rhode Island. State planners argued that a healthy population should use hospital services at a rate below the state average. The alternative interpretation that the existing level of hospital services was responsible for the improved health status of the community was not considered. The state's implicit decision rule for this and all other hospital bed need assessments is based on the belief that Rhode Island has enough acute care beds. The CON staff was willing to allow the 50-bed addition at SMH if other hospitals in the state were willing to reduce their bed complement by an equal number. After an initial disapproval, the state reversed itself and approved the 50-bed expansion to avoid a threatened legal challenge. (See the SMH case description in Part Two for details of this decision.)

In Rhode Island the State Health Department has held a long-standing position that the relatively low 3.7 acute beds per 1,000 residents is sufficient. Since the 1970s, the state has opposed any effort among the hospitals to expand bed supply. While local bed need may be insufficient, as admitted by state planners in the SMH case, expansion in any one hospital will be allowed only if compensatory bed reduction can be effected in other hospitals. Thus, data and analyses relating to local bed need are applied within the context of a fixed (the existing) number of acute care beds in the state.

The examples of bed need determinations presented above demonstrate that similar data on hospital utilization can be interpreted in very different ways by health planners in different states. Existing planning technology does not allow an unequivocal solution to the question of bed need assessment. While we have concentrated on the complexity of needs assessments of acute hospital beds, similar problems occur in determining need for new technology and long-term care beds (see Chapter 7).

Bed Need Assessment in the Plan Development Process

The problem of assessing acute hospital bed needs arises not only in the facilities review process described above, but also in the development of the health plans mandated under PL 93–641. In this section we shall describe a very different approach to assessing bed need which has been applied to the development of acute bed standards included in health plans.

PL 93–641 requires that each Health Systems Agency develop a Health Systems Plan (HSP) and a related Annual Implementation Plan (AIP). The HSPs and AIPs are to be reviewed, updated, and amended annually. The HSPs are to be integrated into an overall State Health Plan (SHP). Final responsibility for preparation of the SHP is vested in the statewide Health Coordinating Councils. However, the SHPDA plays a key role in the actual development of a SHP, including the preparation of a preliminary SHP. In the past, states have also developed a State Medical Facilities Plan (SMFP) as part of their responsibilities under the Hill-Burton program. Now, however, the SMFP is no longer a separate entity but rather is integrated as the medical facilities component of the State Health Plan.

Health plans have a variety of purposes and serve a variety of functions under PL 93–641. Their most basic and traditional function is to provide an inventory of existing health facilities and services. A second major function is to develop a profile of health status for the relevant population (including death rates, frequency of illness, disability rates and so forth) and to promulgate a series of health status goals and short-term measures ("objectives") for achieving them. A third purpose health plans serve is informational. Through the HSA board and committee structure and the public hearings required at both the HSA and state levels, the plan development process becomes a forum for establishing organizational recognition, for debating policy issues, for building coalitions, and for raising the salience of health planning issues on the community agenda. A fourth purpose the plans serve is to act as a guide to the decision-making process for facilities review, including the certificate of need and Section 1122 review programs. Because we have emphasized the regulatory dimension of health planning, we will focus our attention on this aspect of health plan development.

Health plans provide specific guidance for facilities review through the development of quantitative goals for the medical system ("systems goals") and quantitative standards for current operation designed as steps necessary to achieve them. The underlying notion is that of a plan-driven facilities review process. Plan-driven facilities review is analogous to the much more familiar concept of zoning in land use planning where a master development plan for a geographic area is intended to serve as an overall guide to land use. In practice, of course, this model of planning has not eliminated political and economic influence over development; land use planners have been thwarted frequently by variances, exceptions, and temporary use permits granted for political or economic reasons.[12] A plan-driven facilities review process may minimize such variances, especially if the standards applied to resource allocation decisions can be shown to have some basis in analysis and empirical studies. The burden on health planners, then, is to develop quantitative standards that are logically derived through supportable analytic methods. In practice, the success of plan-driven facilities review depends on local acceptability of the standards included in the HSP and SHP; establishing the empirical legitimacy of the quantitative standards is a necessary condition of winning that acceptance. This is particularly true where compliance with the standards implies some reduction in the level of health resources.

Technical Aspects of Acute Bed Standards Development

As indicated above, the planning technology typically used to develop acute bed standards for HSPs and SHPs is very different from that currently being applied to facility review cases in Maine and Vermont. In this section we discuss the process by which acute bed standards are adopted under PL 93-641. The acute hospital bed standards included in the National Guidelines for Health Planning provide a useful starting point for this discussion.

Section 1501 of PL 93–641 requires HEW to issue national guidelines for health planning including:

(1) Standards respecting the appropriate supply, distribution, and organization of health resources.

(2) A statement of national health planning goals . . . which goals, to the maximum extent practicable, shall be expressed in quantitative terms.

The Guidelines were initially issued in draft form by HEW in September, 1977; the final revised Guidelines were published in the *Federal Register* on March 28, 1978. Quantitative resource standards in the following areas were included in the Guidelines: general hospital bed supply and occupancy rates, obstetrical services, neonatal special care units, pediatric inpatient bed supply and occupancy rates, cardiac catheterization services, megavoltage radiation therapy services, computed tomographic (CAT) scanners, and end-stage renal disease treatment facilities. The discussion here concentrates on the standards for hospital bed supply and occupancy rates.

The final HEW Guidelines included the following standards on general hospital bed supply and occupancy:

General hospitals—Bed supply
(a) *Standard.* There should be less than four non-Federal, short-stay hospital beds for each 1,000 persons in a health service area except under extraordinary circumstances. For purposes of this section, short-stay hospital beds include all non-Federal, short-stay hospital beds (including general medical/surgical, children's, obstetric, psychiatric, and other short-stay specialized beds. . . .)

General hospitals—Occupancy rate
(a) *Standard.* There should be an average annual occupancy rate for medically necessary hospital care of at least 80 percent for all non-Federal, short-stay hospital beds considered together in a health service area, except under extraordinary circumstances . . . . From the *Federal Register,* March 28, 1978

The Guidelines referenced a 1976 Institute of Medicine policy statement[13] and a 1976 InterStudy report,[14] both of which call for a nationwide 10 percent reduction of nonfederal hospital beds from 4.4 to 4.0 beds per 1,000 population, over the next five years. The implicit assumption of the Guidelines and the Institute and InterStudy reports is that significant cost savings can be realized through a combination of bed reduction and maintenance of high occupancy (greater than 80 percent) in the remaining beds.

Where Do the Standards Come From?

Earlier in this chapter, we described the complexity of determining need for acute hospital beds. In the face of the uncertainties surrounding bed need determination, planners have traditionally sought convenient proxies for need to be applied in allocation decisions. For acute hospital beds such proxies have been used nationally since the passage of the Hill-Burton Act in 1946. As the current proposed standards for acute hospital beds derive in large measure from Hill-Burton formulas, it is instructive to chronicle the history of hospital bed standards from the early Hill-Burton days.[15]

The purpose of the Hill-Burton program was to survey the adequacy of hospital resources nationally (via state facilities plans) and to support the construction and modernization of hospitals where necessary. The initial Hill-Burton formula for setting priorities among applicants for federal construction grants and loans was based on bed-to-population ratios and included adjustments for population density. A national overall goal of 4.5 acute, nonfederal beds per 1,000 population was set in 1945.[16] This initial target figure was based on providing enough acute bed capacity to accommodate 1,400 hospital bed days per 1,000 population, assuming an average occupancy level of 80 percent.[17] Table 6.2 shows the original Hill-Burton formula for maximum and minimum acute bed levels.

The maximum level applied to whole states. The minimum levels applied to hospital service areas within the states designated as base, intermediate or rural, depending on their role in an overall hospital care system for the state (see Figure 6.6). When the sum of the beds allowed for each service area fell below the maximum allowable level for the state, a reserve bed pool could be established to meet special local needs beyond the minimum figure. The formula clearly shows a rural bias which was characteristic of the initial Hill-Burton effort to support construction of small rural acute hospitals.

As a response to criticism that bed-to-population ratios were inflexible and did not allow for local differences in the "need" for acute hospital services,[18] the approach to determining bed need was changed in 1965 to a demand-based formula. The modified Hill-Burton formula calculated the projected acute hospital bed need by the following method:

1. $$\frac{\text{Number of Patient Days}}{\text{Current Population/1,000}} = \text{Use Rate}$$

2. $$\frac{\text{Use Rate} \times \text{Projected Population/1,000}}{365} = \begin{array}{l}\text{Average Daily} \\ \text{Census (ADC)}\end{array}$$

3. $$\frac{\text{ADC}}{0.80 \text{ occupancy}} + 10 = \text{Projected Hospital Bed Need}$$

This formula, which is heavily weighted for current demand, corrects for increasing population and permits an 80 percent occupancy rate. The additional 10 beds in the formula were added to buffer small, rural hospitals from day-to-day fluctuations in patient census.

In 1972, in response to increasing concern over the cost of inpatient medical care, the Hill-Burton formula was again modified; the permissible occupancy level was changed to 85 percent and the 10 bonus beds were left to state option. In 1973 the Hill-Burton agency suggested that hospitals calculate bed need for service, allowing a 90 percent occupancy factor for obstetric and pediatric beds. It is interesting to note that as of

Table 6.2

The Initial Hill-Burton Formula for Acute
Hospital Bed Need

Maximum and Minimum Bed/Population Ratios		
State Population Per Square Mile	Maximum State Allowance (Beds per 1,000 Pop.)	Minimum Area Standards (Beds per 1,000 Pop.)
12 persons or more	4.5	Rural 2.5
		Intermediate 4.0
		Base 4.5
7–11 persons	5.0	Rural 3.0
		Intermediate 4.5
		Base 5.0
6 persons or less	5.5	Rural 3.5
		Intermediate 5.0
		Base 5.5

Source: Evaluation of the Hill-Burton Bed Need Formula: Short-Term General Hospital Beds, DHEW, Health Care Facilities Evaluation Project 71-4, August, 1972.

Figure 6.6

Coordinated Hospital Service Plan[16]

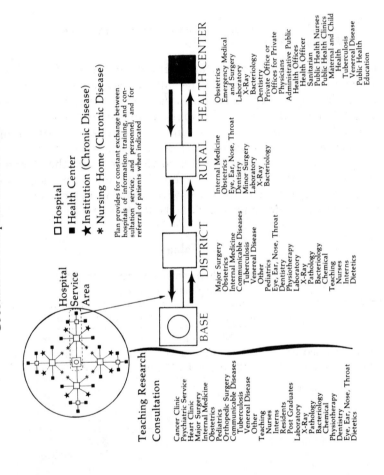

□ Hospital
■ Health Center
★ Institution (Chronic Disease)
* Nursing Home (Chronic Disease)

Plan provides for constant exchange between
hospitals of information, training, and consultation service, and personnel, and for
referral of patients when indicated

Hospital
Service
Area

Teaching Research
Consultation

BASE

Cancer Clinic
Psychiatric Service
Heart Clinic
Major Surgery
Internal Medicine
Obstetrics
Pediatrics
Orthopedic Surgery
Communicable Diseases
    Tuberculosis
    Venereal Disease
    Other
Teaching
    Nurses
    Interns
    Residents
    Post Graduates
Laboratory
    X-Ray
    Pathology
    Bacteriology
    Chemical
Physiotherapy
Dentistry
Eye, Ear, Nose, Throat
Dietetics

DISTRICT

Major Surgery
Obstetrics
Internal Medicine
Communicable Diseases
    Tuberculosis
    Venereal Disease
    Other
Pediatrics
Eye, Ear, Nose, Throat
Dentistry
Physiotherapy
Laboratory
    X-Ray
    Pathology
    Bacteriology
    Chemical
Teaching
    Nurses
    Interns
    Dietetics

RURAL

Internal Medicine
Obstetrics
Eye, Ear, Nose, Throat
Dentistry
Minor Surgery
Laboratory
    X-Ray
    Bacteriology

HEALTH CENTER

Obstetrics
Emergency Medical
    and Surgery
Laboratory
    X-Ray
    Bacteriology
Dentistry
Private Office or
    Offices for Private
    Physicians
Administrative Public
    Health Offices
    Health Officer
Sanitarian
Public Health Nurses
Public Health Clinics
    Maternal and Child
        Health
    Tuberculosis
    Venereal Disease
Public Health
    Education

1975 most health planning agencies were calculating bed need based on the 1972 Hill-Burton formula.[19]

It is important to emphasize that the changes over time in the bed need formulas in the Hill-Burton Program did not result from improvements in the methodology of facilities planning, but rather reflected programmatic policy changes. They were not empirically derived.

The Legacy of the Hill-Burton Standards

Although most writers in the field of hospital bed supply are quick to point out that the Hill-Burton formulas cannot be relied on as accurate reflections of bed need, nonetheless, virtually all published reports decrying the cost of the excess supply of acute care beds in this country are based on some modification of these formulas. Certainly, the simplest arguments on the cost of unused hospital beds are exemplified in the monograph by Ensminger,[20] who employed straight-line extrapolations of operating costs to calculate the burden of maintaining unused beds. Such calculations offered by Ensminger apply an ideal occupancy rate to existing bed capacity (à la Hill-Burton). Any example of local or national occupancy rates below the ideal level is offered as evidence of excess, unneeded bed supply. "Unneeded" beds thus calculated are assigned a cost figure in direct proportion to the total bed complement of the area under consideration. An example of such a calculation of the costs of unused beds based on 1974 national hospital data[21] is provided below for purposes of illustration.

In 1974, there were 931,172 acute, nonfederal hospital beds in the U.S., with an average occupancy rate of 75.3 percent. The total operating expenditures for these hospitals were $32,751,000,000, or $35,172 per hospital bed per year. If this cost per bed per year were applied to the number of "excess" beds calculated by the difference between the minimal accepted occupancy rate of 85 percent (as per Ensminger) and the actual average occupancy rate, 75.3 percent, a cost of maintaining "unneeded" beds can be imputed thus:

931,172 beds x (0.85 - 0.75.3) + 90,324 "unneeded" beds
90,324 x $35,172 + $3,176,876,000

Thus, using a straight-line extrapolation approach, the operating cost of maintaining "excess" hospital beds would be represented as over $3 billion per year. Such an analysis of course implies that:

1. the 85 percent ideal occupancy rate is an accurate and immutable figure.

2. savings in direct proportion to the total cost of hospital care would accrue from closing down 90,324 beds.

Both these assumptions are, of course, incorrect. We have seen that the 85 percent figure was introduced by Hill-Burton for pragmatic reasons, and is not based on any concept of need or efficiency. Moreover, even if 90,000 acute beds were closed, the cost savings would fall far short of the figure indicated because much of the cost of running hospitals is fixed and certainly would not be reduced in direct proportion to total expenditures.

Any potential cost savings from closing hospital beds must be calculated using a complex, stepwise function. As pointed out by McClure,[22] only if bed reduction were accomplished by closing entire hospitals would anything approaching a straight-line extrapolation of hospital costs reflect true cost savings and, even then, savings would depend on the costs incurred when patients seek care in other medical facilities. Nonetheless, as fanciful as the above example may appear, much of the current argument for potential cost savings in the acute hospital sector is based on some modification of these basic calculations.

To be sure, there have been a variety of refinements of estimated cost savings potentially achievable through closing unused beds. Some estimates attempt to separate fixed and variable hospital costs on a per bed basis.[23] Others attempt to refine the definition of ideal occupancy using queuing theory.[24] Whatever the refinements in the methodology, it is important to emphasize that estimates of cost savings from closing beds rest on some concept of ideal occupancy levels.

The Institute of Medicine policy paper[25] referred to in the Guidelines, acknowledges the problem of estimating the number of excess hospital beds in the country:

> The committee finds that, although the accuracy of various aggregate national estimates of hospital bed surpluses is debatable, the evidence clearly indicates:
>
> that significant surpluses of short-term general hospital beds exist or are developing in many areas of the United States and that these are contributing significantly to rising hospital care costs; and
>
> that, although shortages of such beds still exist in some areas, these have been rapidly diminishing in recent years.[26]

The Institute of Medicine committee recommended a 10 percent reduction of acute hospital beds. A similar recommendation appears in the 1976 InterStudy report by McClure.[27] It is important to emphasize that both of these recommendations, upon which the acute bed standards in the Guidelines are based, emerged from considerations of actual hospital occupancy rates in comparison to "optimal" rates as defined by the revised Hill-Burton bed need formulas.

The 4.0 standard contained in the Guidelines represented an attempt to reduce bed supply below current levels and to achieve reductions (from 4.4 to 4.0) within admittedly arbitrary, but rationally defensible parameters. In fact, the Guidelines were clear that 4.0 represented a starting point for bed reductions:

> . . . 4.0 beds per 1,000 population is a ceiling, not an ideal situation. . . . It is anticipated that in subsequent plans HSAs will be required to indicate how they will reach a bed to population ratio of less than 3.7 per 1,000 population except under extraordinary circumstances. HSAs whose areas are currently below the 4.0 per 1,000 level are urged to attempt to decrease bed to population ratios below 3.7 per 1,000 population. . . .[28]

Thus, the 4.0 and 3.7 standards were the product of a series of related assumptions and policy decisions: that the medical system is overbedded; that reductions in bed supply will bring substantial cost savings; and that a process of successive and limited reductions was rationally defensible, particularly if the specific numerical standards adopted fell within the bounds of existing capacity at the upper level and demonstrated HMO experience at the lower level. Thus conceived, the next step for HEW was to win acceptance for the Guidelines at the local level—from the medical profession and from the HSAs and SHPDAs whose policies the Guidelines were intended to influence. Once accepted and incorporated in local health plans, in order to be effective the standards had to function as a useful guide to local regulatory policy and decisions.

Standards Development at the State and Local Levels: The Significance of the Guidelines

When first issued as proposed rules in September, 1977, the Guidelines produced an immediate furor. HEW received some 55,000 written comments on the Guidelines, an unprecedented number. Providers marshaling considerable community and political support both locally and nationally, protested that the proposed Guidelines were too stringent, unsubstantiated by empirical evidence, and represented an unequal burden on smaller and rural hospitals[29]. As a consequence, in December, the House of Representatives unanimously passed a resolution designed to soften the blow to rural hospitals and a majority of the Senate signed a letter to Secretary Califano with similar intent. In response, Congressman Paul Rogers, then the key health figure in the House and a proponent of health planning, conveyed a conciliatory interpretation of the proposed Guidelines to the members:

> I know that many of my colleagues have received expressions of concern from their constituents regarding the recently issued health planning Guidelines. . . .
>
> The primary misunderstanding is that the Guidelines will be used to force hospitals, particularly in rural areas, to close. . . .
>
> I am saying that the Guidelines are simply guidelines. It is a goal to be reached. Hopefully they can be reached and hopefully they will be adhered to.

Secretary Califano sent a similar message to Congress in a letter reading in part:

> The Guidelines are directed at guiding the development of local plans. . . .
> They do not involve any federal authority to close any hospitals or to eliminate any services.

Both the Secretary and the Congressman succeeded in comforting critics by removing from the proposed Guidelines something they (or health planning generally) never had, the authority to close hospitals and services. Now unencumbered by the initial national protest, HEW turned to the primary task of the Guidelines, to bind HSAs and SHPDAs to federal policies through influencing the quantitative standards adopted in local health plans.

Section 1513(b) (2) of PL 93–641 requires HSAs to give "appropriate consideration" to the Guidelines, and to "take into account" and "be consistent with" the specific standards contained in them. Each health systems plan established after December 31, 1978, and each state health plan established after June 30, 1979, is to be consistent with the standards. Despite HSA protest that the Guidelines violate the spirit of "bottom up planning," HEW has successfully utilized its control over HSA and SHPDA funding and designation to ensure at least rough conformance to the Guidelines. It is expected that the 11 standards will be addressed as core elements of each Health System Plan. As explained in guidelines for plan development issued by the Bureau of Health Planning, it is expected that HSAs will use the standards as a starting point in their analyses and that departures from the standards be fully documented:

> ... The HSP must be consistent with the quantitative levels set forth in the resource standards or adjusted to meet specific local circumstances on the basis of sound and well documented analysis. . . .[30]

Indeed, the plan development guidelines issued by the Bureau also contained a "Suggested Analytical Process" to be used by HSAs utilizing the standards as a starting point and as a reference point for plan development.[31]

In a recent request for a proposal to evaluate the performance of HSAs, the Health Resources Administration made it clear that the standards are to serve as one benchmark against which to compare HSA performance:

> This performance evaluation program will provide Bureau (and higher level) program managers and policymakers with information on the success (or failure) of health planning agencies in achieving the goals and objectives of PL 93-641, including progress in achieving the resource standards defined in the National Health Planning Guidelines, the National Health Planning Goals, and goals and objective identified at the state and local level.[32]

Thus, the standards are used by HEW as a boundary-setting device intended to speed the diffusion of federal policy to state and local agencies by encouraging approximate repetition of federally stipulated targets by the 205 HSAs and 56 state agencies.

The strategic significance of plan and standards development can be seen not just in HEW-HSA relationships, but as a key element in HSA-SHPDA relationships as well. The development of quantitative standards is a prime issue addressed in the bargaining that characterizes the planning process. In Massachusetts, for example, resource standards were developed at the initiative of their Commissioner of Public Health (Dr. Jonathan Fielding) independent of the SHP and HSP development processes. The Acute Care Standards and criteria were drafted by a task force composed of representatives from the six HSAs, state agencies, the Massachusetts Hospital Association, and Blue Cross, and subsequently adopted formally by the Public Health Council. Once written into regulations by the Council, the standards formed the basis for the acute care section of the State Health Plan, and were intended to serve as guidelines for HSA plan development and facilities review as well.

In addition, the six HSPs in Massachusetts were developed in accordance with guidelines for uniform format, content, and process developed at the initiative of the Office of State Health Planning by an overall plan development coordinating committee. In their HSPs, the six

HSAs in Massachusetts responded to the Acute Care Standards and Criteria much as they responded to the National Guidelines, promulgating standards that fit comfortably within the overall policy of reduction while maintaining organizational independence by not repeating the state or federal targets exactly. Each of the six HSAs performed the bed need calculations as prescribed in the standards and criteria, but each also amended the methodology or substituted their own approach entirely.

We studied the Boston and Central Massachusetts HSAs most closely.[33] The Central Massachusetts HSA, with a current bed/population ratio of 4.48, projected bed need at 3.67, a target that stands almost midway between the state goal of 3.4 and the federal goal of 4.0. The Central Massachusetts target was set for 1982, rather than for 1985 as were the state and federal targets. In addition, the Central Massachusetts HSA named names, recommending that medical/surgical services at one hospital be completely phased out, that three hospitals consider a merger, and that another be converted to an alcoholic rehabilitation facility. The Boston HSA, with a current ratio of 5.0, rejected the standards and criteria for its area, and did not endorse a specific target. It did, however, advocate occupancy targets of 85 percent for "small" hospitals and 90 percent for "large" hospitals.

Whatever their empirical basis, and whatever the bargaining processes that produce specific quantitative targets, to what extent do standards allow a "plan-driven" facilities review process? To what extent can health plans reinforced by clear priorities and quantitative targets serve as a surrogate for a limit on capital investment or aid in making individual facilities review decisions?

In practice, quantitative standards can strengthen facilities review programs where they are set below existing resource levels. Since planners currently do not have sufficient authority or ability to close beds or to retire capital generally, the presence of such standards will reinforce efforts to remain at existing capacity, whatever it may be. It will not necessarily enable planners to achieve the lower than current capacity target itself. For example, in areas with more than 4.0 beds per 1,000 population, the adoption of a 4.0 standard may assist planners in their efforts to hold the line on bed expansion. It will not necessarily enable them to achieve the 4.0 goal. Obviously, the wider the disparity between the bed goal mandated in a plan and the level that actually exists, the greater the planners' ability to make a strong argument for blocking expansion. However, in areas (or sub-areas) that fall below the bed goal (for example, areas with fewer than 4 beds per 1,000) the presence of the standard and the degree of disparity between it and what actually is the case in the community may strengthen the bargaining position of providers who attempt to add beds.

There would appear to be widespread opportunity for stringent numerical standards to serve this supportive function for facilities review. For example, 98 of the nation's 100 largest cities now have more than 4 beds per 1,000 population; 244 of 287 SMSAs currently exceed the 4.0 figure; and, according to the Institute of Medicine report, 81 percent of the Health Services Areas in the U.S. now exceed 4.0.[34] In practice, the opportunities are fewer than this profile would indicate. This is because HSA areas that exceed 4.0 in the aggregate often contain empirically defined sub-areas which fall below 4.0 and which are represented through sub-area planning councils.

Our data indicate that 4 of the 11 largest hospital service areas[35] in Massachusetts (state average 4.3) fall below the 4.0 goal (Massachusetts has 6 Health Systems Agencies). In Maine, a single-HSA state with an average of 4.0 beds/1,000 population, 6 hospital service areas fall below the line. In Rhode Island (a waiver state with a 3.7 average) 7 of the 11 largest health service regions[36] fall below the 4.0 line.

In order to obtain a bargaining advantage from a bed standard, some HSAs would have to lower the target for the HSA area as a whole or generate different targets for each sub-area. Moreover, targets like 4.0 are systemwide; they apply to large geographic areas and may not be easily applied in individual facilities review cases. Providers may be expected to argue that current utilization or a host of other factors justifies approval in their case, irrespective of the fact that an HSA area in the aggregate exceeds some numerical standard. Thus, attempts to use quantitative standards to "drive" facilities review decisions may be countered by the precedent of a case-by-case facilities review process. Obviously, where quantitative standards speak to individual facilities rather than large geographic areas, such as standards for minimum occupancy, minimum deliveries, minimum CAT scans, and so forth, they are most useful in the facilities review process. It is here where plan-driven facilities review, if not gutted by exceptions and adjustments, is most achievable.

Summary

In this chapter we have contrasted two methodologies applied to acute hospital bed need determination—that used in some facilities review programs in New England and that developed nationally for inclusion in state and local health plans. Very different approaches to bed need determination have been applied in these two instances. In three New England states (Maine, Vermont, and Rhode Island), population-based hospital use data are available for virtually all state residents, allowing comparison of the pattern of hospital use among communities. Analyses of those data are being used to supplement more traditional studies of institutional statistics in facilities review cases in Maine, Vermont and Rhode Island. Such data, however, are not available in most states.[37] Thus, convenient proxies for bed need such as included in the Hill-Burton demand formulas have been widely used by planners throughout the country.[38]

The Hill-Burton formula shown on page 89 assumes that existing hospital use patterns are appropriate and simply applies an ideal occupancy rate. Population-based analyses, in contrast, provide an added dimension to bed need assessment; they allow comparisons of the amount and kinds of hospital services received by residents of similar communities through a state or region. But there are technical diffi- culties with applying either approach to hospital planning. As we described above, population-based analyses of hospital use patterns do not yield unequivocal solutions to the bed need question. Planners and regulators are still left with the question of what level of hospital use is appropriate for each community in their state. And the Hill-Burton formula approach, which with modifications has been the basis of the planning targets included in the National Health Planning Guidelines, ignores the stickier issues associated with the uncertainties of bed need assessments.

The importance of the discussion of bed need methodologies lies in the fact that hospital planning decisions do not emerge unequivocally from technical analyses. Even in states where sophisticated data and analytic resources are available, the technical aspects of hospital re- source planning require considerable value-laden interpretation. The fact that technical solutions to planning problems do not exist explains, in part, why planning decisions are made primarily through political bargaining processes.

Notes

[1] Milton I. Roemer, "Bed Supply and Hospital Utilization: A Natural Exper- iment," *Hospitals*, 35 (November 1, 1961), p. 36.

[2] Martin S. Feldstein, *Economic Analysis for Health Service Efficiency* (Chicago: Markham Publishing Company, 1968), Chapter 7.

[3] Keith Stevenson, SM Thesis, Massachusetts Institute of Technology, 1979.

[4] John E. Wennberg and Alan Gittelsohn, "Small Area Variations in Health Care Delivery," *Science,* 182 (1973), p. 1102. See also American College of Surgeons and the American Surgical Association, *Report of the Study on Surgical Services for the United States* (Chicago, 1976).

[5] American College of Surgeons, ibid.

[6] See Codman Research Group, Final Report, DHEW Contract No. 291-76-0003, May, 1980.

[7] Ibid.

[8] John E. Wennberg, "Using Localized Population-Based Data in Evaluating Health Problems," in *Papers on the National Health Guidelines,* No. HRA-77-641 (Hyattsville, MD: Health Resources Administration, 1977).

[9] A.L. Cochrane, *Effectiveness and Efficiency—Random Reflections on Health Services* (London: Nuffield Provincial Hospital Trust, 1972). See also Thomas McKeown and C.R. Lowe, *An Introduction to Social Medicine* (New York: Oxford University Press, 1974, 2nd ed.) and H.G. Mather, D.C. Morgan, et al., "Myocardial Infarction: A Comparison Between Home and Hospital Care for Patients," *British Medical Journal,* 1 (1976), p. 925.

[10] This case is described in detail in Part Two.

[11] Robert H. Brook and Francis A. Appel, "Quality-of-Care Assessment: Choosing a Method for Peer Review," *New England Journal of Medicine,* 288 (1973), p. 1323

[12] D.E. Ervin, et al., *Land Use Control—Evaluating Economics and Political Effects* (Cambridge, MA: Ballinger, 1977).

[13] Institute of Medicine, *Controlling the Supply of Hospital Beds* (Washington, D.C.: National Academy of Sciences, 1976).

[14] Walter McClure, *Reducing Excess Hospital Capacity,* InterStudy report on HRA Contract No. HRA-230-76-0086, October 15, 1976.

[15] We are indebted to Mr. Robert Lauber of the Division of Planning Methods and Technology of HRA for his help in clarifying Hill-Burton policy changes over time.

[16] J.W. Mountain, E.H. Pennell, and V.M. Hoge, "Health Service Areas—Requirements for General Hospitals and Health Centers," *Public Health Bulletin,* No. 292, Washington, D.C. (1945).

[17] Ibid.

[18] Judith R. Lave and Lester B. Lave, *The Hospital Construction Act: An Evaluation of the Hill-Burton Program, 1945-1973* (Washington, D.C.: American Enterprise Institute for Public Policy Research, 1974). See also M. DuBois, "Areawide Planning: Where It Came From, Where It's Going," *Hospitals,* 40, No. 23 (1966).

[19] M.M. Melum, *Assessing the Need for Hospital Beds: A Review of Current Criteria* (Minneapolis: InterStudy, 1975).

[20] Barry Ensminger, *The $8 Billion Hospital Bed Overrun* (Washington, D.C.: Public Citizen's Health Research Group, 1975).

[21] American Hospital Association, *Hospital Statistics*, 1975 ed. (Chicago, 1975).

[22] McClure, op. cit.

[23] F.L. Sattler and M. Bennett, *A Statistical Profile of Short-Term Hospitals in the United States as of 1973* (Minneapolis: InterStudy). See also McClure, op. cit.

[24] See Robert M. Crane, "Methods Used in Determining Health Service and Facility Requirements," in H.H. Hyman, editor, *Health Regulation* (Germantown, MD: Aspen Systems Corporation, 1977), p. 118.

[25] *Controlling the Supply of Hospital Beds*, op. cit.

[26] Ibid.

[27] McClure, op. cit.

[28] National Guidelines for Health Planning, *Federal Register*, March 28, 1978.

[29] Of the 11 standards contained in the Guidelines, the acute bed supply and occupancy standards, and the standards for occupancy and a minimum annual number of deliveries for obstetrical services elicited the most response.

[30] Guidelines for the Development of Health Systems Plans and Annual Implementation Plans," Health Resources Administration, February 12, 1979, p. 17.

[31] Ibid., p. 17.

[32] Request for Proposal HRA 232–BHP–0070(j) CM:mm.

[33] For a thorough discussion of all six Massachusetts HSPs, see Ronald Hollander, *Review of the First Generation Health Systems Plan in the Commonwealth of Massachusetts* (Burlington, MA: Massachusetts Hospital Association, April, 1978).

[34] Institute of Medicine, *Controlling the Supply of Hospital Beds* (Washington, D.C.: National Academy of Sciences, 1976).

[35] Hospital service areas are empirically defined sets of towns whose residents receive most of their hospital service from one or more hospitals located in the area.

[36] In Rhode Island census tracts are grouped into 18 health service regions.

[37] In addition to Maine, Vermont and Rhode Island, New Jersey and Iowa maintain hospital discharge data files for most resident hospitalizations.

[38] M.M. Melum, op. cit.

Chapter 7

Policies

Consistency is not one of the virtues of American health care policies. Nationally, we have not chosen decisively among conflicting policy objectives. Some agencies have a mandate to restrain health care costs while others hold a mandate to enhance the quality and accessibility of health care services, charters that are necessarily contradictory. The federal system adds to the likelihood of policy inconsistencies. States pursue their own policy interests, acting independently of one another and often of the federal government as well. At no level of government are regulatory and planning decisions well coordinated. We lack, some would say fortunately, a tradition of administrative centralization.

Political changes contribute to the variability that characterizes health care policies. During the course of our study, the national administration changed, New Hampshire voters replaced a conservative Republican governor with a moderate Democrat, Maine voters chose a liberal Democrat as the successor to a nonparty Independent governor who decided not to seek reelection, and Massachusetts voters substituted a conservative Democrat for a liberal Democrat as their governor. One of the HSAs we observed had three executive directors in as many years, while another was headless for a considerable time. If policy consistency requires continuity in political leadership as one would suspect it does, it is understandable why consistent policies are difficult to find.

Congress, when designing what are supposedly national programs, is sensitive to the requirements for obtaining winning legislative coalitions and insensitive to the requirements for achieving policy coherence. As a result, policy inconsistencies are often guaranteed within and among programs enacted. Consider, for example, health sector capital controls established under PL 93-641. Nonfederal hospital investments are regulated, but federal hospital and physician training investments are not. Capital projects are reviewed individually by local councils, locally selected. Regulatory decisions are made by state agencies according to their own procedures and policies. Attempts to impose federal standards are resisted both by consumers and by providers. Little coordination exists between this program and others that control related aspects of the quality, cost, and availability of health services. PSRO boundaries do not match HSA boundaries. Veterans' Administration hospitals, renal treatment, emergency medical systems, and blood resource regions match neither nor each other.

What we have is not a coherent set of national health care policies, but rather dozens of different and changing policies for each national health care program established. In essence, each program produces a series of policy experiments, sometimes state-by-state, sometimes even more fragmented. The interesting analytic problem then is to discern the policy patterns that do develop and to describe their effect on the structure and distribution of health services.

The first step in the analysis is the identification and labeling of the policy patterns. In this chapter we examine four planning and regulatory programs to determine the policies actually being pursued and attempt some categorization. These policies are in effect the administrative output of the political and technical processes described in the preceding chapters. The four policies selected for examination are rate setting, long-term care, capital investment controls, and the regulation of acute care services. Although these are not the only policies that we monitored, they are the most important in terms of potential impact on the cost of health services.

Rate Setting

Rate setting is a form of health care regulation that limits the amount of revenue a hospital can earn. It is as yet not a national program. Of the eight states that have mandatory statewide programs, three are in New England—Massachusetts, Rhode Island and Connecticut—and thus are part of our study sample. The other mandatory statewide programs are in New York, New Jersey, Maryland, Wisconsin, and Washington. A number of other states, but none in New England, have rate-setting programs operated by Blue Cross which directly affect only Blue Cross rates paid to hospitals or by state hospital associations. There are 22 programs of this kind, all differing as do the other eight in structure, scope, sophistication and experience.

The rationale for rate setting is similar to that for capital control programs, but the focus is on operational, rather than capital budgets.

Since the major third-party payers (particularly Medicare, Medicaid, and Blue Cross) provide hospitals with retrospective, cost-based reimbursement, there is little incentive for hospitals to act as prudent purchasers of labor or capital. On the contrary, expanding in the name of quality medicine, hospitals have incentives to increase their cost base. While CON and 1122 reviews can theoretically constrain unneeded, major capital outlays, rate setting seeks to constrain inflation in operational budgets. The potential synergism of linking the two approaches into a unified cost containment strategy has been explored by Katherine Bauer and her colleagues.[1]

Historically, the stimulus for implementing rate-setting programs has come from the pressure on state budgets caused by growth in the Medicaid program and/or Blue Cross rate increases reflecting hospital cost inflation in the private sector. In most states, Blue Cross simply passed on its increased hospital costs through premium adjustments. In a few states, however, the insurance commissioner refused to condone a simple pass through of costs and Blue Cross was forced to engage in negotiations with the hospitals over allowable cost increases. Rising Medicaid costs were the dominant factor in the adoption of rate-setting programs in Connecticut and Massachusetts; in Rhode Island, Blue Cross cost increases led to the rate setting effort.

The experience of the rate-setting programs in New England and their relationship to CON offer important insights into the hospital regulatory process. Although each of the three New England states operating a rate-setting program has developed somewhat different procedures for deciding allowable hospital rate increases, there are some factors common to all three programs and to most other rate-setting programs in the nation.

All programs develop allowable revenue increases from some earlier year's costs. Thus, each is incremental. In no case is the more radical approach taken of setting future rates de novo, according to some calculation of appropriate total costs. The only item under consideration in rate-setting programs is the increase from a base year onwards. With the exception of hospital-salaried physicians, who represent only a small fraction of the total physician bill, no rate-setting program includes physician fees.

All New England programs accept the notion that a hospital has to recover its operating costs, which implicitly means that rate-setting bodies have no tools with which to squeeze "inefficient" or "unnecessary" hospitals out of business. There is thus a commitment to maintain the structure of the industry in its present form. Although the primary programmatic thrust is to contain the rate of increase in hospital revenues, several other arguments are also made in support of rate setting. The process is said to be educational for both regulator and regulated. Management capability in hospitals may be strengthened by the rate-setting process which requires compilation of financial and statistical data according to a uniform format. Rate regulators hope that the process may engender a greater degree of cost consciousness in hospital administrators.[2]

The major rationale for rate setting, however, lies in the hope that hospital budget increases will be contained somewhat, and that some savings will accrue to those payers to whom the rates apply. The higher the percentage of hospital revenues which fall under the approved rates, the more likely it is that overall hospital cost containment can be realized. Obviously, if the rates only apply to a small proportion of revenues (as in the case of the early program in Massachusetts where only Medicaid rates were set) the potential exists to shift costs to noncovered payers. Now, the New England rate-setting programs control the majority of hospital revenues. Thus, even noncost (charge) payers—commercial insurers and selfpay patients—benefit from the budgetary limitations.[3]

Connecticut

After several years of study, and two abortive efforts to pass rate-setting legislation in 1971 and 1972, the Connecticut State Legislature created the Commission on Hospitals and Health Care in 1973. The 17-member Commission is an independent regulatory body responsible for both CON and rate-setting activities.

Through the original legislation and subsequent amendments, the scope of the Commission's authority includes review and approval or disapproval of:

1) requested rate increases of health facilities and institutions
2) new functions or services
3) capital expenditure proposals of $100,000 or more (including leasing of equipment or facility); at this level, the review must include a public hearing
4) hospitals' proposed operating and capital budgets for the following year

The initial definition of a health care facility and institution covered hospitals, nursing homes, mental health and rehabilitative facilities, home health care agencies, clinical laboratories, central service facilities serving health care institutions, and diagnostic and treatment facilities. Recently, state facilities were added to the Commission's jurisdiction.

The Commission is composed of 12 appointees of the governor and an appointee each of the Speaker of the House, the President Pro Tempore of the Senate, and the Commissioners of Health, Mental Health, and Insurance.

In the first years of its operation, the Commission concentrated on controlling the rate of increase of hospital charges. These charges were held to a rate of increase considerably below the national—8.3 and 9.6 percent in fiscal years 1975 and 1976, respectively. But, in the same years Blue Cross had filed rate increases between 15 and 25 percent per year. Fiscal audits subsequently showed that hospitals had been generating excess revenues in spite of the relatively mild increase in patient charges; in fact, Connecticut hospitals had accumulated $17 million in excess revenues in fiscal 1975, the bulk of which could be accounted for in increased volume of special services (e.g., x-rays and laboratory service). The failure of the charge-oriented approach became apparent at the time that the new Grasso Administration, committed to controlling hospital costs, was elected. A new Commission Director was appointed with a mandate to slow the rate of cost inflation in the hospital sector. The new Director was an experienced hospital budget analyst from another state and had a reputation as an aggressive hospital regulator.

The Commission adopted revised procedures for rate review for the 1977 budget cycle in an effort to plug the regulatory loopholes of previous years. The new procedures:

1) substituted a new mechanism to review the total patient revenue budget of a hospital rather than charge increases alone to ensure appropriate review of volume as well as price increases.
2) eliminated the loophole which permitted hospitals to generate $17 million in excess revenue in fiscal 1975. In closing this loophole the Commission did not in any way limit the number of tests performed. Instead, it limited hospital excess revenue to the cost required to provide the additional services.
3) reviewed current year expenses for the first time to determine appropriate productivity levels of hospitals and provide incentives for good management.
4) established limits on the inflationary growth of hospital services based upon factors outside the hospital industry.
5) established criteria for financial requirements of hospitals.[4]

When applied to the 1977 budget cycle, the new procedures and strengthened regulatory resolve of the Commission resulted in an approval of less than half of the revenue increases requested by the hospitals: a 7.4 percent increase was approved as compared to the requested 16.9 percent increase. In reaction to the budget cuts, every hospital in the state immediately instituted appeals.

The first step in the appeals process was public hearings before the Commission.[5] The statute required that the hearings be held within ten days of the Commission's initial decision and that the Commission's final budget order be made within five days of a hearing. As a result 35 hearings had to be arranged within a three-week period. The Commission gave ground, but not enough to satisfy most hospitals. Even though the Commission restored $22 million of the hospitals' requests, permitting an average 10.5 percent rate increase over the preceding year, 31 of 35 hospitals sought judicial relief.

Nearly a year passed before the Court ruled on the first of the cases, deciding strongly against the Commission on the grounds that its methods and criteria were arbitrary. The remaining hospitals were given most of what they had sought in the out-of-court negotiations that followed the initial ruling. Urged on by the Connecticut General Assembly, which was by then amending the enabling legislation to force a more favorable attitude toward the hospitals, the Commission revised its procedures so that a more cooperative atmosphere would govern future rate setting. The rates determined for 1978, for example, though lower than the hospital submissions, engendered none of the hostility of the previous year. The Commission had apparently learned that effective regulation must take place within boundaries acceptable to the industry and that compromise rather than dictation is the only appropriate methodology.[6]

Massachusetts

The Massachusetts Rate Setting Commission was created in 1968 and is headed by three Commissioners appointed by the Governor for staggered terms. Initially the Commission held jurisdiction over the Medicaid portion or 15 percent of hospital revenues. Whatever fiscal relief this may have provided the state government, it did not do much to diminish overall hospital inflation as hospitals were allowed to pass on disallowed Medicaid costs to other payers. Today the Commission sets prospective rates for Medicaid hospital payments and charges to self-pay and commercial insurance carriers. These activities are performed according to different regulations and result in two rate structures, one for Medicaid and another for all remaining payers.

Serious rate regulation began in 1974 when the Commission obtained a waiver from HEW to deviate from the prescribed Medicaid principles of reimbursement. In 1975 the state legislature was persuaded to enact a law requiring all hospitals to submit proposed changes in charges to the Commission for review. The law also mandated the development of a system that would review all hospital budgets annually. In 1976 the legislature passed the Hospital Charge Control Act or Chapter 409, requiring budget review for all hospitals regardless of whether a change in charges is planned. Chapter 409 directly affects only commercial insurers and self-pay patients, although Medicare, Medicaid, and Blue Cross rates are affected indirectly.[7]

Until October, 1978, the Commission set an overall revenue ceiling for each hospital based on an allowed ratio (0.95) of costs to charges. But Chapter 409 also mandated that this charge approval system (the ratio of costs to charges) be revised. The statute specified that the Rate Setting Commission develop a definition of "total patient care charges" which would reflect actual revenue received by each hospital for all patient care services, supplies, and accommodations and a definition of total patient care costs which would reflect the reasonable financial requirements of each hospital for providing patient care services, supplies and accommodation.

To determine "allowable" costs for revenue limits and setting charges, a three-year cycle is used. A hospital's base year costs are listed, consisting of costs reimbursable by Medicare plus bad debts and free care. The base year for FY 79 was FY 77. The costs are divided into 15 categories. An inflation factor for each category is added to yield the "intermediate" year allowable cost due to inflation. However, if actual costs for the intermediate year are lower, that figure would be used. The intermediate year cost categories are then augmented using another inflation factor to produce the budget year's allowable cost due to inflation. As before, if actual costs are lower, they are substituted for the estimates.

Two other factors are considered in estimating allowable costs: a volume factor and costs beyond the control of the hospital. The volume adjustment factor permits modifications in the allowed costs and charges when certain corridors of utilization (e.g., +3 percent and -5 percent) are exceeded. Costs beyond the control of the hospital are also recognized. Examples of such allowable costs are those relating to requirements by government to bring the hospital into compliance with new regulations or to written warning from the Joint Commission on Accreditation of Hospitals (JCAH) that accreditation will be lost.

The State Medicaid program operates under a separate cost-based, prospective rate-setting process. The Commission has a waiver from the federal government exempting it from the federally mandated reimbursement system. The basis for Medicaid rate setting is the hospital's end-of-year cost report. In this case, the base year is two years prior to the rate year, e.g., for FY 79, FY 77 would serve as the base year. Allowable inpatient costs in the base year are projected forward two years and adjusted for inflation. Other administrative adjustments are made to take into account current expenses not reflected in base year data.

Once rate year allowable inpatient costs have been determined, the total figure is divided by allowed inpatient days to derive an all-inclusive per diem rate, applicable to all Medicaid patient days. Outpatient visits are reimbursed according to a ratio of costs to revenues computed for the base year. This ratio generally runs between 0.90 and 1.00.

The cost-based prospective rate-setting process just described is generally employed for Medicaid reimbursement. Exceptions to this would occur if these rates were higher than the "charges to the general public" computed under Chapter 409. In this case, Medicaid would reimburse at the lower rate.

Most hospital budgets are sent to the Commission by August 1. Fifteen budget analysts work for two months, following a specifically developed audit program, analyzing the budgets, checking estimates and utilization factors, and reviewing special requests (e.g., cost beyond control). Staff reviews and suggestions then are given to the Commissioners for final decisions. Hospitals have appeal rights. Although there is a decline in the number of hospitals protesting and appealing rate decisions, it is clear that Massachusetts hospitals are not at one with the Rate Setting Commission. A recent publication by the Massachusetts Hospital Association (MHA) documents the increase in hospital deficits in the state, contending that the regulatory strategy is threatening the financial viability of the hospital industry. MHA argues that hospitals are increasingly forced to use up their endowments and reserves to compensate for operating losses resulting from tight revenue controls.[8] The struggle between the Commission and the hospital association is far from over, and it can easily be predicted that the atmosphere will remain a contentious one for some time to come.

Rhode Island

Unlike Connecticut and Massachusetts, Rhode Island has rejected a formula-based approach to hospital rate setting. The unique feature of the Rhode Island rate-setting program is an annual ceiling on total operating expenses for all short-term hospitals. Within the overall ceiling or Maxicap as it is called, the operating budget of each hospital is set by direct negotiations.

The origins of the program go back to 1969 when for the third consecutive year, Blue Cross of Rhode Island requested a substantial premium increase. The Director of Business Regulation for Rhode Island refused that year to grant the request in full, virtually ordering Blue Cross and the hospitals to restructure the reimbursement system to include cost saving incentives. The result was a system of prospective rate setting with incentive payments, referred to as prospective reimbursement.

Blue Cross, faced with serious financial difficulties, negotiated an agreement with the hospitals whereby they would reduce their proposed rate of cost increase and guarantee their projected budgets for fiscal year 1970–1971. During that same year a pilot prospective rate-setting experiment was carried out with the state's largest hospital. The following fiscal year all hospitals participated in a full experiment which included cost saving incentives. In 1972 the experiment was suspended when it became administratively difficult to synchronize the prospective reimbursement experiment with the Economic Stabilization Program.

The first two experimental years were evaluated by Rhode Island Health Service Research (SEARCH) under a contract with the Social Security Administration (SSA).[9] Although empirical data would not support a conclusion that prospective reimbursement alone reduced the rate of hospital cost inflation, SEARCH argued that the combination of prospective reimbursement with wage and price controls had held down costs relative to other states.

A second experiment, begun in 1974 after the end of the Economic Stabilization Program, was conducted under contract with SSA under the provisions of Section 222 of PL 92–603. As in the earlier experiment, participants included Blue Cross, the State Budget Office (representing the interests of the state as a third-party payer through Medicaid and Title V), all 16 of the state's voluntary hospitals and the Hospital Association of Rhode Island (HARI). In addition, SSA "observed" the process and paid agreed-upon hospital rates for Medicare patients as well as half the administrative expenses of the experiment. When the three-year experiment ended at the close of fiscal year 1977, a new proposal to continue the Rhode Island experiment was submitted to the Health Care Financing Administration, the successor agency to SSA for the management of the Medicare program, but was not approved. The proposal was disapproved because the Rhode Island program was not considered generalizable due to the complexity of the negotiating process and the absence of a formula for establishing allowable increases in hospital budgets. The subjectivity of the decision making process was viewed as a disadvantage; the program's effectiveness was seen to be highly dependent on the leadership of key individuals whose counterparts could not be guaranteed in other states. The prospective reimbursement program has continued without Medicare participation.

The Maxicap idea, the key feature of the Rhode Island program, developed from a belief that line-by-line controls would be too inflexible to work. Outside limits though, it was thought, might protect the third parties while providing some opportunities for purchase of equipment or service expansion if needed. The Maxicap each year limits aggregated gross operating expenses for all voluntary hospitals. Excluded from controls are expenses associated with professional components (e.g., Medicare Part B) and activities financed by grants and contracts.

It must be stressed that the Maxicap is not a target for expenses, but a ceiling within which hospital budgets are negotiated with a reserve maintained for unforeseen expenses. Its purpose is to "CAP" hospital operating expenses for each year. This does not mean that each hospital is given an across-the-board increase reflective of the increase in the Maxicap. The parties are free to negotiate hospital budgets above and below the percent increase of the CAP. However, in the aggregate when budget negotiations are complete, the Maxicap is supposed not to be exceeded. Although the goal is to place a ceiling on total expenses, the process allows for recognition of problems, programmatic development, and unusual circumstances at a given hospital.

Each spring Maxicap negotiations take place with representatives from the State Budget Office and Blue Cross jointly presenting their position and HARI presenting the hospital's position. Both sets of negotiators use national and local economic indicators, anticipated or known factors such as capital spending applications approved by health planning agencies, labor contract experience and other factors that affect hospital costs, to develop a rationale for their position. When negotiations are completed the agreed-upon percentage increase for the following year is applied to the expense base for the current year to give the total budget increase to be distributed by negotiation with each of the 16 voluntary hospitals in the state.

Prior to individual bargaining sessions each hospital submits detailed information on its cost and utilization on prescribed formats for analysis by Blue Cross and state staffs. The focus of the negotiations, though, is on exceptions to predetermined ranges or unexplained increases rather than a review of each line item. Although both sides might prefer the application of a methodology for quantitatively determining all required adjustments, they recognize that it does not exist and are prepared to accept bargained compromises.

After completion of budget negotiations, rates are set for individual hospitals by processing each budget through a cost finding procedure. Rates for Blue Cross, Medicare and Medicaid are derived from total costs according to each purchaser's principles of reimbursement. Because in each of these cases the allowable rate is lower than a hospital's actual expenditures, self-pay patients and commercial insurers are charged at a rate greater than cost. The relationship between cost and charge is expressed as the ratio of costs to charges which Medicaid and Blue Cross guarantee prospectively for one year from the date of implementation by the hospital. The hospital also guarantees not to exceed these charges with certain exceptions.

When volume corridor adjustments are brought into use both the budgeted expenses and the revenues of the hospital may be affected. As volume increases the hospital retains a percentage of revenues collected. The hospital also adjusts budgeted expenses by a similar amount, therefore in aggregate it is possible to exceed the Maxicap.

Adjustments to negotiated expenses can also be made for a change in the intensity of care, subject to agreement between the hospital and Blue Cross and the state. However, since it is difficult to document changes in patient mix or intensity of service, no hospital to date has been able to persuade the third-party payers that a change has occurred.

In contrast to Massachusetts and Connecticut where litigation and acrimony have been observed, relationships between hospitals and rate setters in Rhode Island appear to be amicable. In spite of its acceptability, such a process may be difficult to replicate in other states, particularly those with large numbers of hospitals. The mechanics of standardizing the negotiation process when large numbers of hospitals are involved could easily deter wider implementation.

Discussion

Although hospital rate setting has taken a variety of forms in New England, all programs aim to contain the annual rate of increase in hospital operating budgets. In Connecticut, rate setting is seen as the major regulatory instrument for containing hospital cost inflation; the rate-setting process in Connecticut annually reviews both proposed operating and capital budgets. Because the Commission on Hospitals and Health Care is the decision-making body for both CON and rate setting, these two regulatory instruments have been effectively coordinated in Connecticut. In Massachusetts and Rhode Island, where the regulatory review processes for CON and rate setting are performed by different agencies, these regulatory programs have not been as closely linked.

The experience of rate setters in New England is instructive in considering the limitation of regulatory power. The tough regulatory stance of the rate setters in Connecticut in the 1977 budget review cycle exceeded the boundaries of regulation acceptable to the hospitals. After considerable legal challenge to the process, both sides agreed to a more moderate approach. The Rhode Island approach to rate review has always taken place in an atmosphere of relative cooperation between the hospitals and regulators and a willingness to bargain and negotiate. Some critics have argued that the regulators have yielded too much to the hospitals to achieve an amicable process. The most recent Massachusetts rate-setting program is still relatively new, but there have been serious recent charges by the Massachusetts Hospital Association that past and current budget controls are threatening the financial viability of the hospital industry in that state. Unlike past circumstances in Connecticut where hospitals had accumulated impressive revenue surpluses, Massachusetts hospitals claim that regulation has forced them to deficit financing.

Regulating Medical Technology: The CAT Scanner

The CAT scanner is a sophisticated diagnostic device that provides the physician with an image of selected anatomical structures. The development of CAT scanner policy offers perhaps the best example of how the analytical and political components of health planning interact to determine regulatory policy. And more specifically, the CAT scanner example allows us to assess the capacity of the current planning system to deal effectively with the proliferation of new and costly medical technology. As with rate setting, there is considerable variation in the dynamics of CAT scanner policy in the New England states.

One lesson of the CAT scanner experience is that in the absence of conclusive research and hard data on the diagnostic value, clinical efficacy, and cost effectiveness of CAT scanning, policy will be made in the more prosaic grounds of political bargaining and compromise between interest groups. A more important lesson, however, is that even if much better data become available, the difficulties of choosing between benefits and of trading off various costs and benefits will consistently elevate value judgment and political bargaining to the level of first importance. For CAT scanners in particular and for medical technology in general, the data are unlikely to yield clear policy decisions. In this section we will introduce the CAT scanner problem, look at the analytical difficulties of determining need, and explore the allocation strategies developed by health planners in New England in the absence of clear, analytically determined answers.

The CAT Scanner Problem

In most industries, new technology is introduced because it is expected to enhance the profitability of the firm. There is no desire to invest in new technology in the absence of the promise of improved operating efficiencies or some other advantage affecting profits. Indeed, there is currently a growing concern that various forms of regulation have reduced the potential profit contribution of new technology in industry, resulting in a national rate of innovation lower than necessary to maintain acceptable levels of productivity and a favorable balance of trade and thus to hold back inflation.

The health care industry, by contrast, operates under a different set of incentives; profits in the traditional sense are irrelevant for most industry participants and efficiency improvements are only rarely the purpose of technological innovation. The availability of capital financing for purchasing new technology and third-party reimbursements for its clinical use, and the receptivity of physicians, hospitals, and patients to new and more sophisticated diagnostic and therapeutic techniques all guarantee a ready market for new medical technology. Moreover, in health, regulation occurs after the fact. Technology, the CAT scanner for example, is researched, developed, manufactured, and marketed without any significant input from health regulators except those concerned with safety. The first important opportunity for regulatory intervention comes at the time of purchase and then only where the capital investment involved is high enough to trigger a Certificate of Need review.

Health planners are hard pressed to control the pace of medical technology. Although new technology typically promises diagnostic and clinical advantages, efficacy is seldom fully established prior to actual widespread clinical experience. And as we will discover shortly, there is seldom universal agreement on what standard of "efficacy" to apply. Despite the lack of hard data on benefits, diffusion (even with regulation) occurs rapidly. But if the benefits are sometimes unclear to health planners, the costs are often crystal clear. Capital costs can be substantial; the latest CAT scanner costs more than one million dollars.

And although capital costs can be high, operating costs are even more important. The long-term "effect" of capital investment for resource intensive technology is of primary concern to health planners. This, then is the CAT scanner problem: what posture should health planners take towards the spread of a costly new technology given inadequate and inconclusive information and the need for quick action? Before moving ahead to look in depth at the analytical difficulties of formulating CAT scanner policy, it is useful to say something about the magnitude of the problem planners face, the role of scanner producers in exploiting a ready market, and the speed and the extent of the scanner's diffusion.

CAT scanner producers have achieved rapid market penetration in the United States. The CAT scanner was first developed in England by EMI Inc. in the early 1970s. The first CAT scanners manufactured by EMI and other companies produced images of the head. By 1974, second generation scanners were available providing transverse section images anywhere in the body. The first CAT scanner in the United States was installed at the Mayo Clinic in mid 1973. After that, diffusion of CAT technology occurred rapidly. By 1977, almost 800 CAT scanners produced by nearly a dozen manufacturers were in operation or had been ordered by U.S. hospitals, clinics, and physicians.[10] At present there are more than 1,000 CAT scanners in operation in this country, the great majority of which are distributed among the nation's 7,000 hospitals.[11] Table 7.1 shows that there are significantly more CAT scanners in the United States, both per capita and in absolute numbers, than in other countries.

There is now some evidence that the scanner market in the United States has reached maximum growth. In 1978, the scanner industry sold 120 new machines in this country, compared with 400 in 1977 and 600 in 1976.[12] By some estimates, the scanner market has shrunk by 75 percent.[13] Some manufacturers have already pulled out of the U.S. market altogether, while EMI, once the largest manufacturer of U.S. scanners, is reported contemplating merger or withdrawal.[14] General Electric, which currently claims almost 50 percent of the U.S. market, is busily pursuing overseas sales, with Japan regarded as GE's most promising new market. Varian Associates has joined GE in the search for foreign markets. Technicare Corporation, one of the early scanner giants, reported earnings for its Ohio Nuclear Division down 31.2 percent in 1978. G.D. Searle and Company has abandoned the scanner business entirely.[15] And American Science and Engineering, an innovative but small manufacturer, has sold the rights to its machines to Pfizer, a major pharmaceutical firm, after suffering major losses.[16] The

Table 7.1

Number of Installed CAT Scanners by March 31, 1978

Country	Head	Body	CAT Scanners Totals	Total Scanners/ Million Inhabitants
US	—	—	933 (+150)	4.4 (5.1)
Japan	180	112	292	2.6
UK	36	16	52	0.9
West Germany	51	42	93	1.5
France	10	2	12	0.2
Sweden	8	5	13 (+ 2)	1.6 (1.8)
Norway	2	4	6 (+ 2)	1.5 (2.0)
Denmark	2	1	3 (+ 2)	0.6 (1.0)
Finland	1	0	1 (+ 3)	0.2 (0.8)

Figures in parentheses indicate the number of CAT scanners ordered for installation before end of 1978. These figures were not available for Japan, West Germany and France.

Source: New England Journal of Medicine, September 21, 1978, p. 666.

implication of this for health planners, however, is not necessarily that the problem has passed, but that it is now more complicated. Rather than deal exclusively with the problem of initial market entry, planners will face three kinds of decisions: proposals for initial purchase, as before; proposals for modernizing and upgrading existing machines; and proposals for new and more sophisticated scanners to replace existing CON approved units. Industry too is gearing up for the current market situation. EMI, for example, is banking the future of its medical operations on the reception of a new $1.1 million full body scanner.[17] Technicare's Ohio Nuclear Division has adjusted by developing an inexpensive scanner which, at $96,500, does not currently require CON review in most states.

Planning for CAT Scanners: The Limits of Analysis

CAT scanners have held a special attraction for health planners. They recognize that new medical technologies, scanners included, may represent potentially significant advances in diagnosis or treatment. They know that imperfections in the health care market—primarily the prevalence of third party reimbursements—lead to overinvestments in all medical technologies, not only scanners. But as CAT scanning technology and the planning system developed at approximately the same time and as scanners were especially costly and visible pieces of equipment, the control of CAT scanners became viewed as a device by which the planning system could establish its early credibility. For this reason they were of great symbolic importance to planners.

Ideally, in order to perform their function as gatekeepers for medical technology, planners would assess the costs and benefits of CAT scanning. In practice, however, planners find that cost/benefit analysis is not often a useful analytical tool in any circumstance. The two main problems are the measurement of costs and benefits, and the difficulties of reaching consensus on what the trade offs between them mean.

The cost side of the equation is easier for planners to get a handle on, but not without measurement difficulties. The capital costs for CAT scanners include the costs of purchasing the machine and the costs of related renovation and construction to house it. Capital costs for CAT are easily determined, with the exception of those instances where it is difficult to disentangle CAT-related renovation and replacement from a larger renovation replacement project. The magnitude of the capital costs involved has been a primary reason why planners have paid close attention to the CAT issue. The current average price for a CAT scanner is over $500,000, with a range of $96,500 to more than one million dollars. Thus, the more than 1,000 scanners now in operation in this country represent a capital investment well in excess of one-half billion dollars.

The operating and secondary costs of CAT scanning are also of concern to planners. The operating costs include the salaries of technical staff, maintenance, insurance, supplies, allocated overhead, and so forth. Annual operating costs generally fall in the $300,000 to $500,000 range, depending on the setting in which the CAT scanner operates. Different methods used by providers for allocating administrative and overhead costs to various services and procedures for purposes of reimbursement make it difficult for planners to compare the relative efficiency of proposed CAT installations. The secondary costs of CAT scanning, for example a related increase in surgery or chemotherapy resulting from improved diagnosis, are the most difficult to determine.

Taken together, the capital costs, operating costs, the possible secondary effects of CAT scanning, and the added costs of professional fees for supervision and interpretation, represent the total dollar cost of CAT scanning on the health system. These costs are only partially reflected in patient charges for CAT scanning which, including both technical and professional components, range approximately from $120 to $550 per procedure.[18] Thus, from the health planner's point of view, the various costs of CAT scanning are known, although not perfectly known, and they are regarded as significant.

Determining the benefits of CAT scanning poses a more difficult problem. Possible benefits fall into the following categories.

Technical Accuracy: The CAT scanner provides an accurate and reliable image of the area scanned.

Diagnostic Information: The CAT scanner provides information useful in making a correct diagnosis.

Substitutability: The CAT scanner replaces the use of other techniques, including invasive imaging procedures, exploratory surgery, and biopsy. The CAT scanner allows for diagnosis on an outpatient rather than an inpatient basis.

Clinical Impact: The information provided by the CAT scanner may lead to a change in patient therapy.

Patient Outcome: The CAT scanner has an impact on patient morbidity and mortality including the psychological effect of more rapid and certain diagnosis.

The first problem for planners is the availability of data. While the technical accuracy and diagnostic value of CAT scanning are accepted across a wide range of applications based on available data, there is no consensus as yet with regard to substitutability, clinical impact, and impact on patient outcome. A related problem is measurement. Here clearly the outcome category is the most difficult, particularly with regard to morbidity and psychological effect. Some cost/benefit analysts have developed techniques for assigning different numerical values based on the "quality" of the impact on patients' lives. Thus, the benefit of a CAT scan where surgery resulted in complete recovery would be greater than the benefit where surgery resulted in only partial or temporary cure.[19] To date, health planners have been unable or unwilling to apply such techniques. Thus, the measurement of benefits for purposes of comparing them with costs remains an obstacle to the use of cost/benefit analysis.

The most important problem, however, is not the measurement of benefits, but choosing among benefits. Here there simply is no agreement among health planners. Some regard improved diagnostic information alone as verification of the efficacy of the technology. Others, however, insist that given the costs involved, an acceptable return on investment requires not just better information, but a resulting change in therapy. Still others insist that an acceptable return on investment requires improved information, change in therapy, and some positive impact on patient outcome.

In summary, then, cost/benefit analysis is of uncertain utility to planners in addressing the scanning issue. Insufficient data and problems of measurement make it difficult to compare costs and benefits. Even if costs and benefits could be measured, there is no agreement on what to use on the benefit side of the equation. Finally, even if these obstacles could be overcome, giving planners a general sense of the costs and benefits of CAT scanning, there is no automatic link between general knowledge and specific decisions. In effect, the analytical validity and value judgments in the cost/benefit analysis would be debated each time planners applied cost/benefit analysis in a CON case.

Regulating CAT Scanners in New England

Given the difficulties of determining a comprehensive CAT scanner policy based on cost/benefit analysis, planners have opted for a strategy that is both expedient and realistic. Generally, the CAT scanner planning strategy common in New England is one of incremental addition and adjustment. Planners take the existing number of scanners in their area as a starting point and allow phased additions over time. Thus, each review of a Certificate of Need or 1122 application for a CAT scanner is different, since it occurs in the context of a situation altered by the impact of the previously approved machine. The policy focus, then, is short term and adaptive. The advantage of this is that it allows planners to minimize health cost impact while adjusting policy as further needs become apparent and as new information is more available.

The strategy of incremental addition and adjustment is often formalized in a set of general policies regarding the addition of new CAT scanners. These are usually expressed as numerical standards. The most common standard is a minimum level required for "efficient utilization" of a CAT scanner. Three New England states, Vermont, New Hampshire and Connecticut, apply the utilization standards contained in the National Guidelines for Health Planning developed by HEW. The relevant standards are:

1) A computed tomographic scanner (head and body) should operate at a minimum of 2,500 medically necessary patient procedures per year, for the second year of its operation and thereafter.
2) There should be no additional scanners approved unless each existing scanner in the health service area is performing at a rate greater than 2,500 medically necessary patient procedures per year.

In the case of New Hampshire, these standards were used informally, pending the completion of a State Health Plan. In Maine a formal standard of 1,000 procedures per year was established in 1976. Massachusetts and Rhode Island take a slightly different approach. In Massachusetts planners have adopted flexible "guidelines" to accommodate differences and changes in CAT technology. Formal utilization guidelines range from 2,000 to 4,000 depending upon the kind of CAT scanner (head or body, early or late model). According to the state guidelines, no additional scanners are to be added until existing units have operated at capacity for six months. In Rhode Island, planners eschewed numerical standards for scanner utilization. They have preferred to operate with maximum flexibility and are wary of the incentive for inappropriate utilization implicit in tough utilization standards.

In addition to scanner utilization standards, all New England states have adopted a variety of standards related to staffing and service intensity and sophistication. For example, in order to qualify for a scanner, a hospital might be required to have a full-time neurologist, neurosurgeon, and neuroradiologist, a minimum census for neurology and neurosurgery, a minimum number of neurological procedures including nuclear brain scans, angiograms, pneumoencephalograms, and so forth. It is important to emphasize that these utilization, staffing and service mix standards represent attempts to formalize and codify a general policy of containment. There is no agreement among analysts regarding a precise "break even" point for utilization (estimates range from 1,700 to 4,000 procedures annually), nor is there consensus on staffing and other quality requirements. This holds true for a variety of other standards often used by state agencies and HSAs such as those based on population, bed size, patient discharge data, and so forth. Thus, the formal standards all reflect a general CAT scanner planning strategy—to check proliferation, add slowly, and adjust policy over time.

Although planners in New England states have generally adopted this policy of containment, there are differences in the degree to which they recognize the CAT scanner control issue as a major problem, with corresponding differences in state regulatory response. Because the CAT scanner has achieved special status as a "cause celebre" in health planning, policy positions taken on CAT should not necessarily be regarded as reliable indicators of overall state regulatory posture in health.

In Maine, New Hampshire, Rhode Island, Connecticut, and Vermont, the major battles involving CAT scanners have already been fought. In each of these states, scanners are currently operating in major hospitals and the CAT scanner issue is no longer at the top of the health planning agenda. Although it is impossible to determine how many CAT scanners would be operating in these states in the absence of controls, it can be observed that there is a rough, although not perfect equilibrium between what planners are willing to accept and what providers in the current regulatory environment are demanding.[21] In Maine, for example, five of the six largest hospitals in the state currently operate CAT scanners. Although there have been discussions of a mobile scanner in Northern Maine and a letter of intent to purchase a scanner was filed by a small southern Maine hospital, no formal applications have actually been filed nor are any expected.

A similar equilibrium between provider demand and planning policy exists in the other four states. Two CAT scanners are currently in operation in Vermont, a head scanner at Vermont's major medical center, and a privately owned full body scanner in the northern part of the state. Although there has been some informal discussion regarding a second at Vermont's largest teaching hospital and the addition of a new scanner at another hospital, no applications have been filed. Pressure for the addition of new scanners is not anticipated nor is CAT scanning an important agenda item in Vermont. Three scanners are currently in operation in Rhode Island, one head and two full body scanners. Planners in Rhode Island are satisfied with the current distribution of scanners in the state. As with Maine and Vermont, CAT scanning is no longer a hot planning issue in Rhode Island. In Connecticut there is at least one CAT scanner operating in each HSA area and a total of 13 scanners in the state (11 full body and 2 head). Although the addition of new scanners in eastern Connecticut is anticipated in coming years, no CON applications have been filed. There are three full body scanners currently in operation in New Hampshire. No immediate additions are expected although population growth in southern New Hampshire and along the seacoast may result in the addition of scanners in those areas at some point in the future.

Despite the fact that these states utilize very different approaches to health regulation, the pattern of scanner proliferation in each is similar. Major hospitals have been able to obtain CAT scanners, although often after protracted conflict with planning agencies. The regulatory environment created during the initial period of rapid proliferation is undoubtedly one reason why demand for new scanners has subsided. A more probable explanation, however, given the very different approaches to regulation among New England states, is that the CAT scanner market has approached its saturation point. In other words, at current purchase and operating prices, and given the constant change in

scanner technology, the majority of hospitals in New England interested in acquiring CAT scanners have already done so. Those hospitals
currently leasing scanners may represent the pool of potential additional customers when prices come down further and the technology
stabilizes. In this respect, these five New England states may not be
unique. With over 1,000 CAT scanners now in operation in this
country, roughly one out of every seven hospitals already has acquired
CAT scanners.[22] It is certainly plausible that states like California (177
CAT scanners), Florida (80), Illinois (66), Texas (56), and New York (57)
may have begun to approach market saturation. There are more CAT
scanners in these states than in New England as a whole. At the very
least, it is understandable why in many states the CAT scanner issue is
no longer at the top of the health planning agenda.

In Massachusetts, with a larger, more sophisticated and competitive
hospital industry than the other New England states, there is a different
CAT scanner situation. In the early years of CON in Massachusetts,
from 1972 to late in 1975, CAT scanner policy resembled that of the
other five New England states—the gradual addition of scanners for
major hospitals. In February of 1976, however, the state's Public Health
Council adopted review criteria that amounted to a moratorium on the
addition of new CAT scanners pending the accumulation of new
information on the efficacy of CAT scanning and the development of
accompanying guidelines. The moratorium, enacted during the administration of a governor and a commissioner of public health committed to
tight fiscal management, reflected the intense early pressure for CAT
scanners from Massachusetts hospitals. It also reflected the belief of the
Director of the State Office of Radiation Control that the cost/benefit
value of CAT scanning had not yet been fully documented.

In October of 1978 the Public Health Council adopted new CAT
scanner guidelines. In February of 1979 Burbank Hospital, a community
hospital not far from the New Hampshire border, received approval for
a $159,000 reconditioned body scanner, the first CAT approval in
Massachusetts in over two years. Since that time, an additional scanner
has been approved at the Berkshire Medical Center in the western part
of the state. These scanners, however, represent somewhat unique
cases. Both scanners were justified on the basis of the "geographical
isolation" of the hospitals involved. Nevertheless, by the spring of 1979
the logjam had obviously been broken. By April of 1979, 15 additional
scanner applications had been filed, nine in the Boston HSA area alone.
Because of the tough regulatory posture previously adopted in Massachusetts there is still apparently a sizeable market for CAT scanners in
the state; the antiregulatory reputation of the King Administration may

also have encouraged new applications. As a result, CAT scanning has once again become a health planning issue. Moreover, for health planners in Massachusetts, the CAT problem may be more difficult than for health planners in other New England states. The size, sophistication, and competitiveness of the hospital industry is such that there is not likely to be convergence between what hospitals will demand and what planners feel they can accept. The CAT scanner situation in New England and the formal regulatory policy currently in effect in New England states is summarized in Table 7.2.

Analysis of the Dynamics of Scanner Planning

The policy pattern we have described—incremental addition and adjustment—is a product of a complex bargaining process among interest groups. It is not, however, the result of any single or discrete bargaining transaction, but rather of a series of ongoing and over-lapping bargaining relationships between different planning agencies and between planners and providers. The clearest example of this policymaking process comes from Boston.

As described briefly, in 1970 the Massachusetts Public Health Council adopted scanner guidelines developed by Department of Public Health planners. These guidelines produced what in effect was a moratorium on new CAT scanners. (Although the guidelines called for one CAT scanner per HSA, each HSA in the state already had at least one scanner.) The guidelines were intended as a mechanism to contain expansion pending the arrival of more reliable cost/benefit information. Under the guidelines, however, the Boston HSA had no significant role to play in scanner planning. The HSA had been preempted by the state-created moratorium.

When the moratorium was imposed, the Boston HSA was in the process of developing a scanner strategy of its own, one based in part on an HSA study conducted in 1975 showing a need for additional head scanners in the Boston area.[23] The HSA proposed a plan for the phased addition of new scanners. And more significantly, the HSA plan called for the hospitals themselves to determine the priorities for placement of new scanners. Under the plan, the Metropolitan Boston Hospital Council, one of the six hospital councils conterminous with HSA areas, would oversee the ranking process. After the hospital with the highest rank received a scanner, the second hospital on the list would be approved only after a series of volume and waiting time criteria had been met. The same conditions would then apply to the hospital ranked third, and so forth.

Interestingly, both the hospitals and the state accepted the HSA plan.

Table 7.2

CAT Scanners in New England, 1979

	CATs in Hospitals	CATs Privately Owned	CATs Approved and Not in Operation	Head Scanners	Full Body Scanners	Total	CAT Applications Pending	Standards and Criteria
Massachusetts	20	4	2	6	20	26	15 (9 in HSA IV)	Flexible State Guidelines
Maine	3	1	1	2	3	5	0	1976 State Guidelines in effect
Vermont	1	1	0	1	1	2	0	Use of Federal Guidelines
Connecticut	11	0	2	2	9	13	0	Use of Federal Guidelines
Rhode Island	2	1	0	1	2	3	0	Flexible—No numerical standards used, state or federal
New Hampshire	3	0	0	0	3	3	0	Plan will reflect Federal Guidelines

Source: New England Journal of Medicine, September 21, 1978, p. 666.

The hospitals' motivation was clear: under a moratorium they would get nothing; under the HSA plan they would get something, albeit over a period of time. To signify acceptance of the plan, six Boston hospitals with pending CAT applications withdrew them. For the state, the plan meant a modification of the moratorium, but not a drastic modification. Moreover, acceptance of the HSA plan relieved the state of some of the political problems its hard-line stand had engendered while still offering the benefit of considerable delay in the acquisition of new scanners. It also allowed the state to permit a scanner planning role for the HSA at little cost. The HSA plan, then, represented a compromise between the interests of the HSA, the state planners, and the Boston area hospitals.

Not surprisingly, the hospitals were unable to agree on numerical rankings. In the end, the Metropolitan Boston Council formally gave equal endorsement to three applicants, Children's Hospital, Mt. Auburn Hospital, and Framingham Union Hospital. The three other applicants, Waltham Hospital, Deaconess Hospital, and St. Elizabeth's Hospital, were simply not endorsed. Soon after the Hospital Council's action, all six original applicants resubmitted their CON applications. Then, as described earlier, the moratorium continued in effect until new and more flexible guidelines were issued by the Public Health Council late in 1978.

The major accomplishment of the early scanner in Boston then was delay. It was a policy based on a compromise between the different organizational interests of planners and providers, one that is visible only by looking at scanner policymaking in the Boston area over time. The ultimate impact of the policy will depend upon the next set of compromises made between planners and providers operating, this time, in a political atmosphere transformed by the election of a governor publicly opposed to stringent regulation of health care facility investments.

Perhaps the key factor emerging from the Boston CAT scanner story is the political contest between planners and hospitals. This may be described as the conflict between REGIONALIZATION and REGIONALISM. Regionalization refers to the efforts of planners to organize what, from their point of view, are rational delivery systems, i.e., systems linking together acute care, ambulatory care, long-term care, primary care, and care in specialty settings. In theory, each regional system would be built around a sophisticated medical center. Regionalization would allow CAT scanners only at these major high-technology centers. Regionalism refers to the claims made by hospitals to status as major area referral centers. Where the goals of planners and the claims staked by hospitals coincide, political conflict over CAT scanners is minimal. This has been the case, for example, in Rhode Island, New Hampshire, and Vermont. Where regionalization and regionalism conflict, however, CAT often becomes a difficult political issue. This is precisely what is happening currently in Massachusetts. But the conflict between regionalization and regionalism is best illustrated by events in Maine.

By 1976, when PL 93–641 was first being implemented in Maine, hospitals in three of the four largest population centers in the state, Portland, Bangor, and Waterville, had already acquired scanners. For these hospitals, the scanners represented successful claims to primacy as area referral centers. The first territorial claim had been pressed in March of 1975 by a hospital in Waterville, only recently appropriately renamed the Mid-Maine Medical Center. Almost immediately, hospitals in Bangor (Eastern Maine Medical Center) and Portland (Maine Medical Center, the state's largest hospital) submitted CAT applications. In July of 1975, the Maine Department of Human Services authorized the purchase of a single scanner to be located in Portland. Within six months, while state planners were hastily drafting scanner guidelines, Waterville and Bangor had acquired scanners as well. Waterville had obtained formal approval. In Bangor, a group of physicians had purchased a scanner without submitting an application and had leased scanner services to Eastern Maine Medical Center.[24]

In 1976, a hospital in Lewiston, the state's second largest population center, also submitted a CAT application. The application coincided with the renaming of the hospital from Lewiston General to Central Maine Medical Center. In its application, Central Maine had argued that a denial "might well result in changing the character of our institution from that of a community hospital and a regional referral center to that of a community hospital only."

By this time changes in the 1122 review process, occasioned in Maine by the passage of PL 93–641, had occurred. Maine had both a single statewide HSA and a State Health Planning and Development Agency. The staff at the HSA recommended denial, basing its recommendation on the claim that population patterns, referral patterns, and cost data did not indicate the need for a scanner in Lewiston. Blue Cross and Lewiston's other hospital joined the HSA in opposing the scanner. Nevertheless, the full HSA board voted in an acrimonious and emotional meeting to approve the Lewiston application. The State Health Planning and Development Agency, on the other hand, recommended denial, hoping to eventually centralize scanner referrals in Portland. In October of 1976 the Commissioner of Human Services denied the Lewiston application, temporarily preventing the hospital from acquiring a scanner. In December the SHPDA issued guidelines designed to limit and centralize scanner services. The Lewiston hospital, however, was exempted from the guidelines, with the exception of certain minimal stipulations regarding utilization at the other hospitals with already operating scanners. By late 1978, Central Maine Medical Center in Lewiston had acquired its scanner. In addition, a fifth scanner had been acquired by Augusta General Hospital, located in Maine's capital.

The scanner decisions show the importance of regionalism in Maine health planning. In each region a hospital had sought and gained primacy. Despite the fact that there is but one HSA in Maine, there are now five CAT scanners. However, with the five major hospitals having successfully pressed their claims, there appears to be little interest among other hospitals in acquiring a CAT scanner. Thus, there is a rough (but not perfect) equilibrium between regionalization and regionalism in Maine. At the time the Central Maine scanner represented the degree of difference between what planners would allow and what hospitals attempted to obtain.

Thus, in general, policy formulation for CAT scanning reflects the pulling and hauling that occurs among planning agencies and between planners and providers. Typically, the key issue to be resolved is the tension between planners' efforts to centralize technology and hospital pressure to decentralize it. In addition to policy formulation, another key problem is the implementation of scanner policy. Put simply, implementation is complicated by a variety of provider efforts to evade scanner regulation. Because private physician purchases do not currently require a CON or 1122 application in New England, private physician purchase of a scanner combined with leasing to a hospital is not uncommon. Often the leased scanner is physically located within the hospital to which it technically is leased. There are currently seven privately owned CAT scanners in New England. Indeed, the sole full body scanner in operation in Vermont is privately owned. Health planners have little leverage over private purchase. Where control is exercised, it generally comes from rate setters or third-party payers. In Rhode Island, for example, Blue Cross will not reimburse for non-approved scanners. In Maine, Medicaid withholds reimbursement for capital costs associated with the Bangor scanner. In Massachusetts, rate setters have succeeded in containing private ownership by negotiating charge levels for privately owned scanners comparable to those for hospital owned units.

A second evasive technique is the purchase of scanners at prices below the trigger levels for CON and 1122 review. Manufacturers have encouraged this loophole by offering a line of scanners in the

$96,000-$99,000 range. In Massachusetts, Waltham and Newton Wellesley Hospitals purchased scanners via this route despite a clause in the law requiring a CON for a "major change in service." Eventually both hospitals were allowed to keep their scanners, although a court did rule that in the future even inexpensive scanners would be regarded as a major change in service.

There are still other and more subtle and ingenious methods available. For example, in 1976 when the Massachusetts General Hospital learned that the Peter Bent Brigham was in line for the one new full body research scanner authorized by planners for Massachusetts, it arranged to "borrow" a scanner for a one-year "demonstration" project from the manufacturer, EMI Inc.[25] Since neither MGH nor EMI had made a capital expenditure in excess of $100,000, no CON was required.[26] The MGH operated its scanner during 1977 and 1978. In 1979, as planners expected, MGH applied for a CON for its "borrowed" scanner. One further twist: during 1978 the MGH scanner experienced mechanical problems. As a result, rather than request a CON for a repaired scanner (estimated at between $300,000 and $400,000), MGH applied for a new $800,000 full body scanner. In the meantime, despite their belief that only one full body scanner was necessary in Boston at the time, in what was regarded as a major decision planners rewarded the Peter Bent Brigham with an approval for working within the planning process.[27]

Summary

The CAT scanner issue is perhaps the perfect example of the interaction between the analytical and political aspects of health planning. Planners are faced with a problem, the rapid proliferation of technology that is both expensive to purchase and to operate. Demand is guaranteed; the manufacturers market aggressively and physicians, patients, and hospitals act as eager, affluent consumers. Although health planners need to act quickly, cost/benefit data and information are insufficient and inconclusive. Indeed, given the value questions involved in assessing benefits, the data are likely to remain inconclusive. Planners adapt by adjusting the regulatory response incrementally, attempting to slow the introduction of new scanners while soliciting further information. Their policy of gradualism is formalized in numerical standards and guidelines. Within this overall pattern of response, the specific policies that are developed and the review decisions that are made reflect an accommodation between the organizational interests of different planning agencies, and of planners and providers. Typically, planners attempt to centralize services, while the providers, acting individually, pressure for decentralization. The success planners achieve depends upon the point at which they intervene in the expansion process, the match between planning goals and the inclinations of the hospital industry, and the frequency with which providers are able to circumvent the regulatory policy that develops.

Long-Term Care

Since the passage of Medicare and Medicaid, states have been increasingly concerned with the regulation of long-term care (LTC) facilities. By 1977 40 percent of Medicaid payments were made for services in LTC facilities; in some states over half of Medicaid dollars became nursing home dollars.[28] Only a few years after the implementation of Medicare and Medicaid it became clear to many planners and regulators that if they were to control state health care costs they must control LTC services.

The policy instruments available to state governments to exercise authority over the delivery of long-term care services would appear to be formidable. The states license and inspect all long-term care providers. They determine the rates at which providers will be reimbursed for services rendered to recipients of state aid. Through Certificate of Need and 1122 reviews the state can control entry into the market to provide institutionalized long-term care services.

In few aspects of state health activities has the rationale for action been more carefully drawn than it has for long-term care policy. Task forces have been formed. Consultants have been hired. Procedure manuals have been prepared. Gubernatorial white papers have been issued.

The desire in New England, as elsewhere, is for less institutionalized care and for more community-based services. The white papers talk about the need for the appropriate placement of patients and for the elimination of low-quality providers. Innovative service delivery modes, especially for the elderly, are always praised.[29]

And yet, long-term care policy would appear to be in disarray. The cost of care continues to rise, as does dissatisfaction with the quality and distribution of services provided. Hospitals report the accumulation of administrative bed days due to inability to transfer patients in need of long-term care to more appropriate facilities. Nursing home operators complain about the inadequacy of the rates the states offer. Auditors reviewing nursing homes continually cite the existence of poor care and dangerous conditions. The shift to community-based services has not occurred. Innovation proceeds with primarily private initiative and at the slowest pace.

This policy paradox—the states showing great interest in long-term care but meager policy results—stems from at least two factors. First, the many studies and white papers notwithstanding, there is usually disagreement within state government as to the preferred direction for long-term care policy. Jurisdiction for this policy is often split among several agencies. In Massachusetts, for example, the Departments of Public Welfare, Public Health, and Elder Affairs, the Rate Setting Commission, the Commission of Administration and Finance and the local health planning system share responsibility for long-term care policymaking. Each agency views the problem from its own administrative perspective and tends to champion a particular policy value such as cost control, service quality or service access. As in the federal government, there exists no uniform ranking among these values that is acceptable to all relevant agencies.

Second, even if there were agreement on a priority ranking, say one that would place greatest emphasis on noninstitutionalized care, the states in reality have only limited policy flexibility. On the one hand, they are very much bound by the structure of federal programs, for none among them can afford to bypass the maximum available amount of federal reimbursements. On the other hand, the states must ensure the financial viability of existing providers in order not to threaten the continued availability of services for the thousands of elderly for whom the states have become the permanent guarantor of care. No matter what their policy preference, the states can ignore neither federal guidelines nor the financial interests of long-term care providers.

State planners and regulators are faced with two major issues relating to LTC services: determining the need for and appropriate distribution of LTC facilities and developing reimbursement strategies that are at the same time fair and frugal. As we shall see, the reimbursement issue has been by far the most complex one, in part because the LTC industry is primarily composed of for-profit nursing homes.

Determining the Need for Long-Term Care Facilities

Operating in an environment without a clear federal regulatory policy for nursing home care, the New England states have taken several different approaches to setting targets for LTC beds. In Maine, for example, until recently there has been an intense dispute between the State Department of Human Services and the Maine Health

Systems Agency over the appropriate number of intermediate care facilities (ICF) that should be constructed. The Department advocated the application of loose review criteria so as to increase substantially the availability of ICF beds in the state. It argued that effective control over the cost and quality of nursing home care could be exerted only when the market to supply this care was thoroughly saturated. The HSA had a different perception. It believed that unless rigorous quality and distribution criteria were applied to the review of nursing home expansion proposals, the state would be burdened eventually with the need to support an inefficient and overly large industry. Moreover, the HSA resented being bypassed in the formulation of long-term care policy, as would occur if only the most blatantly inappropriate nursing home proposals were to be turned down.

The Department justified its position on the basis of its own experience. The increase in demand for nursing home services which accompanied the implementation of the Medicaid program during the late 1960s made it impossible, the Department believed, to enforce quality standards in the delivery of these services. Every threat to enforce standards was met by an implied threat on the part of the operators of homes to close down and essentially "dump the old people onto the streets." Admittedly, the situation then was exacerbated by the state's initial policy of reimbursing nursing homes on a flat rate basis. Under the flat rate scheme the simplest way for nursing home operators to maintain profits was to cut patient services (i.e., "water the soup").

In 1972 the Department altered its reimbursement policies to permit operators to receive straight cost reimbursement for the care of state-aided clients. The guidelines for calculating allowable costs, particularly depreciation, were such that very attractive returns could be earned on nursing home investments. This in turn provided a large incentive for the construction of long-term care facilities. Though the cost to the state of maintaining the elderly in nursing homes has increased, so too has the number of modern, code-conforming beds. The Department's expectation was that the competition of new facilities would force the conversion of older, less desirable facilities into lower levels of care. The hope was that there would be a large increase in boarding beds, a category of care thought to be in short supply.

The HSA professed the same goals as the Department, but it believed that quite different methods were necessary to obtain these goals. It too wished to decrease the emphasis on skilled nursing care, but the HSA preferred a regulatory strategy to what it termed the Department's market strategy. The clash between these strategies was most visible in the Ledgeview Memorial case.

Ledgeview Memorial is a West Paris, Maine nursing home owned and operated by the Northern New England Conference of Seventh Day Adventists. In late 1975 Ledgeview applied for permission to construct a 44-bed addition to its existing 80-bed unit. Ledgeview justified the expansion on the basis of the fact that it served coreligionists in New England and that it had a waiting list for vacancies. The review of the application by the Tri-County Health Planning Agency, the relevant "b" agency, though praising the quality of services Ledgeview offered, denied the expansion request on the grounds that no additional beds were needed in its region. The denial was subsequently confirmed by the newly established Maine HSA. Based on the application of need projection formulas, the HSA concluded that the West Paris region was overbedded.

Although the Ledgeview management appeared to accept this judgment, the Department of Human Services did not. Without consulting with the HSA, the Department approved the project, citing as justification its policy of encouraging the construction of low-cost, quality ICF beds. When challenged by the HSA, the Department supported its decision by offering its own need formula which the HSA claimed only confirmed the judgment that the region was overbedded. The HSA then appealed the Department's decision to HEW. Both the HEW Regional Office and Secretary's Office, where a subsequent appeal was lodged, were sympathetic to the HSA's position, but refused to override the state's action.

The Maine Department of Human Services' conscious use of market strategy to encourage investment in ICF beds is unusual. Most states have developed optimal ratios of long-term care beds to elderly population for use in guiding facilities review of nursing home applications. A highly sophisticated approach calculating such optimal LTC bed ratios was developed in Massachusetts in 1976.[30] Bed-to-population ratios were calculated based on data from several studies of the appropriateness of existing placement of patients in four levels of chronic care— chronic disease hospitals, Level II (skilled nursing facilities), Level III (intermediate care facilities) and Level IV (rest homes).* These studies indicated that significant numbers of patients through the LTC system could be cared for in lower level and less costly facilities (see Table 7.3). Based on the data on inappropriate patient placements, bed to population ratios for each level of care were developed for application to the facilities review process at the HSA level.

In Rhode Island, the supply of nursing home beds has increased by 23

*These designations are unique to Massachusetts.

Table 7.3

Massachusetts Patient Placement as Measured by the 1973
Department of Public Health
Long-Term Care Patient Surveys

1973 Placement	Proper Placement			
	Chronic/Rehab	Level I/II	Level III	Level IV and Community Place.
Chronic/Rehab Hospital (6,280)	1,054 (17%)	2,350 (37%)	1,695 (27%)	1,181 (19%)
Level I/II (12,902)	0	11,612 (90%)	1,290 (10%)	0
Level III (26,220)	40	5,566 (22%)	12,074 (46%)	8,540 (37%)
Level IV (6,950)	9	145 (2%)	1,173 (17%)	5,623 (81%)
Rehab Unit in Acute Hospital (172)	151 (88%)	18 (11%)	2 (1%)	1
Long-Term Unit in Acute Hospital (326)	64 (19%)	207 (62%)	48 (?)	7 (5%)
Awaiting Placement (1,705)	132 (8%)	771 (45%)	556 (33%)	246 (14%)

Note: In Table 7.3, the column headed "1973 Placement" lists the various levels of long-term care available in the system. The rows under the heading "Proper Placement" display the actual patient mix within the levels of care shown in the "1973 Placement" column. For example, the 1973 surveys found 6,280 people placed in chronic/rehab facilities. Of these 6,280, 1,054 (17%) belonged in chronic/rehab; 2,350 (37%) belonged in Level I/II, etc. The numbers 1,054, 2,350, 1,695, and 1,181 sum to 6,280.

Source: Proposed Interim Standards and Criteria for the Allocation of Long-Term Care Beds, Massachusetts Department of Health and the HSAs, November 1, 1976.

percent between 1971 and 1976. Assuming existing bed levels, planners expect nursing home utilization in Rhode Island, currently at 22 days per 1,000 persons age 65 and over per year, to continue to increase substantially over the next five years. They estimate that total state expenditures for nursing home care will triple by 1985. Accordingly, they have determined that "there is currently no need for additional nursing home development in Rhode Island."[31] They have also established a projected 1983 level of 26 days/1000 persons 65+/year as the utilization target. The 26 days/1,000 persons 65+/year target was selected because it fell between the current Massachusetts standard of

22.1 and the 27.1 standard used in Rochester, New York. The 1983 target of 26 days/1000 persons 65+/year was also chosen because it approximates the current utilization average for New England of 26.5.

Reimbursement of Nursing Homes

The fact that the great majority of nursing homes in this country are for-profit entities complicates the design of a fair reimbursement system for long-term care of publicly supported patients. Under the tight state budgetary pressures, public funds which contribute to windfall profits of some investors are especially visible and potentially embarrassing to state administrators.

In the early days of Medicaid, states had great flexibility in their arrangements for payment of institutional providers. At first New England states, like most states, chose a flat rate of reimbursement for nursing homes; one rate applied statewide. This system contained incentives to the operators to provide minimal care. The flat rate was therefore periodically negotiated upward by nursing home operators who needed to upgrade facilities and staff to meet licensing requirements. The result was financial hardship for some operators and windfall profits for others. The federal government, states, and many nursing home owners, therefore, sought an alternative to the flat rate approach. In 1968, Massachusetts was one of the first states in the country to adopt a cost-based reimbursement system for ICF care. Maine and Rhode Island followed in 1972, New Hampshire in 1975.

These cost-based systems were patterned after the Medicare system of payment to hospital and skilled nursing facilities. All states were required by regulation to adopt "cost-related" payment to ICFs under Medicaid by January, 1978.

Although an improvement over flat rate systems of payment, the use of a cost-based reimbursement contained unanticipated incentives that encouraged some operators to rapidly turn over the ownership of facilities, realize large profits, and significantly increase the cost of nursing home services to Medicaid. How different states dealt with this problem presents an interesting comparative study of regulation.

The Medicare principles of reimbursement for institutional care, adopted by most states when they moved to cost-related payments to ICFs under Medicaid, pay all operating costs attributable to enrolled patients. With the exception of land, the historical costs of either purchase or construction of a nursing home are reimbursed through straight-line depreciation. These cost reimbursement principles treat profit as an allowable cost; a rate of return on owner's equity of between 10 and 11 percent has been allowed in recent years. The concept of an allowable percentage profit for institutions heavily reliant on public funds is well-established in the area of public utility regulation.

When a nursing home is sold, Medicaid establishes a new "allowable basis" for cost reimbursement that incorporates the sale price. Obviously, under cost reimbursement, the higher the sale price, the higher the rate Medicaid will pay for nursing care. Two factors contribute to inflating the resale price of ICFs. First, in the absence of regulation, a purchaser had little incentive to drive a hard bargain, since the price paid could be recouped through Medicaid payments. Second, the sale price of nursing homes reflects the increased expense of building a similar facility at today's higher construction costs. Indeed, the Medicare principles of reimbursement allow the sale price to reflect the cost of replacing the facility at the time of the sale.[32] For the seller of an older nursing home this means substantial capital gains.

However, capital gains represent only part of the economic attractiveness of selling an ICF. Payment through cost reimbursement coupled with tax benefits afford considerable cash flow advantages in the first years of operation, which are significantly reduced if the home is owned for a longer period of time.

One such cash flow advantage results from the fact that interest and depreciation are reimbursable costs under Medicaid, and in the early years of operation the yearly sum of the interest payment on the mortgage plus depreciation are greater than the annual payments to the financing institution. Thus Medicaid reimburses more than is actually paid out; moreover, the owner is being paid depreciation for an asset that is actually appreciating.

Another economic advantage of the early years of nursing home ownership derives from the difference between the income a facility reports to Medicare and the income it reports to federal and state income tax authorities. There are two primary tax incentives which apply to proprietary owners—the investment tax credit and accelerated depreciation. The nursing home owner/investor can obtain a ten percent income tax credit on the purchase of all movable equipment. This tax credit provides an incentive to purchase equipment. Accelerated depreciation allows the operator to minimize reportable income in the early years of operation.

The two tax advantages provide additional incentives to proprietary owners to sell the facility after a short period. Indeed, there are few business reasons, if any, for long-term proprietary ownership of nursing homes in an unregulated market. Since a proprietary provider may judge his investment by its ability to generate cash, the investment may be sold if more cash is realized through sale than through continued ownership. With less and less cash being generated each year and the value of the physical plant escalating, the sale of the facility is an attractive means of maximizing monetary return. Moreover, the same incentives apply to subsequent purchases of the nursing home. These incentives contributed to an active market in nursing home sales in the pre-regulatory days. Four New England states responded to this problem in different ways, applying different regulatory instruments to avoid uncontrolled inflation in the cost to Medicaid for nursing home care.

In 1972 the Rhode Island Department of Health adopted cost reimbursement as the means by which Medicaid would pay for ICF care. Under this plan facilities were reimbursed for depreciation and interest on related debt and were paid a return on owner's equity as a profit. When a nursing home was sold at a profit, the seller was required to repay to Medicaid that portion of past payments attributable to depreciation. This depreciation recapture provision, adopted from the Medicare principles of reimbursement for SNFs, eliminated one factor contributing to windfall profits at resale. Nonetheless, in 1977 the Department of Health had to modify the reimbursement principles in an effort to limit the still substantial cost impact on Medicaid resulting from the large rise in the capital base produced from the sale of nursing homes. The new reimbursement principles limited the buyer's "allowable basis" for cost reimbursement to the original "basis" plus five percent per year for the period of the seller's ownership. The new principles of reimbursement modified the original recapture of depreciation—an amount that increases each year of ownership. Thus, reimbursement principles limited the capital gains in quick resales and provided a financial incentive (depreciation credit) to encourage long-term ownership.

The major thrust of regulating nursing home sales in Rhode Island is through the reimbursement system. The direct mechanism by which sales are monitored is through the licensing program; all nursing home transfers require relicensing of the facility. When applying for a new license, the prospective purchaser is made aware of the limitations on the "allowable basis" for reimbursement under Medicaid. The transaction is carefully scrutinized by the Medicaid Audit Division, the Fire Marshal's office, and the sanitation department. If all departments agree, the prospective buyer is given an assurance that a new license will be granted. This mechanism avoids retroactive adjustments in the "allowable basis" for reimbursement.

Thus, in Rhode Island, the cost impact on Medicaid of nursing home sales has been effectively regulated by a combination of limiting capital gains at resale and providing incentives for continued ownership through a depreciation credit provision. The regulatory process does not involve the CON program, but is tied to relicensure of the facility.

As described previously, the Maine Department of Human Services has had a long-standing policy of encouraging the construction of additional ICF beds to both meet the nursing needs of Maine residents and to drive out existing poor quality beds through competition. To encourage new ICF construction, the Maine Medicaid program in 1972 adopted a cost reimbursement plan which included, in addition to the economic incentives described above, an inflated rate of depreciation of the facility. The incentives to operators resulted in a significant amount of new ICF construction, consistent with the Department's objectives.

In July, 1976, the first of a series of nursing home resale cases came to the attention of the Department. It appeared that the same incentives which successfully encouraged ICF construction were about to stimulate early resales which would not provide additional beds, but would merely inflate the cost of nursing home care to Medicaid. The Department at first tried to counter the resale incentives by introducing a modified reimbursement strategy which would freeze the "allowable basis" for cost reimbursement to that level appraised at the time of original construction. Under such a plan resales would not result in an increase in the cost of nursing care. Because of overwhelming opposition to this type of plan from nursing home operators, the proposal was never implemented.

Having failed in an effort to apply regulation through reimbursement controls, the state invoked Section 1122 review of nursing home sales as a vehicle through which the price of resale could be scrutinized. The following example illustrates how the state became a party to the negotiation of the price of resale through the 1122 review process. Oceanview Nursing Home, a 72-bed ICF, was constructed in 1973-1974 at a cost of $547,000. The cost of land, fixed and movable equipment plus minor renovations added $110,000 to the owner's investment. In September, 1976, an offer was made to purchase Oceanview for $1,080,000. It was calculated that the cost per patient day would be increased from $20 to $24 per day. The sale was reviewed by the state under Section 1122 and denied on the basis that it would unreasonably increase the cost of nursing home care. Had the home been sold for the proposed sale price, the return on the original owner's equity would have been approximately 280 percent.

A second application for sale of the Oceanview Nursing Home for

$900,000 was submitted to the 1122 Agency in September, 1977. In reviewing this application, the 1122 staff raised several issues in addition to the actual sale price, particularly the fact that the transaction was not at arms length by Medicare definition; the financial interests of the buyers and sellers were intermingled. Moreover, the proposed transaction did not involve any cash changing hands but would have resulted in a considerable increase in the cost to Medicaid for ICF care. The State Department of Human Services, through discussions with the buyers and sellers, made known that it would adhere to Medicare regulations applying to arms length transactions and would agree to a transfer of ownership only if no change in the allowed basis for reimbursement would occur. Moreover, the state insisted on recapturing depreciation paid to the seller at the time of the transfer. Faced with a second 1122 denial, the owners agreed to the state's conditions; the amended application for transfer of ownership at $600,000 was approved.

Thus, in Maine the Section 1122 review process has been invoked as an instrument by which the price and nature of ICF sales are regulated. Although it is arguable whether Section 1122 was intended as an instrument to control the sale price of nursing homes, no court test of this regulatory application has yet occurred. In January, 1978, Maine's Medicaid program amended its reimbursement principles to include a provision limiting the profit on ICF sales. This provision is similar to that in Rhode Island; the buyer's "allowable basis" for reimbursement is calculated by inflating the seller's historical cost at acquisition by the consumer price index. The formula will provide a clear basis on which to assess the price of future nursing home sales.

Massachusetts, in 1968, was one of the first states in the country to adopt a cost reimbursement formula for paying ICFs. Unlike the Medicare formula, the one adopted by the Rate Review Commission did not provide for recapture of depreciation reimbursement at the time of the sale, but did limit the increase in "allowable basis" to the estimated original construction cost inflated by the construction cost index. The Rate Review Commission made public the new method of determining the "allowable basis" after sale, and thus may have assured that subsequent sale prices reflected the allowed ceiling.

Through the 1970s the increasing Medicaid budget, and specifically that portion which paid for long-term care, became a major political issue in Massachusetts. As one approach to controlling further increases in the Medicaid budget, the Rate Setting Commission revised its original cost reimbursement formula in 1977, stipulating that the original basis for reimbursement for interest, depreciation, and return on equity would not be increased in the event of a sale, i.e., they "froze the basis" at the existing level. This radical step clearly eliminates the major incentive for nursing home sales—the previously assured market for services at a guaranteed price reflecting costs.

The impact of the Commission's action may be more than was anticipated. No longer is there a viable market for nursing home properties within the state as banks wonder about the ability of owners to repay loans. With mortgage principal and interest costs exceeding depreciation reimbursements, owners face inevitable bankruptcy after about ten years unless they have created appropriate reserves (which few apparently have done).

The Department of Public Welfare fears that owners will abandon their properties as bankruptcies occur. The Commission's effective solution will then become the Department's nightmare as it will have to arrange for the refinancing and professional management of the homes in order to protect the interest of their residents and the reimbursements the state receives from the federal government for the residents' care. Seeing the nursing home financial crisis approaching, the Department laments the failure in interagency coordination.[33]

Unlike the other three states described above, to date New Hampshire has not experienced speculation in the nursing home market. A description of Medicaid's strategy for ICFs payment in New Hampshire provides an interesting comparison to that of the other three states.

New Hampshire reimbursed ICFs on a $16 per day flat rate basis until 1975. The flat rate system was inexpensive and provided little incentive to nursing home operators to either accept Medicaid patients or to provide anything but minimal care to those who were accepted. The switch to cost reimbursement in 1975 was occasioned by concern in some state offices with the deteriorating condition of many nursing homes coupled with the uncertainty of a future federal mandate requiring all states to use cost reimbursement for ICFs. However, because cost reimbursement resulted in an increase in the state's outlays for ICF care in excess of its budget, a decision was made to reimburse ICFs at only 95 percent of cost. A year later, continued budgetary concerns occasioned a further reduction to 91 percent of cost. The New Hampshire Nursing Home Association brought suits against the state on the grounds that their reimbursement system did not comply with the federal requirement of cost-related payments.

As a result of the legal challenge, in 1977 New Hampshire adopted a new set of principles of reimbursement for ICFs which has been approved by HEW. Under these principles, nursing homes are divided into three bed-sized classes. For the capital component of cost (interest, depreciation and return on equity) all homes are reimbursed 100 percent. Operating costs are reimbursed up to the 75th percentile in each bed class; nursing homes with operating costs below the 75th percentile receive a 10 percent bonus payment. Thus, the formula contains an incentive to control operating costs. The nursing home owners are content with this formula as most of the proprietary homes are below the 75th percentile. Those above the limit are mostly publicly run institutions which appear to have higher operating costs.

However, notably absent from the formula is any control on the capital base for reimbursement. This contrast with other states reflects the fact that New Hampshire has not experienced speculation in nursing homes; no resales resulting in an increased capital component base have occurred to date.

Unlike other states which had to adapt regulatory instruments to contain nursing home sales, New Hampshire avoided the problem by making nursing home ownership relatively unattractive through strict limits on reimbursement. The new principles of reimbursement may change the climate for speculation, making New Hampshire one of the only states without a mechanism for regulating the capital component of nursing home sales. Although the 1122 program does review nursing home sales, without guidelines on allowable profits denials under 1122 may be vulnerable to legal appeals. Thus, New Hampshire, which lagged in moving to cost reimbursement, may soon discover the need to specifically target regulation toward containing profits in nursing home sales.

Summary

In three New England states cost reimbursement formulas for ICF payment resulted in speculation in nursing homes and increased costs to Medicaid. The differences in state response to this problem are notable. Rhode Island attempted to regulate unreasonable profits through a reimbursement mechanism which provided some incentives for continued ownership of nursing homes. Massachusetts, after a considerable period of time without a regulatory strategy, finally invoked a radical device which allowed no profit in the event of a sale. Maine at first regulated on a case-by-case basis using the 1122 review, then moved to a formula-based 1122 review. New Hampshire has avoided speculation in nursing homes through low rates of payment. Its recent cost reimbursement formula may result in the same problems faced by the other states.

The method of payment to ICFs under Medicaid has been left

essentially to the states; regulation of ICF payment reflects individual state health care objectives and regulatory philosophy. New England affords a useful set of examples of state-level coping with the costly resale phenomenon, ranging from a carefully defined reimbursement strategy in Rhode Island to the blunt instrument of freezing the basis in Massachusetts.

Acute Care

The public's awareness of local health planning and regulatory activities centers almost exclusively on attempts to control the distribution of acute care services. Whenever there appears to be even the slightest threat to a community's access to obstetrics, pediatrics, emergency care and the other basic acute services, hearing rooms are jammed, petitions are prepared, and the politicians are aroused. The chronicle of health facility regulation, usually filler material in local newspapers, becomes then a front page story.

The federal government too is intensely interested in the distribution of local acute services, but for a different purpose. As the HEW planning guidelines indicate, the federal government hopes to limit the growth in health care capital stock, especially that which is devoted to the delivery of hospital services. The standing of the health planning system among the mechanisms to be used in the federal effort to control health care costs depends largely on the system's ability to restrain the enhancement and proliferation of acute services.

Local regulators are well aware of the threat to their own survival that lies in these conflicting perspectives. They attempt to limit their risk of offending either local voters or federal officials by encouraging regionalization in acute care services, hoping that regionalization will tame the desire of hospitals to intensify or expand services and thus reduce the need to make tough regulatory decisions.

The ability of regulators to affect an increased regionalization in acute care services depends greatly on the degree to which hospitals are satisfied with the status they have obtained in the local hierarchy of health facilities. As we have observed in New England there are states in which an accepted, traditional hierarchy exists among local hospitals and others in which leadership positions are intensely disputed. Where hospital status is in doubt, facility regulation is a source of continual political controversy.

Stable Hierarchies, Quiet States

Rhode Island, Vermont, and New Hampshire, the three least populated states in New England, have the most stable hospital systems in
our study. In each, the dominance of particular hospitals is accepted and
the patterns of service growth are predictable and generally unthreat-
ening to the prevailing provider hierarchy. Although not always exhibit-
ing great elegance, health facility regulation in these states generates
minimal conflict.

Practically a city-state, Rhode Island has but 14 general hospitals.
Over the years, these hospitals evolved a pattern of mutual relationships that each apparently has found comfortable. Neither the establishment of the federally mandated health planning system nor the
transformation of the two-year Brown University medical program into
a full-scale medical school has jeopardized the relationships among the
hospitals. Rhode Island Hospital, the most sophisticated of the hospitals,
is modest in its dominance. State officials, intimately familiar with the
structure of the local medical community, apparently find no need to
seek drastic alterations. Only one hospital geographically isolated from
Providence has felt threatened by a state regulatory decision and it won
a reversal in the political arena (see the Suburban Memorial case in Part
Two).

Vermont's hospital system is not untroubled, but its problems are
largely externally caused. Still very much a rural state, Vermont has
barely the population to support the medical school it maintains in
Burlington at the State University. Two other medical schools with
their attendant teaching hospitals are located close to the state's
boundaries, one in Albany, New York, and the other in Hanover, New
Hampshire, and both treat many Vermont residents. The small community hospitals scattered about the state have only limited aspirations.
Only the Burlington teaching affiliates of the State University claim
major league status. State regulators have the appropriate loyalties to
the Burlington hospitals, but can do little to alleviate their perpetually
precarious situation.

Despite the loose regulatory environment that prevails in New
Hampshire, the state's hospitals have not pressed for significant expan-
sions. The opportunity for expansion exists, particularly in the southern half of the state which is experiencing rapid population growth.
(New Hampshire is the second fastest growing state east of the
Mississippi with the counties adjacent to Massachusetts attracting most
of the in-migration.[34]) As Manchester and Nashua are the only com-

munities in New Hampshire with more than one hospital and as both are in the region of rapid population growth, it is unlikely that hospital expansion when it does occur will generate much interhospital rivalry.

Unstable Hierarchies, Conflict-Ridden States

Two controversial issues fill the agenda of hospital regulators in Maine. One is the unresolved question of what is the minimum number of regions that providers would find acceptable. The other is the need to discover a mechanism to improve the quality of care available in Maine's dozens of small rural hospitals, given that their closure is a politically impossible option.

The regional issue has its roots in the state's relatively large (for New England) size. Portland, the state's largest city, is closer to New York City 450 miles to the south than it is to points in Aroostook County on the state's northern border with Canada. The state's other cities have a tradition of asserting their independence from one another and Portland. Reflecting this preexisting political and economic fragmentation, Maine's initial health planning system was composed of five "b" level agencies. In each of the "b" regions one or more hospitals sought primacy and the status of a regional referral center.

The implementation of the new planning law required a choice be made as to the number of local health planning regions (health systems areas) that would continue to be recognized. Five was an apparently impossible number because the new law mandated relatively large minimum populations for each area and Maine is a sparsely populated state. Not surprisingly, most of the "b" agencies favored retaining as many areas as the federal government would permit while the state's largest hospital (Maine Medical Center in Portland) and the only hospital within the state to qualify as a specialty center preferred the designation of a single statewide health systems agency. Alternative plans for one, two, three, and five health systems areas were presented to Governor James Longley.[35]

Longley, newly elected as the nation's only Independent governor, was intent on fulfilling a campaign pledge to cut the cost of state government in health as well as other policy arenas. One of his first actions was to veto a bill establishing a state medical school (a school that was to be shared among the several "medical centers" in the state) on the grounds that it was too costly a venture for Maine to undertake. Another was to order cuts in the budget of the state's Medicaid program. When considering the plans for the number of health systems areas, the Governor was advised that less federal money would be available for local health planning activities under the new law than had been available under the old and that the state needed coordination of health planning activities in order to reduce waste and duplication in health services. The Governor chose to designate a single statewide HSA for Maine.

Several of those who advised Longley in his decision later came to wish he had selected either the two or the three HSA option instead. Despite the designation of a single HSA, Maine has what is in essence five health planning regions. In order to placate local interests, the Governor urged the formation of local sub-area councils and permitted the old "b" agencies to dominate the selection of the HSA board. A regionalism conforming to the "b" agency regions' boundaries pervades the HSA board's thinking about planning, though not all of the sub-area councils have actually been established. In three of the five sub-areas a single hospital clearly dominates. The attempt of these hospitals and the state to limit the diffusion of specialized medical services and advanced technologies to the three regional centers is being opposed by hospitals in the other sub-areas. The Lewiston area hospitals, in particular, though beset by their own rivalry, have been unwilling to accept subordinate status (see the Lewiston case in Part Two). The politics of the situation is such that facilities review decisions have had to concede the existence of five regions when many involved, including providers as well as state officials, believe a smaller number to be more reasonable.

The rural hospital issue presents planners with an even more delicate political problem. Scattered about Maine are many less than 50-bed hospitals including several still housed in wood frame buildings. Applications from these hospitals for facility modernization often accompanied by requests for additional beds are repeatedly being presented. Planners, doubtful that quality care can be provided in these institutions even if they are upgraded, prefer the closure or merger of the rural hospitals. Public articulation of such quality concerns, however, is nearly impossible. One official who did openly mention the desirability of reducing the number of rural hospitals, the first director of the HSA, was said to have been forced from his position for his indiscretion.[36] Attempts to utilize planning methodologies to achieve a reduction in beds in rural facilities have failed (see the "A" General Hospital case in Part Two). Regionalization, either through mergers or linkages with referral centers, is not seen as viable alternative policy. Given the power of rural communities in the Maine legislature, it certainly is not a policy for which the urban hospitals would be willing to risk their own political capital to obtain. Inefficient rural hospitals are likely long to remain a fixture in Maine.

In Massachusetts the important conflict is the competition between the major teaching affiliates of the state's four medical schools and large community hospitals in the Boston and Worcester areas over a declining and shifting patient base. This competition is particularly intense in metropolitan Boston where the dozen or so major tertiary and speciality care centers located in Boston proper are surrounded by a ring of ambitious community hospitals. The recent upgrading of medical facilities throughout New England which has reduced the flow of referral patients into the Boston teaching hospitals coincided with an acceleration in the movement of Boston's population to the suburbs. Attempts by the Boston hospitals to retain patients conflict with the desires of community hospitals to expand their facilities in order to take advantage of new clinical opportunities.

A somewhat similar situation exists in Worcester where the University of Massachusetts chose to locate its new medical school and to build its own teaching hospital. Worcester's other hospitals with ambitions of their own now compete for patients with the University's hospital in a severely overbedded city. One or more of the hospitals is certain to fall victim in the competition. The most likely candidate for closure though is Worcester City Hospital, an underfunded, publicly owned institution with strong political if not community ties (see the Worcester City Hospital case in Part Two).

The rest of the state is immune to this sort of instability. In the Western Massachusetts–Springfield area the 1,000-bed Bay State Medical Center, the product of a recent merger, has an obvious dominant position. The Merrimac Valley and North Shore HSAs have successfully isolated themselves from the Boston hospital market. The South Shore-Cape Cod area has the advantage of a growing and relatively evenly dispersed population.

State officials are at a loss for a method to achieve their desired regionalization of acute care facilities in Boston and Worcester. The movement of Lahey Clinic and the Harvard Community Health Plan, an HMO, into the western suburbs of Boston will intensify the competition for patients, as will the growth of the Fallon HMO Plan in Worcester, but it will not end it. Given the prevalence of insurance coverage, hospital rivalry frequently takes the form of a contest to obtain the latest in medical technology. As officials discovered in their attempt to allocate scanners though, there is little regulators can do to control these competitive urges or to direct their outcome (see the Body

Scanner case in Part Two). Order will not prevail in Massachusetts acute care services until the relationship between teaching facilities and community hospitals is resolved by the hospitals themselves.

Connecticut like Maine has too many health planning regions. But unlike Maine's governor, Connecticut's governor chose to have five HSAs. In 1975 when it was time to outline HSA boundaries, the governor received recommendations for every number between one and six as to the number of HSAs that would be desirable to designate. The state's Council on Human Services, for example, favored the designation of only one health systems agency on the grounds that a single agency would facilitate coordination with existing administrative and planning units, while the state's Regional Medical Program which worked closely with Connecticut's two medical schools favored the establishment of two agencies with boundaries approximating the boundaries of the medical schools' patient service areas.[37] Governor Grasso apparently preferred the advice of the legislature which advocated the creation of the maximum number of HSAs that federal officials would permit so as to maximize community involvement in health planning.[38]

However, as three of Connecticut's five HSAs lack a major teaching hospital there is uncertainty about which of the available hospitals will have primacy within the region. Rivalry has developed as the hospitals strive for specialty service prominence. Even the major teaching institutions in New Haven and Hartford face uncertain futures as their referral areas shrink due to the growth of facilities in the other cities within the state.

Acute care policy then, like the other policies reviewed in this chapter, is highly dependent upon the particular political alignments that develop within a state and among the state's health care providers. Federal programs merely provide the opportunity for these forces to express themselves. Variation in health policies reflects the diversity that exists in American society.

Notes

[1] K.G. Bauer, "Hospital Rate Setting—This Way to Salvation" in *Hospital Cost Containment*, M. Zubkoff, E. Raskin, and R.S. Hanft, editors, Milbank Memorial Fund, New York, 1978; K.G. Bauer, *Cost Containment Under PL 93–641: Strengthening the Partnership Between Health Planning and Regulation*, Final Report, Contract No. 230-76-0222, January, 1978; M. Sweetland, *How Links and Gaps Between PL 93–641 Planning and Regulatory Functions Affected One Connecticut Hospital: A Case*

Report, Harvard University Center for Community Health and Medical Care, Report Series R 58–2, December, 1977.

[2] Hospital administrators have a different perspective on rate regulation. See Emily Friedman, "State Rate Review: The High Cost of Savings," *Hospitals* (March 16, 1980), pp. 67–70, 118.

[3] Charge payers generally pay higher rates that include cost items disallowed by cost payers (e.g., bad debts). The charge payers, however, still benefit when a hospital budget increase is held to a predetermined level by the rate regulation process.

[4] From the *Third Annual Report to the Governor and General Assembly,* Commission on Hospitals and Health Care, January 1, 1977.

[5] M. Sweetland, *How Links and Gaps Between PL 93–641 Planning and Regulatory Functions Affected One Connecticut Hospital: A Case Report,* Harvard University Center for Community Health and Medical Care, Report Series R 58–2, December, 1977.

[6] For another view of the Connecticut experience see Gary Gaumer, et al., "Prospective Reimbursement in Connecticut," *Topics in Health Care Financing,* Vol. 6, No. 1 (Fall 1979), pp. 51–57.

[7] S. Rubin, *Hospital Reimbursement Methodologies in Use at the Massachusetts Rate Setting Commission,* October, 1977.

[8] L.E. Seck, *Impact: Diagnosing the Financial Illness of Massachusetts Hospitals,* Massachusetts Hospital Association, June, 1978.

[9] H. Thornberry and A. Zimmerman, "Hospital Cost Control: An Assessment of the Rhode Island Experiment with Prospective Rate Setting," prepared for the Office of Research and Statistics, Social Security Administration, June, 1975. It should be noted that Hellinger interpreted the data in the above report as evidence that the prospective budget review systems had not showed the rate of increase in hospitals' costs (F.J. Hellinger, *Inquiry* 13, 309, 1976).

[10] Institute of Medicine, *Computer Tomographic Scanning,* April, 1977.

[11] The Congressional Office of Technology Assessment has reported that in 1977 15% of operating CAT scanners were owned by physicians and located in private offices or clinics, and 6% owned by private physicians but located in hospitals.

[12] *Standard & Poor's,* March 2, 1978, p. H21.

[13] "Why EMI Seeks a Merger in the U.S.," *Business Week* (April 9, 1978).

[14] Ibid.

[15] *Standard & Poor's,* op. cit.

[16] 1978 Annual Report, American Science and Engineering, Inc., Cambridge, MA.

[17] *Business Week,* op. cit.

[18] If we combine the lowest price ($120) with the federally recommended minimum number of 2,500 procedures per year and multiply by 1,000 CAT scanners (roughly the number now in place), the result is $300,000,000 per year.

[19] See, for example, Richard Zeckhauser's concept of Quality Adjusted Life Years.

[20] *Federal Register,* March 28, 1978, Part N P 13049.

[21] It can be noted that the scanner manufacturers believe that the increasingly stringent regulatory environment under PL 93–641 bears a major responsibility for falling sales and profits in the U.S.

[22] Survey conducted by Center for Analysis of Health Practices, Harvard School of Public Health, November, 1977.

[23] The HSA Study, "A Systems Study of Computerized Axial Tomography," showed that head scanning was of significant diagnostic value, that utilization of existing scanners was appropriate, and that waiting times for nonurgent scans were significant.

[24] Private physician purchases are not covered by Section 1122 review requirements.

[25] At the time of the Peter Bent Brigham application, two body scanners were already in operation in Massachusetts, one at St. Vincent's Hospital in Worcester (only used for head scans), the other at New England Medical Center in Boston.

[26] The Massachusetts CON trigger cost is now $150,000.

[27] The Peter Bent Brigham-MGH Scanner Decision, see Case 8, Part Two.

[28] See Table 2.2 in Chapter 2.

[29] Memorandum to Karen Quigley from Dennis Beatrice, titled Rate Setting Issues, April 28, 1978, Department of Public Welfare, Commonwealth of Massachusetts. Not all reviewers of long-term care policy proposals believe that enough emphasis is placed on innovative approaches. They want even more stress placed on alternatives to current practice. See Stanley J. Brody and Anna Belle Woodfin, "Long-Term Support Systems: An Analysis of Health Systems Agency Plans," Issue Paper No. 5, National Health Care Management Center, University of Pennsylvania, Philadelphia, PA, November, 1979, and Saul Spivack, "New England Health Systems Plan Technical Review: Long-Term Care," Center for Health Planning, Boston University, Boston, MA, 1979.

[30] *Proposed Interim Standards and Criteria for the Allocation of Long-Term Care Beds,* Intergency Task Force: Massachusetts Department of Public Health and the HSAs, November 1, 1976.

[31] Preliminary State Health Plan, Rhode Island Department of Health, 1979, pp. 7–120.

[32] Under Medicare Principles of Reimbursement, the new "allowable basis" to

the buyer of a nursing home can be the cost of replacing the facility minus the depreciation factor which is a function of the facility's age.

[33] Memorandum to Karen Quigley from Dennis Beatrice, op. cit.

[34] Table 22 "Estimates of the Population of the States," U.S. Bureau of the Census, Population Profile of the United States: 1978, Current Population Reports P-20. No. 338, April, 1979.

[35] "Health Planning in Maine," First Annual Report, Codman Research Group, September, 1977. Contract No. 291-76-0003/HRA, HEW.

[36] Interviews.

[37] "Recommendation of Connecticut Regional Medical Program to the Governor of Connecticut for the Designation of Health Service Areas Under PL 93-641," April, 1975.

[38] Ibid, p. 7.

Chapter 8

Conclusions

Analysis

PL 93–641, like any ambitious federal legislation, has multiple and sometimes conflicting goals and objectives. Some of these are explicitly stated in the language of the statute; others are hidden or implied. Moreover, emphasis on particular goals changes over time; guidelines and regulations are developed that balance what is stated in the statute against the practical lessons of implementation. Amendments are proposed in Congress, administrations change, and the mood of the country towards government intervention shifts. Always, there is a significant element of interpretation involved in weighing the objectives of legislation and of government programs; the purpose of major government programs cannot be inferred simply by reference to the language of the enabling statute.

We have argued that the implementation of PL 93–641 should be considered primarily in the context of federal policy to contain the rate of inflation in medical care costs. Coming in 1974, soon after the 1972 enactment of the Professional Standards Review Organization Program (professional self-regulation) and the Health Maintenance Organization Act in 1973 (market competition), PL 93–641 signaled the choice of a regulatory direction in federal health policy. With the failure to pass the Carter Administration's hospital cost containment legislation, PL 93–641 remains at the leading edge of the federal government's regulatory efforts to contain costs in the health sector.

Facilities review under CON and 1122 review, plus health plan development, are the primary mechanisms for accomplishing cost containment under the planning law. In practice, facilities review attempts to limit capital expansion, particularly for new hospital beds and technology. Health plans describe the current resources of the medical care delivery system and suggest changes in the level and organization of health care resources that might result in an improved future medical care delivery system. In effect, health plans provide the analytical rationale and the underlying policy for the specific decisions that are made to limit growth or reallocate resources. In practice, the distinction that is often made between "planning" and "regulatory" activities of the PL 93-641 agencies breaks down. Based on our observations in New England, we perceive both plan development and facilities review as interdependent activities designed to achieve what is essentially a regulatory goal—cost containment at acceptable levels of quality and access. Both plan development and facilities review seek to establish a more efficient allocation of health resources based on a regionalized medical care delivery system and multi-institutional sharing.

The processes by which both plan development and facilities review are accomplished are very similar. Each involves participation by consumer and provider representatives and each is characterized by extensive bargaining and negotiation among contending parties. If planning and regulation cannot be distinguished with regard to purpose, neither can they be distinguished on the basis of process. Indeed, the often-used characterization of the current planning program as "planning with teeth" testifies to the blurred distinction between planning and regulatory functions under PL 93-641.

Although we believe that the familiar distinction between planning and regulation makes little sense in the context of current health planning programs, a distinction between the resource containment and resource development purposes of the program is meaningful. There are many areas of the country where access to health care is inadequate and certainly HSAs and SHPDAs in such areas are addressing this issue. But improved access can be catalyzed under PL 93-641 only by the instruments currently available to health planners—facilities review and health plans.[1] Facilities review ("regulation") and plan development ("planning") can be used as a mechanism for either resource containment or expansion; neither goal is the exclusive purpose of one activity or the other. But in practice in New England, and we suspect throughout the country, planning and regulatory instruments have been used much more often under the current planning program to contain, rather than promote, growth. Thus, in our view the central purpose of PL 93-641 is regulatory and both facilities review and plan development are first and foremost means towards a regulatory objective.

The regulatory aspects of the health planning program were given special attention by the Congress when it considered amendments to the planning law in 1979. Controversial issues considered by the Congress concerned the CON program including an exemption of HMO facilities, antitrust implications, potential inclusion of major capital equipment in physicians' offices, and an exemption of projects aimed at complying with life safety code regulations. The most persuasive evidence presented to Congress in support of the planning program was the estimated dollar savings achieved by CON and 1122 review programs nationally.[2]

The attention given to the regulatory aspects of PL 93–641 is not surprising. With the failure of passage to date of the Carter Administration's hospital cost containment legislation, the regulatory functions of PL 93–641 are the mainstay of the federal health cost containment strategy. And controls on hospital capital formation through CON and Section 1122 review, along with the standards developed for local and state health plans to guide facility review decisions, are by far the most visible and politically sensitive instruments of hospital regulation. Although PSRO concurrent review and state hospital budget review take place in the privacy of a hospital or conference room, health plan development and facilities review programs involve public hearings, media coverage, and open debate. As public phenomena, the activities of health planning under PL 93–641 have been the most controversial of the new hospital regulatory initiatives.

Our studies in New England have shown that the regulatory intent of the health planning program to limit hospital capital formation through CON runs counter to the desires of many providers and consumers of health care. As a regulatory program it is unusual in that it benefits the federal government most directly (in containing Medicare and Medicaid hospital cost inflation), but relies on the state governments for administration. In spite of increasing outlays for hospital care and insurance, not all states and few health care consumers and providers accept the regulatory objectives of PL 93–641.

The essential stress in health planning derives from the conflict between the regulators' desire to limit health cost increases and the widely held belief that access to the latest medical technology *could* mean the difference between life and death for a given individual. Community residents want access to the "best," certainly the latest, medical technology in the event that they or their family members are seriously ill. Investment in health resources is in a sense an insurance policy; it will cost the community (and thus the individual) a little now for a potentially big benefit should a critical need arise. In one sense local opposition to health planning goals reflects a difference in interpretation of probabilities between planners and community residents and physicians. The planners and regulators wish to "rationalize" the system, using as a guide what has been called "statistical compassion." Such reasoning would lead to centralization and the elimination of inefficient services and institutions. But residents of communities whose hospitals would lose OB services or would be denied CAT scanners are not comforted by the improved efficiency promised for the system as a whole. Their concerns are with potential access in case of critical need, even if this need is unlikely, and inefficiencies result. "Statistical compassion" provides much less comfort to individuals than the local availability of a modern, well-equipped intensive care unit.

The goals of cost containment and system rationalization further conflict with one of the basic tenets of medical practice, the tenet that the physician must do everything possible to diagnose and treat each patient. The worst kind of failure in medicine is the failure to recognize and appropriately treat a curable illness. Errors of commission (doing too much) in diagnosis and treatment are generally forgivable (and frequently undetectable), while errors of omission in diagnosis and treatment are not only unforgivable, but frequently actionable. A rational, planned health care system, however, would have some physicians who serve some communities operate below the state-of-the-art, unable to provide all diagnostic and therapeutic services required by their patients. Sending a patient on a journey for a CAT scan or to an intensive care unit is often unpalatable to both physician and patient and has led to a frequently encountered argument for medical self-sufficiency at the community level.

The polarity of positions on hospital regulation was repeatedly observed in New England in the debate over local CON and 1122 applications. Typically, a coalition of community residents and providers sought improved access to a new or improved facility or service. Their motivations included the comfort of knowing access would be available should the need arise, as well as pride in local institutions and the convenience of obtaining or providing hospital services locally. While the cost containment position of the federal government is embraced with varying degrees of vigor by state regulators in New England, HSAs, who look for full designation and financial support from HEW, have emerged as vocal cheerleaders for the federal position. Indeed, the HSAs in New England have in many cases advocated more stringent planning targets than either the states or HEW. Their arguments against specific capital projects or for stringent planning targets are frequently in conflict with the desires of community residents (e.g., see the Leonard Morse case in Part Two) and contradict early predictions that HSAs would lack enthusiasm for rational planning and cost containment.[3]

Given that the positions of the planner/regulator and the facility proponents develop from different premises, it is not surprising that technical analysis of need cannot resolve the underlying philosophical debate. Although planners in some areas have been applying increasingly sophisticated studies to the CON and 1122 processes, such analyses are never determining; they only add one bargaining chip to the side of the planner in the ensuing political struggle to resolve the conflict over specific facilities (see the "A" General Hospital case in Part Two).

What most often determines the outcome of any CON or 1122 application is the relative political strength and finesse of the applicant in comparison to the regulators. In most cases, capital projects can eventually be approved, although often with substantial modifications, if the applicant has the appropriate level of patience, political allies, legal resources, and community support.

The bargaining surrounding the planning process is complex, involving many participants. But while bargaining takes place among all possible combinations of agencies, institutions, and groups (HEW, SHPDA, SHCC, HSA, community residents, and individual hospitals), the key bargaining determining the outcome of CON or 1122 applications takes place between the applicant and the state regulators. A state administration committed to restraining capital formation in hospitals can successfully deny a CON or 1122 approval for a major capital project (e.g., see the Baptist case). Yet, even in pro-regulatory states, locally popular projects proceed over the objections of the regulators through a variety of mechanisms: marshalling political support (e.g., exemptive legislation in Massachusetts); legal challenges to the regulatory process (Suburban Memorial Hospital); bypassing the system of review through loopholes (body scanner in Boston); and purchasing equipment through exempt facilities (e.g., physician groups that purchased CAT scanners in Maine and Vermont).

State administrations change and new governors have different commitments to hospital regulation. In Massachusetts, there are signs that the King Administration will relax the CON process; in New Hampshire the new administration may move closer than its predecessor to the federal goals of PL 93–641.

We stress that even the greatest successes claimed for CON and 1122 review cannot necessarily be attributed to the implementation of PL 93–641; the majority of states currently operating CON programs were engaged in CON review before the planning law was signed.[4] In New England, for example, little impact can be claimed for PL 93–641 on the degree of hospital regulation in Connecticut, Massachusetts, and Rhode Island, states engaged in active CON and rate-setting programs well before passage of the planning law. In New Hampshire, capital controls are still in their infancy (in spite of seven years of 1122 review). Only in Maine and Vermont can one make a strong case that the movement toward hospital regulation was stimulated by the implementation of PL 93–641.

The existence of HSAs has certainly improved the quality of the debate surrounding hospital cost containment in general and individual CON and 1122 applications in particular. But the debate at the HSA level results in an advisory opinion to the states: used to support the state position if it agrees, often ignored if the state differs with the HSA.

The HSAs in New England have been more supportive of the HEW hospital regulatory strategy than had been predicted by most early observers. The HSA pro-regulatory position can be understood by considering the motivations of HSA staff and board members. *HSA staff* is committed to the continued operation of an agency that receives its funding and certification from HEW. Repeating the HEW planning guidelines in the HSP (or better yet, adopting more stringent guidelines) and making a record of opposition to CON and 1122 applications is thought to please the funding agency. Moreover, the staff are generally trained as planners and believe in the tenets of planning—centralization of services and efficiency of resource use. And a staff member who gains a reputation as a "tough" and knowledgeable regulator at the HSA level has future employment opportunities with hospitals, SHPDAs, and HEW.

The consumer representatives on the HSA board are also motivated to support a regulatory stance toward the hospitals. They, too, adopt organizational survival goals and frequently come to board membership from previous experience in organizations committed to public interest goals. Many consumer representatives, particularly in urban areas, have negative views of local hospitals that come into conflict with local communities. The size of the HSA areas also helps explain the support of consumer representatives for regulation. The HSA areas are sufficiently large so that it is rare that the personal interest of a consumer representative or of the group or neighborhood he/she represents is perceived to be at stake in any facilities review decision. The noninvolvement of parochial interest frees consumer representatives to pursue public interest goals. Consumer representatives also learn on the job. They are influenced by staff efforts at board education. In addition, faced for the first time with a host of applications covering a wide geographic area, they learn to develop informal criteria for weighing the relative merits of different provider claims.

For their part, *provider representatives* on HSA boards seldom present a unified challenge to the regulatory decisions and policies made by the staff. Provider representatives are typically either disinterested or divided. Where providers are not competing with the applicant they remain uninvolved—unwilling to use up political capital of their own, they leave the applicant to confront the regulatory system alone. The substantial differences in the interests of providers represented on the HSA board (e.g., hospitals, nursing homes, HMOs, clinics, and physicians) ensure that behavior of this kind is the rule. Where providers do recognize competing interests (say between two teaching hospitals) they are divided, with the applicant opposed to regulation and the competitor(s) inclined to support it.

The effect in either case is that there is seldom a unified challenge from the medical profession to regulatory decisions and policy. In this sense, the representational structure on HSA boards works effectively to support the purposes of the planning program. Only in those controversial instances where providers expand the scope of conflict by mobilizing community residents in support of their claims is this support in the HSA board room likely to be overwhelmed (e.g., the Leonard Morse case).

But while many factions vie for supremacy in the HSA board room, the outcome of these often heated debates is a recommendation: to HEW on the proposed use of federal funds; to the states on CON and 1122 applications and appropriateness review; and to the SHCC on the State Health Plan. Although the HSAs in New England have taken their missions seriously, their net effect on the short-term objective of controlling capital growth of hospitals has been minimal. The state governments frequently do not rely heavily on HSA recommendations when making CON and 1122 decisions.

Options

Policy options for long-term health planning are difficult to develop.[5] The basic issue to be addressed is the appropriate role of HSAs in the future. It could be argued that the federal govenment can use the local planning network as a forum for debate on cost containment and as a conduit for the diffusion of information to support more rational strategies for health resource allocation. Regulators, informed that there are low-cost beds, cost-saving investments, and quality improvements worthy of rapid adoption might avoid challenging effective projects and thus save scarce regulatory resources for the important battles. Some believe that if communities were aware of the ways higher health care costs are distributed throughout society in the form of higher taxes and product prices, they might be more self-restrained in presenting their demands. Providers knowing the impact various capital expenditures have on long-term operating costs might seek better designed projects. At least one can hope that these would be the results of diffusing more information on the local level.[6]

However, in spite of these potential benefits, it is our judgment that to remain as advisory organizations to HEW and the states and to serve as echoes of federal regulatory policy would relegate HSAs to a trivial role and would represent an inefficient allocation of resources. The functions of HSAs will either have to be strengthened or the agencies will eventually lose their credibility. Surely future versions of the planning law will occasion debate over the costs and benefits of maintaining the HSAs rather than using their budgets to strengthen the hand of state regulators.

Whatever the future of the HSAs, it is clear that there are a number of policy alternatives which would meet the short-term objectives of controlling the rate of growth of health care institutions in a more effective and efficient manner than the current planning and regulatory programs. We discuss below some short-term mechanisms for strengthening the facilities review process.

Many regulators engaged in CON review have expressed frustration with the process which forces analysis of absolute "need" in each case rather than allowing relative assessments of priorities among competing applications. The complexity of defining need for medical services has been the subject of numerous recent papers[7] and relates to the observation that the local supply of medical resources strongly influences the pattern of services received by local residents. Since great variations exist in the amount and kinds of medical and hospital services consumed by residents of similar communities without an obvious impact on health status,[8] it is difficult to identify those services which are truly needed. One way to avoid the hazards of attempting to assess absolute need for each CON application is to evaluate the merits of a set of applications relative to one another. Although absolute need for a capital project may be difficult or impossible to establish, relative priorities among projects can be established with a higher degree of confidence. Based on this argument, two mechanisms have been devised to move CON review toward a priority-setting process—batching and capping. Batching, which is grouping similar applications for capital expenditure, appeals to regulators because similar projects can be analyzed at the same time and in competition with one another.[9] A companion strategy for tightening CON regulation is capping, limiting the annual capital expenditures for hospitals (and other health care institutions) to a preset, and presumably low, level by state or region of a state. This mechanism, like batching, emphasizes the relative merits of applications for capital, but forces trade offs and priority setting among different kinds of applications.[10] A CAT scanner in Portland could receive a higher priority than a new surgical suite in Bangor.

The Carter Administration first proposed a national ceiling on hospital capital expenditures in 1977 as Title II of the proposed Hospital Cost Containment bill.[11] Under Title I of this bill, revenue limitations would have been imposed on virtually all hospitals in the country. Under Title II, capital spending would have been placed under a nationwide annual cap of $2.5 billion, initially to be allocated among the states in proportion to population. Adjustments would be made later for such variables as the age and condition of local hospital capital stock. Only those HSA areas with bed-to-population ratios of less than four beds per 1,000 and hospital occupancy rates greater than 80 percent would have been permitted to expand their hospital bed supply. All other areas would be required to close two beds for any new bed opened. The penalty for exceeding these standards in states operating 1122 review programs was to be ten times the amount of depreciation and interest attributable to federal patients for any capital project which went forward in spite of 1122 disapproval. Moreover, any state or local government bonds issued for such disapproved projects would be denied tax-exempt status. These were indeed tough regulatory conditions, but they made little headway in the 95th Congress leery of increasing federal regulatory power. The Administration's current hospital cost containment bill omits the capital cap provision. In its place former HEW Secretary Califano advocated a voluntary limit of $3 billion annually for hospital capital projects costing more than $150,000. Reference to a $3 billion cap is included in the Carter Administration's National Health Plan. But the political viability of a mandated national cap on hospital capital formation in the short run is problematic given the reception such a program received recently in Congress. One possibility for a nationwide program might be to issue a cap with state specific allocations as a National Guideline for Health Planning, thus requiring planners to conduct facilities reviews in terms of relative need and to document and justify departures from federal policy as they are currently required to do under the guidelines.

Although a nationwide cap does not appear feasible in the near future, some states are considering the establishment of caps. Capping bills have been introduced in state legislatures in Maine and Maryland, and this approach is being studied by Rhode Island health planners and regulators. New York State has given this approach intensive study, developing a regional allocation system of capital ceilings based on an analysis of existing capital stock, population trends, construction costs, and other relevant variables. But even in New York, support of a capital ceiling was considered a political liability; a statewide approach was adandoned by the Administration in anticipation of the recent gubernatorial election. A limited demonstration program is currently being implemented.

Given the difficulties of passing a national cap and the variations among states in their commitment to hospital cost containment, one obvious federal strategy is to provide incentives and support to those states that wish to tighten the loopholes of CON through adopting batching and capping. Federal resources and energy might better be spent on efforts to encourage receptive states to go further in their cost control programs rather than forcing recalcitrant state bureaucracies to "get tough." Along these lines, the federal government might also consider allowing aggressive states greater control over health planning policies and funding in their jurisdictions. For example, in return for a plan of action, one that meets the overall intentions of the law and a substantial new commitment of state dollars for planning, states might be granted greater policy flexibility and control over the flow of federal support for health planning in their areas.

Another approach to containing hospital costs included in the 1979 amendments to the health planning act (PL 96–79 Title III) provides loans and grants to encourage hospitals in overbedded areas to close or convert acute beds to ambulatory care or long-term care units. Such a program is already underway in Michigan and offers a new instrument to planners enabling them to actively encourage the reduction of beds, rather than simply opposing further bed expansion through CON. Concentrating the resources of the closure/conversion program in a few selected, pro-regulatory states would provide an opportunity to demonstrate a major impact on hospital costs of the new legislative authority contained in PL 96–79.[12]

Taken together, a program of demonstration grants to selected states for capping and/or closure and conversion represents the *short-term* policy option we prefer. Regulatory resources would be focused on those states willing to take action. The cost containment results would most likely exceed those under the current untargeted system of allocation of regulatory resources.[13] And the planning program, it is hoped, would record some much needed success stories.

None of these mechanisms for strengthening hospital regulation requires any modification in the organization of hospital planning and regulation; rather the policy change suggested here would be one of emphasis and concentration of federal resources in those states whose cost containment goals approximate that of HEW. Though the current political climate will not permit the establishment of a nationwide program to cap health care investments, much headway could be made in selected states.

Given the failure of recent Administration efforts to pass a national hospital revenue cap and a national ceiling on capital investments, the replacement of the PL 93–641 planning program with a comprehensive federal regulatory system is not a politically viable option at this point. Nevertheless, the gradual assumption of regulatory responsibility by the federal government remains a possible intermediate and long-range goal. Instead of trying to influence others to save federal revenues, the federal government could impose cost savings directly, through a program similar to the 1977 version of the Carter Administration's hospital cost containment program. But the passage of such legislation awaits a much wider acceptance of the federal concern with cost containment in the health sector.

Notes

[1] The Area Health Services Development Fund which to date has not received an appropriation could be a useful mechanism for improving access when it is sufficiently supported.

[2] American Health Planning Association, "Survey of Health Planning Agencies," Alexandria, VA, September, 1978. The survey findings were challenged by the General Accounting Office, see "GAO Disputes AHPA's Savings Study," *Washington Report on Medicine and Health/Planning Letter,* March 31, 1980, p. 4. The planning bureau's approach to the issue of efficacy was a report on seven HSA success stories, Health Resources Administration, *Health Planning in Action,* DHEW No. 79–14030 (Hyattsville, MD: PHS-HRA, 1979).

[3] For example, Bruce Vladeck, "Interest Group Representation and the HSAs: Health Planning and Political Theory," *American Journal of Public Health* (January,

1977), pp. 23-29, and Aaron Wildavsky, "Doing Better and Feeling Worse: The Political Pathology of Health Policy," *Daedalus* (Winter 1977), pp. 105-124.

[4] State health policy priorities seldom shift to match federal priorities no matter what the inducement or sanction. Note Health Resources Administration, *Evaluation of the Impact of PHS Programs on State Health Goals and Activities* prepared by Miller and Byrne, Inc., DHEW No. (HRA) 77-604 (Hyattsville, MD: PHS-HRA, 1977).

[5] Penny Hollander Feldman and Richard J. Zeckhauser, "Some Sober Thoughts on Health Care Regulation," in C. Argyus, editor, *Regulating Business* (San Francisco: Institute for Contemporary Studies, 1978), pp. 93-120 offer a similar observation regarding all health policy changes. Note also Eli Ginzberg, "Health Reform: The Outlook for the 1980s," *Inquiry*, Vol. XV (December, 1978), p. 326.

[6] Basil J.F. Mott, "The New Planning System" in A. Levin, editor, *Health Services: The Local Perspective* (New York: Academy of Political Science, 1977), pp. 238-254.

[7] A.L. Cochrane, *Effectiveness and Efficiency—Random Reflections on Health Services* (London: Nuffield Provincial Hospital Trust, 1972); T. McKean and C.R. Lowe, *An Introduction to Social Medicine* (New York: Oxford University Press, 1974), 2nd ed.

[8] John E. Wennberg and F.J. Fowler, "A Test of Consumer Contributions to Small Area Variations in Health Care Delivery," *Journal of the Maine Medical Association* (1977), p. 275.

[9] Elizabeth G. Mulcahy, *Batching: An Alternative Methodology for Certificate of Need Review*, MS thesis, Massachusetts Institute of Technology, 1979.

[10] Drew Altman, "Health Planning" in S. Altman and H.M. Sapolsky, editors, *Federal Health Care Programs* (Lexington, MA: Heath/Lexington, forthcoming).

[11] For a discussion of the origin of the cost containment bill see David S. Abernethy and David A. Pearson, *Regulating Hospital Costs: The Development of Public Policy* (Ann Arbor, MI: AUPHA Press, 1979). Its status in the 1980 Presidential campaign and that of other health policy issues is described in Elizabeth Wehr, "Health Policy is Low Priority Political Issue," *Congressional Quarterly*, March 8, 1980, pp. 657-659. Critiques of the cost containment bill are contained in Martin Feldstein, "Limiting the Rise in Hospital Costs Without Regulation," Summary of Testimony Before the Senate Health Subcommittee, March 15, 1979, processed, and Congressional Budget Office, *Rising Hospital Costs* (Washington: Government Printing Office, 1979).

[12] The need for concentration is evident in studies that show at least a 20 percent reduction in capacity would be required to affect hospital costs significantly. Sheila L. Simler, "Closing Hospitals Won't Generate Any Savings," *Modern Healthcare* (February, 1980), p. 36.

13 For a statistical analysis of their weakness see David S. Salkever and Thomas W. Bice, *Hospital Certificate-of-Need Controls: Impact on Investment, Costs, and Use* (Washington: American Enterprise Institute, 1979). Note also Health Resources Administration, *Certificate of Need Programs: A Review, Analysis, and Annotated Bibliography of the Research Literature*, DHEW No. 79–14005 (Hyattsville, MD: PHS-HRA, 1979) and Harvey M. Sapolsky, "Overview" in S. Altman and H.M. Sapolsky, editors, *Federal Health Care Programs* (Lexington, MA: Heath/Lexington, forthcoming).

PART TWO

Health Planning and Regulation: The Case Studies

Introduction

In this section we present nine case studies illustrating the dynamics of the resource allocation process in New England under PL 93-641. Each case was selected in consultation with key state and local health officials because it exemplified important issues facing health planners and regulators. We emphasize that the cases are illustrative; they are in no sense statistical samples of planning decisions.

Six of the cases presented describe the facilities review processes under PL 93-641—Certificate of Need (CON) and Section 1122 Review. One case describes the interaction among planners, institutional staff, and community residents in the development of a resource standard for local and state health plans. The two other cases present the dynamics of the hospital planning process in the context of competition among local institutions. Our heavy concentration on facilities review cases reflects our interpretation of the emphasis of the current health planning program as primarily focused on limiting capital expansion of health care institutions.

One of the themes that runs throughout the six facilities review cases is that regulation of capital expansion under PL 93-641 can be circumvented by a broad spectrum of strategies including exemptive legislation (St. Joseph Nursing Home), legal appeal of regulatory decisions (Suburban Memorial Hospital and Tufts New England Hospital) and "borrowing" rather than purchasing capital equipment (Body Scanners in Boston). In only one case included in this section (The Baptist Hospital) did the facilities review process successfully stop a proposed capital project. We have emphasized that such denials have been rare in New England.

The acute hospital facilities review cases span a broad spectrum of types of facilities and local circumstances. In the Tufts New England Hospital case, a medical school teaching hospital's attempt to renovate a major service (pediatrics) was challenged by state regulators wishing to decentralize pediatric services to the growing suburban Boston area. Patience and administrative appeal resulted in a victory for the hospital. The Suburban Memorial Hospital case illustrates the point that even in the stringent regulatory environment of Rhode Island a community hospital with sufficient resources and ingenuity can obtain approval for bed expansion. The "A" General Hospital case in Maine demonstrates the limited impact of sophisticated analytic planning techniques in the essentially political forum of facilities review.

The Leonard Morse case is included to illustrate the dynamics of standards development in health planning. In this case a community hospital was able to mobilize local residents to challenge effectively HSA and state-level proposed standards for minimal acceptable numbers of obstetrical deliveries per hospital per year. This is of interest because obstetrical standards provoked heated opposition not only in New England, but throughout the country. Other examples of communities mobilizing to challenge obstetrical standards occurred in response to the draft National Health Planning Guidelines originally published in the *Federal Register* in September, 1977. The proposed standard of at least 500 deliveries annually in any hospital outside a SMSA provoked massive letter-writing campaigns in two rural areas— Sibley, Iowa, and New Braunfels, Texas.* The proposed standard was dropped from the final National Health Planning Guidelines.

The Worcester City Hospital and Lewiston, Maine, cases provide two examples of communities in which hospitals are in competition with one another. In Worcester, Massachusetts, the new state medical school hospital will add 400 beds to an already overbedded city. Planners have looked to a deteriorating public hospital for possible bed closure, compensating for the new university facility. In Lewiston, Maine, two community hospitals of the same size are fighting for regional dominance in an atmosphere of increasingly stringent state CON review.

In two case studies we have disguised the names of the facilities involved ("A" General Hospital and Suburban Memorial Hospital). This was done to comply with our agreements with the Maine Data Service and SEARCH, the Rhode Island data network, concerning confidentiality of hospital use statistics in Maine and Rhode Island.

---

*P. Danaceau, *Health Planning Guideline Controversy: A Report From Iowa and Texas;* HRA 79-647; HEW, 1979.

Case 1

New England Medical Center: Zero-Based Determination of Need?

The New England Medical Center (NEMC) application for a Determination of Need (DON)* was filed on September 2, 1974. On October 11, 1977, three years later, NEMC won approval for its DON application. During this period NEMC engaged in a lengthy cooperative planning process with the Massachusetts Department of Public Health (DPH) and the Boston HSA; received the endorsement of the DON office, the HSA, and a ten taxpayer group; suffered a denial by the Public Health Council engineered by the Commissioner of the DPH; won a subsequent appeal to the Health Facilities Appeals Board remanding the application to the DPH and the Public Health Council for reconsideration, and suffered a second (this time de facto) reversal at the Public Health Council.

The NEMC proposal occurred in the midst of a changing policy environment. The NEMC application coincided with the change from Comprehensive Health Planning to PL 93-641. It also covered a period that saw three different DON office directors and two different DPH Commissioners. During this period, the Governor's office changed hands, the state legislature became the focus of efforts to nullify and to amend the DON process, and state fiscal problems led to the development of an increasingly stringent regulatory strategy that looked to Determination of Need as a means of saving money.

---

*DON = Determination of Need, the name of the Certificate of Need Program in Massachusetts. The Public Health Council has final authority on DON cases.

The NEMC Application

NEMC is a tertiary care facility which emphasizes specialty care, research, and teaching. In September of 1974, at the time of the initial DON application, the hospital had a total of 455 beds, including "Tufts Floating Hospital," a pediatric inpatient unit named for its ship-based predecessor, the Boston Floating Hospital, which operated during the early 1900s.

NEMC proposed substantial renovation and construction. There were six basic elements to the application:

1) replacement of the pediatric facility with the construction of a new 96-bed pediatric service
2) expansion and replacement of pediatric and adult ambulatory services
3) replacement and relocation of operating and recovery facilities
4) replacement and relocation of laboratory facilities
5) replacement and relocation of pediatric X-ray facilities
6) renovation of the administrative services building

In order to accomplish these six goals NEMC proposed construction of a new ten-level building, a three-level connecting bridge, and renovation of other already existing structures. The estimated capital expenditure for the project was put at $51,214,000, of which $32 million represented construction costs.

The Review Process: Cooperative Planning

The initial NEMC proposal submitted in September of 1974 was developed internally in conjunction with a series of development plans finished in 1972 and 1973. These plans represented the culmination of a planning process which began when NEMC was first established in 1965 through the merger of three hospitals. When presented with the application, the Boston area HSA (then the "b" Agency) complained that it had had little input into the pre-submission planning process. When it became clear that a negative review was imminent, NEMC agreed to participate in a coordinated planning process involving both the state agency and the HSA. NEMC also agreed to extend the review period from 90 days to one year in order to accomplish the review.

The three parties to the review process agreed to examine each element of the proposal separately and NEMC agreed to revise its application to reflect the findings of the joint analysis. Over time, the

HSA came to play the major role in the process, acting with state agency concurrence, as staff to the project. Because DON office resources were already strained by the demands of reviewing other applications, the DON Director was happy to let the HSA play the major role in the NEMC review.

Pediatric Beds

The review task force concentrated first on the proposal to replace the NEMC pediatric facility, the "Floating Hospital." The existing pediatric facility was built in 1893, and no longer met federal, state, and local construction codes. Much of the analysis of the pediatric component was based on an HSA planning paper, "Hospital Based Pediatric Services in Metropolitan Boston: Goals, Priorities, and Recommended Strategies for Change, 1975–1985."

The task force review showed that the NEMC request for 96 pediatric beds was reasonable. The task force estimate of pediatric bed need at NEMC was initially set at 105. The 105-bed need figure was derived by statistically determining service area populations, the proportion of the service area population served by NEMC, admission rates, average length of stay, and the occupancy rate. When the bed need projections were corrected to compensate for the impact of inflated population projections, a new bed need figure of 90–95 was set.

An audit of pediatric length of stay at NEMC was also conducted. Using a one-day sample, NEMC patients were compared to length-of-stay norms by diagnosis obtained in the Professional Activity Study (PAS) of the southern United States. All cases exceeding the PAS 75th percentile were referred to the Bay State Professional Standards Review Organization. The PSRO determined that these extended stays were in fact justified by medical necessity. Thus, both the bed need estimate and the length-of-stay review found the NEMC 96-pediatric bed proposal to be justified.

Operating Rooms

NEMC proposed the construction/replacement of 12 operating rooms and the expansion of recovery room services from 11 to 26 beds. The task force agreed with NEMC that the existing operating areas were disjointed (with the scattered location causing duplication in services and supplies) and outdated. To tackle the further question of need, the reviewers utilized an array of quantitative techniques, including "waiting line or queuing theory analysis," and a "probablistic computer simulation model analysis" borrowed from operations research. Both of these techniques utilize two different types of data: macro-level (surgical procedures per year), and micro-level (surgical procedure time per case, recovery room time, etc.). Based on these techniques, the task force found that the NEMC operating room proposal was justifiable using even conservative demand projections.

Pediatric X-Ray Facilities

NEMC proposed the consolidation of pediatric radiology. services previously housed in two separate locations. The new service would include three radiographic rooms, three fluoroscope rooms and one chest X-ray room. The task force agreed with NEMC that existing X-ray facilities were inadequate (there was insufficient space, too much traffic, a dispersed pediatric radiology department). Using a seven-step analysis of inpatient and outpatient volume and actual use rates, the reviewers projected radiographic exam room need in the NEMC area at between 5.98 and 7.21 rooms. The NEMC proposals fell comfortably within these limits.

Laboratory Facilities

NEMC proposed consolidation and expansion of its chemistry, bacteriology, clinical pathology, and amino acid labs. The task force staff agreed with NEMC that the existing labs were inadequate. Using a methodology that calculated total work load hours relative to projected volume of clinical lab procedures expected by 1985, the staff was able to derive estimates of the space needed for clinical laboratories. The NEMC proposal also fell comfortably within these limits.

Ambulatory Care

NEMC proposed the construction of a 36,680 square foot facility for ambulatory care, housing ten pediatric clinics, an oral pediatrics service, eight general specialty services, and offices for full-time physicians. Using a one-week sample of all ambulatory visits to NEMC, a use rate by region was obtained and developed into a projected volume for 1980 and 1985. NEMC projections for 1980 and 1985 matched those made by the task force staff, and the reviewers judged the ambulatory care proposal to be a sound one.

Additional Review Components

Task force staff endorsed a number of other elements in the NEMC proposal. They accepted the proposal to renovate the 87,210 square foot Biewend Building for administrative use. And they accepted the financial feasibility of the NEMC project. They also determined that the proposal would have no significantly harmful long-term environmental effects. NEMC won added support for their project from the local taxpayer group, "Citizens for Better Health Care."

Thus, the review process in the NEMC case was a long and a complicated one. Although staff from the HSA played the most prominent role, there was considerable input from the hospital and the state DON office as well. The review itself was sophisticated. It formally utilized the following technical components:

- Market share analysis
- Analysis of referral network patterns
- Clinical case review of appropriateness of admissions and length of stay by the regional PSRO
- Queuing theory and operations research
- Staffing pattern analysis
- Application of standards to determine appropriate work area size

By agreeing to participate fully in the planning process, the hospital added credibility to its proposal. The NEMC project, originally conceived internally, emerged from the coordinated review relatively unchanged. On September 9, 1975, the HSA recommended approval of the project. A week later, the DON office staff formally concurred, agreeing to submit a recommendation for approval to the Public Health Council.

Rejection by the Public Health Council

On April 4, 1976, the Public Health Council voted 3 to 2, with the Commissioner casting the deciding vote, to deny NEMC its Determination of Need. The Council voted down the proposal despite the fact that NEMC had gained considerable support for its plan by working cooperatively with HSA and DON office planners for over a year.

As had been the case in other DON decisions, the Council was motivated by concern for rising costs, as reflected, in particular, in the state Medicaid budget. The Council, and the Commissioner in particular, did not look favorably on new bed proposals in the Boston area. As a matter of policy, the Council placed the burden of proof in DON cases squarely on the applicant's shoulders. But in the NEMC case, the Commissioner sought to take the Council one step further, denying not only new beds but replacement beds in an effort to redirect the health system.

NEMC had made a strong case that its physical plant (and especially the "Floating" pediatric unit) was obsolete. On this point, NEMC, the HSA, the DON staff, and the Commissioner were in agreement. In addition, the planners' projections showed that there could be sufficient demand in the future for services of the kind and scale contained in the NEMC application. Taken separately and purely on its own merits, the NEMC case for replacement and renovation was a strong one. Normally, the logic and precedent for Determination of Need would have dictated approval. But the Commissioner and the Council sought to bring a broader perspective to bear in the NEMC case. Given what they regarded as overbedding and duplication in the Boston area, they questioned whether it was sound policy to revitalize NEMC in total. They were troubled, in particular, by the pediatric bed component of the proposal. With the Commissioner taking the lead, the Council questioned whether Tufts Medical School should rotate pediatric specialty residents through other hospitals rather than replace its pediatric facility. Ideally, they argued, specialty pediatrics should be encouraged to grow where they believed it was most needed, outside rather than inside Boston.

In effect, the Commissioner and Council attempted to compensate for a weakness inherent in the DON process. Despite the fact that NEMC had made a strong case for replacement of its pediatric beds and that the planners believed that the hospital would be able to fill those beds with some success, the Council sought to apply a regional perspective. Since specialty pediatric care was already available in the Boston area, an approval for NEMC would, in the eyes of the Council, only serve to reestablish duplication. The goals of cost control and regionalization would be better served by multi-institutional cooperation than by modernization at NEMC. Its strong case notwithstanding, the NEMC pediatric facility would be penalized for reaching old age ahead of its counterparts.

The Council looked with favor on some elements of the NEMC proposal, notably those pertaining to operating room and laboratory expansion and renovation. They did not attempt to encourage a general decline at NEMC. But the Council did question whether there should be a new pediatric service at NEMC. Where the pediatric beds were concerned, the Council felt, perhaps obsolescence should be allowed to run its course.

The actual language of the Council decision was carefully worded. NEMC was denied on three grounds:

(1) Alternative program and construction proposals with explicit discussion of the cost and patient care implications of each was not adequately prepared. The applicant failed to clearly distinguish between those elements of the proposal which were clearly essential from those that were merely desirable. While there was some need to improve the facilities of the pediatric unit ("Floating Hospital"), the applicant's plan did not present priorities for the use of both existing and proposed square footage.

(2) Although the applicant made a sizeable effort to work with state and regional planning agencies, the Council felt that further expenditures in the Boston area, without a joint regionalized planning effort, represented a poor allocation of health care resources.

(3) The Council concluded that the lack of priorities and failure to present alternatives did not represent the provision of adequate health care services at the lowest reasonable aggregate cost.

The Appeals Process

NEMC believed that its application was a strong one. Obsolescence had been well-documented. Given the past record in replacement bed cases, NEMC had expected approval. In addition, the hospital had worked with the planners and had won their endorsement. As a result, rather than attempt to circumvent the process through exemptive legislation (which NEMC had contemplated and which, by the time of the NEMC denial, had become common practice), NEMC brought their case to the Health Facilities Appeals Board.

The Appeals Board consists of five members appointed by the Governor for terms of three years. Three members of the Board are "consumers." One consumer member is a lawyer and is designated by the Governor to serve as chairman. The Board, by regulation, deals with procedural rather than substantive DON issues. On August 10, 1976, the Appeals Board ruled in favor of NEMC. The Board set forth its reasoning as follows:

> The burden cannot be placed on any single applicant to undertake joint planning for all hospitals in the region . . . .

> An applicant obviously cannot be expected to raise an infinite number of alternatives before the Council . . . .

> We believe the reasons for the Council denial . . . reflect an abuse of administrative discretion in light of the record considered as a whole. In this case, the "a" Agency, "b" Agency, Department staff and the ten taxpayer groups all participated extensively in the planning and application process, and made findings consistent with their ultimate unanimous recommendation that the NEMC proposal be approved . . . . Any other result in this case would be tantamount to a recognition by this Board that the Public Health Council's discretion to decide policy despite the record is so broad as to be unreviewable.

The effect of the Appeals Board decision was to remand the NEMC case to the DPH and the Council for further consideration.

As a result of the Appeals Board ruling, the DON staff conducted a further review of the NEMC application. Since more than two years had passed since the initial application, new statistics and financial figures were requested and analyzed. Upon reconsideration, the HSA staff and the DON staff again essentially endorsed the original NEMC proposal, although this time revised downward by NEMC from $51,214,000 to $38,200,000. The Public Health Council found itself in the same position as before. It could bow to the record and the logic of Determination of Need and reward obsolescence with approval of replacement beds, or it could repeat its attempts to use Determination of Need procedures to promote the system of regionalized pediatric specialty care it believed more rational. This time, however, the review would occur in the context of increasing tension between the Commissioner and both the HSA and DON staff, and in the context of growing criticism of Determination of Need, including challenges in the courts and the legislature.

On July 26, 1977, the Public Health Council met to reconsider the NEMC proposal. Despite the Health Facilities Appeal Board remand and criticism of the initial Council rating, and despite renewed DON staff and HSA support for the application, the DPH Commissioner continued to oppose the NEMC project. The Commissioner questioned whether Tufts had considered the "option" of locating either the pediatric and/or ambulatory components of its proposal at Boston City or Faulkner Hospitals, in the eyes of NEMC two potentially competing facilities. In the process, the Commissioner reopened the question of need for the proposed NEMC facility. At the Commissioner's insistence, the Council voted to table the application pending the results of a further DON staff analysis of the ambulatory services component (including operating and recovery rooms, lab and pediatric X-ray) of the project.

The Commissioner, interviewed in *The Boston Globe,* cited confusion due to a failure of communication between the Council and the DON staff as a cause of his opposition and the continued delay. He termed the NEMC experience "a massive screw-up." The President of the Massachusetts Hospital Association, on the other hand, blamed the Commissioner. In his words: "The open anti-hospital bias of our Health Commissioner and his flagrant disregard for the DON program's own rules of process leads MHA to reconsider its position on legislation that would remove him as Chairman of the Public Health Council and reorganize the Council itself."

A Third Trip to the Public Health Council

In October of 1977 both the HSA and the DON staff recommended approval for a third time. This time they were recommending approval of the revised ($38,000,000) application minus one pediatric X-ray room, $100,000 in estimated costs. On October 11, 1977, the Public Health Council voted unanimously to approve the NEMC project.

Conclusion

In the NEMC case, the Commissioner and the Public Health Council sought to apply a "zero-based" approach to Determination of Need. The Commissioner and the Council agreed that the existing NEMC pediatric facilities were obsolete. However, they also believed that approval of the NEMC application would seriously damage efforts to regionalize pediatric specialty care in the Metro area, while contributing to rising costs in the process. Thus, the Commissioner sought to evaluate need as if NEMC was proposing an entirely new facility, one that had not existed in the past, much less one from a recognized leader in pediatric care in Boston and New England. This effort to use DON as a broader planning tool stretched the "rules" for Determination of Need, both legal and historical. NEMC had convincingly documented the obsolescence of its physical plant. Using traditional demand-based measures and a variety of sophisticated analytical techniques, NEMC had documented need as well. The Commissioner's effort to use Determination of Need as a broad planning tool eventually brought conflict with both the DON and HSA staff. It also subjected the DON program to strong criticism from the hospital community. The NEMC case offered critics some welcome and visible verification of the vagaries of Determination of Need process, even when hospitals play by the rules. In the end, the NEMC project approved in October of 1977 closely resembled the original project proposed three years earlier.

Case 2

St. Joseph's Manor Nursing Home: The Importance of Lithuania for Health Planning

On December 9, 1975, the Massachusetts Public Health Council voted to deny the St. Joseph's Manor Nursing Home application for a Determination of Need. St. Joseph's Manor, located in Brockton, Massachusetts, had proposed the construction of 64 new beds, consisting of 12 Level I/II,* 60 Level III, and 20 Level IV. The cost of the project was put at $1,039,806. The denial reflected Department of Public Health policy aimed at containing and ultimately reducing the number of long-term care beds in the state. Roughly one year later, however, the state legislature passed a special bill, the first of its kind for nursing homes, exempting St. Joseph's Manor from the DON denial and allowing the nursing home to proceed with its construction plans.

The story of the St. Joseph's application raises a number of issues concerning the way in which planning decisions are made and implemented in Massachusetts. Some of these are specific to long-term care, others are of broader significance. This version of the St. Joseph's story will focus on the various and ultimately successful strategies used by the nursing home in order to evade a very stringent Determination of Need policy for long-term care.

---

*Nursing and rest home beds are licensed in Massachusetts according to four designated levels of care: I & II = Skilled Nursing Care; III = Intermediate or Supportive Care; IV = Rest Care.

The Case For Need

St. Joseph's Manor based its case on the argument that demand for beds at the nursing home far exceeded the available supply. Representatives for the nursing home maintained that it had been functioning at 100 percent occupancy since its early days of operation in 1965. They also cited a waiting list of 80 applicants, indicating that additional prospective applicants were turned away daily over the telephone.

Nursing home representatives argued, in addition, that more beds would enable them to improve upon ("already first-rate") quality of care. This was because the nursing home, which had been approved to provide only Level II care, was proposing the addition of Level III and IV units. They argued in their application that there was a great demand, in particular, for Level IV beds.

> If we are granted permission to add these units, we would then be in a unique position to provide services in a multi-level facility, thereby assuring the patients continuity of care within the same facility . . . changing from facility to facility because of their changing condition can be a traumatic experience which often results in irreparable damage to elderly patients. (From St. Joseph's application.)

Anticipating that their demand and quality of care arguments would not win state planners over to their side, a third argument was added, one that eventually became the pivotal issue in the case. St. Joseph's Manor maintained that its DON application was unique because the nursing home served a large group of Lithuanian-born Americans who could not find similar nursing home care elsewhere. Because of this, St. Joseph's argued that state long-term care bed need methodologies should not be fully applied to their nursing home.

> Because of the fact that there are a substantial number of foreign born Lithuanians in the Commonwealth, and because of the fact that we are the only nursing home in the Commonwealth that does furnish these unique services, we feel we should not be restricted, and hopefully the Council won't view the overbedding issue as restrictively in this context . . . we are serving a very quiet minority that has offered so much to the Commonwealth of Massachusetts, has helped build the Commonwealth . . . and must be served in their own special way. (From Public Health Council Minutes.)

This point was buttressed by the contention that St. Joseph's was, in fact, a "multi-regional" Lithuanian referral center, serving Lithuanians not just from the Brockton area, but from all over Massachusetts. To support its case, St. Joseph's presented data showing that at the time of the application 21 of the 56 patients in the nursing home were of Lithuanian origin. It was apparent that St. Joseph's had discovered its Lithuanian roots.

The "b" Agency Endorsement

The Brockton area "b" Agency, Comprehensive Health Planning, Incorporated, is not a subject of this study. Nevertheless, it is important to describe its endorsement of the St. Joseph's application in order to fully understand the case that was presented to DON staff and to the Public Health Council.

The "b" Agency recommended approval of the St. Joseph's application on the following grounds:

1) It had requested that the DPH conduct a Periodic Medical Review* survey of the nursing home. Of all the Medicaid patients reviewed by the DPH, none were recommended for transfer. Based on that data, the "b" Agency concluded that the utilization of the facility was appropriate.
2) That the initial cost projection of $1,500,000 had been reduced to a "more realistic" $1,153,046.
3) That deviations from state-mandated long-term bed averages were acceptable because (a) the new beds would bring Level II and III capacity up to optimum unit size, at 40 Level II and 60 Level III; (b) strict bed need formulas should not have been applied because the facility was a multi-regional one with ethnic ties to the Lithuanian community; (c) architectural constraints were such that different combinations of beds and levels would have been difficult.

The State Response

Both DON staff and the Public Health Council members rejected all of the major St. Joseph's arguments for need. First, they rejected the nursing home's contention that patient demand for beds proved a need for the project. According to the DPH mandated averages, DON staff

---

*The Periodic Medical Review Program of the DPH performs site visit evaluations of the "quality and appropriateness" of nursing home placements of Medicaid patients. The reviews are based on the judgments of a team composed of a physician, nurse, and social worker.

argued, the Brockton area was "one of the most significantly over-bedded in the state" with more nursing home beds per thousand than all but three of the thirty-six planning areas in the state. Staff reminded the Council that two applications from the Brockton area made prior to the St. Joseph's application had been rejected based on the mandated state averages. Even after adjusting for patient origin, comparative state averages continued to show substantial overbedding. Council members were dubious that a waiting list represented a real measure of demand. One Council member put it this way: "It's always difficult to evaluate what the meaning of an 80 person waiting list is—waiting lists have a way of piling up and names get on and stay on for a period of time. . . ."

Most importantly, the DON staff rejected the St. Joseph's claim to special status based on service to the Lithuanian community. This judgment reflected a staff analysis showing that less than half of the St. Joseph's patients were Lithuanian, and that the nursing home offered no special preferences to admission of Lithuanian patients. In fact, staff argued, there were eleven other nursing homes in the region in which Lithuanian was spoken, and in which some special language, dietary, and religious services to Lithuanians were offered. In her testimony before the Public Health Council, the Director of DON made these remarks:

> The applicant has stated that they feel they are in a unique situation because they are oriented towards the treatment of Lithuanian patients and Lithuanian patients constituted a special population per se . . . . Staff has determined that roughly half of the patients were Lithuanian and half were not, that there are no special preferences in terms of admission of Lithuanian patients, that a Lithuanian who is waiting to get into the facility goes to the waiting list as opposed to any priority treatment . . . rather than exacerbate the oversupply of nursing home beds in the area, it would seem that if the applicant wanted to concentrate solely on Lithuanian patients they could alter their 50 percent current non-Lithuanians and make it solely a Lithuanian home rather than construct new beds.

Much of the Public Health Council session dealing with the St. Joseph's application focused on the Lithuanian issue. Time and time again Council members queried both the nursing home and DON staff regarding the menu at St. Joseph's, the number of Lithuanian-speaking staff, subscriptions to Lithuanian publications, special admissions practices for Lithuanians and so forth. On December 22, 1975, the Public Health Council voted to deny the St. Joseph's application. At that time the Council noted that it might look more favorably on a future application based upon conversion to an exclusively Lithuanian facility or the purchase of an existing Brockton-area nursing home.

The Decision Context

The DON staff and the Public Health Council formally discounted the St. Joseph's application on its merits. Some of the arguments for need, such as the Lithuanian one, required special analysis and refutation. Other issues, however, such as bed need, were decided on the basis of preexisting formulas and policy. It was necessary only to plug the St. Joseph's numbers into formulas that had been designed to contain the growth of nursing home beds in the state.

DPH and Public Health Council policy aimed at containing the number of nursing home beds in Massachusetts had been emerging since the early days of the state's DON program. In fact, for a year and a half prior to the St. Joseph's application, the Council had not approved any nursing home beds in the Brockton area. By the time of the Council's decision in the St. Joseph's case, in December of 1975, a much publicized "fiscal crisis" in the state government had created a decision climate that did not auger well for new bed proposals. The state's Medicaid budget was seen as the main culprit.

From FY 69 to FY 74 (the time of St. Joseph's application) the costs of nursing home care in Massachusetts rose by 118 percent, with total expenditures for nursing home care increasing from $132 million in FY 69 to $288 million in FY 73. By January, 1976, DON approvals had been issued for an additional 7,696 nursing home beds that were scheduled to become operational over a period of a few years, adding an additional anticipated strain on the Medicaid budget.* Indeed, a study completed late in 1976 found that, on a per capita basis, Massachusetts had the third most expensive Medicaid program in the United States. The blame for these costs was placed squarely on payments for institutional care for the elderly. Payments to ambulatory care and for Aid to Families with Dependent Children in Massachusetts were either comparable to, or less than, those in other states. But Medicaid payments for nursing home care were higher than in other states, consuming about 75 percent of the Medicaid budget in Massachusetts, as compared with an

---

* Figures from "White Paper on Health Care Expenditures for Massachusetts," Commonwealth of Massachusetts, Executive Department.

average of 69 percent in other states.* The Medicaid budget had become a source of increasing concern to Governor Dukakis, prompting him to order major cutbacks in state-provided general relief funds in 1976. In fact, a $90 million Medicaid increase in FY 78, from $630 million to $720 million, represented more than half of the total state budget increase of $160 million over the previous year.

Concern for rising Medicaid costs and for nursing home costs in particular led to the development of a formal policy of containment. In the spring of 1976 the Public Health Council declared a moratorium on construction of long-term care facilities pending the development of a methodology for determining need for nursing home beds. Subsequently, "Standards and Criteria for the Allocation of Long-Term Beds" were developed by the DPH and were considered for formal adoption by the Public Health Council. Nursing home officials objected strongly that they were not consulted during the development of the long-term care criteria and maintained that the criteria were both poorly conceived and unfair.

The long-term care criteria projected bed need through 1985 for each of the 36 geographic service areas in the state. The criteria were tied directly to the Determination of Need decision process through a series of statewide mandated averages for long-term care beds. These averages, by level of care, were:

1) *Chronic disease and rehabilitation beds*
   2.4 beds per thousand elderly
2) *Skilled nursing beds—Level I/II*
   34.8 beds per thousand elderly
3) *Intermediate care beds—Level III*
   28.9 beds per thousand elderly
4) *Rest home beds—Level IV*
   25.8 placements per thousand elderly who require
   Level IV or community placement

These planning targets were derived through the use of survey profiles of appropriate placement by level of care of long-term care patients and of those awaiting placement. The mandated averages were adjusted to reflect bed need in each of the 36 service areas. The regional adjustments were based on two variables, the number of elderly in the region and the percentage of the elderly living extrafamilially. By applying the survey profiles and the regional

* The study referred to was prepared for the DPH by the Harvard Center for Health and Medical Care.

modifiers to 1985 population projections, the planners developed long-range nursing home bed targets. Despite the fact that they had not been formally adopted, the mandated state averages served as the basis for Determination of Need decisions for long-term care.

DPH planners believed that the imposition of the planning targets would produce significant savings. They predicted a savings of between $59,030,124 and $87,920,427 by 1980 when compared with projections based on the existing system and its growth patterns. Substantial additional savings would occur, they argued, if changes were made in the reimbursement method for nursing homes. This was because nursing homes were reimbursed according to the level of bed occupied by the patient, rather than on the basis of care actually delivered. Because the frequency of improper bed-level placement was high (by DPH standards estimated as high as 85 percent) nursing homes were thought to have been reimbursed at an artificially inflated rate.

Applying the Mandated Averages in the St. Joseph's Case

The impact of the mandated averages can be illustrated in the context of the St. Joseph's DON application. A comparison of the state mandated averages for the Brockton area with bed need projections promulgated by the "b" Agency underscores the stringent nature of the DPH long-term care bed policy. The final figures for additional nursing home beds are of primary interest (Tables C.1 and C.2).

The Brockton area "b" Agency indicated a need for an additional 40 Level I/II beds; DPH mandated averages called for a reduction of 296 Level I/II beds. On Level III beds, both "b" Agency and DPH formulas called for major reductions (–315 and –320, respectively). For Level IV, the "b" Agency formula showed a need for 683 additional beds; state averages required the addition of only 114 Level IV beds. The state mandated averages, adjusted to consider the Brockton area elderly population and nursing home utilization, projected a need for 88.9 Level I, II, III, IV beds per thousand elderly in the region as of August 1, 1975. Counting construction of the St. Joseph's beds as planned in the application, the Brockton area would run considerably above that figure, with 115 total beds per 1,000 elderly.

Both the Public Health Council decision in the St. Joseph's case and the state mandated averages that served as the basis for the decisions reflected overall state policy. That policy, more than anything else,

Table C.1

Bed Need Projections by Brockton Area CHP Agency

		Level I, II	Level III	Level IV
1.	Total beds licensed and approved by DPH	792	1,220	248
2.	Additional beds approved by "b" Agency	66	–11	25
3.	Total of all beds	858	1,209	273
4.	Total conforming beds licensed and approved	691	708	273
5.	Beds needed per "b" Agency formula	731	393	959
6.	New beds needed	**40**	**–315**	**683**

Table C.2

Bed Need by State Mandated Averages

		Level I, II	Level III	Level IV
1.	Existing & DPH-approved beds	792	1,220	248
2.	Beds needed per state averages (based on 1980 est. pop. 65+)	496	900	362
3.	New beds needed	**–296**	**–320**	**114**

was based on the Governor's interest in holding the line on the state Medicaid budget, and on the belief that long-term care claimed an unusually large share of the Medicaid budget. Operating within this policy context, DPH planners and Public Health Council members would not have been favorably disposed towards any new nursing home bed proposals, much less a proposal from an area that by DPH standards was one of the most overbedded in the state. Indeed, just prior to the St. Joseph's application, the DPH had proclaimed a 30 percent statewide reduction in the number of nursing home beds as a goal to be reached by 1980. The state mandated averages, the earlier moratorium on long-term care beds, and the decision in the St. Joseph's case all reflected that policy.

Challenges to the Determination of Need Process

In December of 1976 the Massachusetts legislature passed a special bill reversing the Public Health Council denial and allowing St. Joseph's Manor to proceed with its construction plans. St. Joseph's thus became the first nursing home in Massachusetts to win exemptive legislation.

Until 1975, the state legislature's role in health policy matters fell within the jurisdiction of the Joint House and Senate Committee on Social Welfare. In 1975, the Committee on Social Welfare was divided into three separate joint committees—Human Services, Elder Affairs, and Health Care. Where Medicaid and other health budgetary issues were concerned, the Joint Committee on Ways and Means played a major role as well. Some members of the Health Care Committee, notably those from the Senate side, including the Chairman of the Committee, were supportive of Public Health Council efforts to contain costs. However, the majority, including the leadership from the House side, were generally sympathetic to provider interests. This was a posture they shared with most of the legislature.

In the St. Joseph's case, the successful attempt to gain exemptive legislation was initiated by Brockton-area Representatives. The Health Care Committee did not formally comment on the St. Joseph's bill (which is tantamount to an adverse report), but the legislature voted overwhelmingly in favor of St. Joseph's. The Speaker of the Massachusetts House, who apparently had been impressed with the care a relative had received at St. Joseph's, played a major role in organizing support for the legislation. In the St. Joseph's case, as generally, the members of the legislature were receptive to provider claims of unique status based on quality of care, long-standing community service, and service to special ethnic or religious groups. Thus, the legislators were impressed with the claim of special service to Lithuanian Americans. Although some legislators at the time had sought Health Care Committee appointments in order to identify themselves with health care cost containment as an issue, the majority saw little political mileage in a pro-regulatory stance.

Health care facilities were viewed as important sources of employment. They often included on their Boards of Trustees key community leaders who would be important in local elections. Those legislators whose self-interest was not involved were unlikely to deny a favor to a Brockton-area legislator whose support they might need in the future. The St. Joseph's case affirmed the well-traveled credo of the state legislature: "all politics is local politics."

In fact, politics had entered the St. Joseph's case right from the start. Just a half hour after the Public Health Council had voted to deny the St. Joseph's DON, the DPH Commissioner was called away from the continuing Council session. The Speaker of the Massachusetts House was on the phone arguing the St. Joseph's case.

The Politicization of Determination of Need

St. Joseph's Manor was the first nursing home to gain exemption from the DON process, but it was not the first case of its kind. In fact, exemptive legislation in Massachusetts dates back to the very early days of the DON program. Precedents for special exemptive legislation were established prior to St. Joseph's by the Bessie M. Burke Memorial Hospital and by Winchendon Hospital.

On December 21, 1971, the Bessie Burke, a chronic care facility located in Lawrence, Massachusetts, filed for a Determination of Need for renovation of buildings housing hospital beds, support services, and administration, at an estimated cost of $1,500,000. On April 11, 1972, the Public Health Council voted to endorse the "b" Agency recommendation and deny the Burke application. The denial was based primarily on the belief that only 21 of the 95 patients at the hospital actually required chronic disease level care, and that a majority of the Burke's patients would be more appropriately placed in nursing home facilities. Rather than take their case to the Health Facilities Appeal Board or seek judicial relief, the Burke took its case to the legislature. On October 17, 1973, a year and a half later, the state legislature enacted a law (ST. 1973, c. 923) allowing the hospital to proceed with its construction plans.

The facts in the Winchendon case were similar. On August 13, 1973, Winchendon Hospital applied for a DON for a construction project including an ambulatory care center, 4 intensive care beds, a 52-bed extended care facility, and a 26-bed acute care facility. On November 13, the Public Health Council voted to approve the extended care facility at Winchendon, but disapproved the acute facility and the 4 intensive care beds. Although Winchendon Hospital appealed the ruling to the Health Facilities Appeals Board, it also simultaneously sought exemptive legislation. On November 19, 1973, the state legislature passed ST. 1973, c. 1053, overriding the Governor's veto and instructing the DPH to issue a Determination of Need to Winchendon Hospital.

Aware that the Burke and Winchendon cases posed a potential threat to the entire Determination of Need process, the DPH went to court to question the legality of the legislature's action. On February 5, 1975, the Supreme Judicial Court of Massachusetts reached a decision in the *Commissioner of Public Health v. Bessie Burke Hospital,* upholding the constitutionality under Massachusetts law of exemptive legislation.

(Ironically, neither Burke nor Winchendon exercised their exemptions. Burke had problems financing its renovation. Winchendon was persuaded after a protracted battle with the Worcester HSA to merge services with another hospital and, in effect, terminate its inpatient acute care.)

Summary

During the Dukakis administration, the Massachusetts DPH took a tough stand aimed at reducing the number of nursing home beds in the state. The nursing home policy was part of an overall effort to hold the line on the state Medicaid budget. The mandated statewide averages operationalized the overall policy, so that, except in special circumstances, decisions followed quickly from pre-set rules. Staff analysis became a part of the decision implementation process rather than a prelude to such decisions.

The policy on long-term care beds, however, left St. Joseph's with little room for bargaining and negotiation. And when the nursing home's claim to special and unique status fell on deaf ears, they shifted their efforts to the legislative arena where, quite clearly, an entirely different set of decision rules applied. In the legislature St. Joseph's was able to press its claim to special status successfully. Such was the importance of Lithuania in health planning.

Case 3

Worcester City Hospital:
The Competition Selects a
Victim for Regulation

Worcester City Hospital* is a decaying 400-bed public institution located in a neglected neighborhood just off Worcester's central business district. Like similar municipal hospitals in other cities, it is the focus of intense controversy. Its residents have recently organized and threatened to strike. Community groups and staff publicly question the quality of its services. Charges of fiscal mismanagement have been made. But worst of all from its perspective, the local health systems agency has recommended that it be merged with the newly opened University Hospital, the prime teaching affiliate of the University of Massachusetts Medical School.

Hospital politics in Worcester have been in turmoil since University Hospital opened in 1975. Worcester is severely overbedded according to planning standards. Not counting any of the 400 beds intended for University Hospital, Worcester has nearly twice the national average of acute care beds per 1,000 population. Though only 200 of University Hosptial's beds have been licensed, the squeeze has already been felt. Occupancy rates are down while institutional tempers are up. A major hospital needs to close. To many among Worcester's hospital administrators and health planners, Worcester City Hospital is the obvious target.

When University Hospital was being planned in the mid-1960s the

---

*Although Worcester City Hospital is a public institution, private physicians can admit private patients. Salaried staff physicians provide service to the poor who have no medical insurance coverage.

expectation was that it would complement the medical services available in Worcester. University officials in charge of developing the medical school were determined to create an institution of the first rank. It was unthinkable in their view that such a school would rely heavily upon the then existing Worcester hospitals for the clinical training of medical students. These hospitals had little experience with teaching programs, were generally considered to be middle- to low-quality, and were located two or more miles from the site selected for the school. An early decision was made to construct a 400-bed treatment center attached to the school's laboratory building.

As a public institution the University Hospital was exempt from the original Massachusetts Determination of Need law. Although the law was broadened to cover public institutions in 1972, University Hospital was protected from review by a grandfather clause applying to all projects of public institutions previously planned. University Hospital officials did submit a letter in 1972 to the then existing "b" Agency apparently promising the Agency the opportunity to review new projects at University Hospital, but the wording was so vague as to leave the matter of what projects would be submitted for voluntary review open to conflicting interpretation. In fact, the fully equipped 400-bed tertiary care facility has successfully avoided the Determination of Need of process.

Initial fears among members of Worcester's medical community that the new hospital would disrupt local referral patterns were dissipated by the stress university officials placed on tertiary care in the plans for the hospital. Rather than siphoning off local patients, University Hospital, it was said, would compete with the Boston teaching hospitals for referrals of complicated cases from throughout New England. The establishment of several affiliations with larger Worcester hospitals and the appointment of leading Worcester area specialists to the medical school faculty also helped to avoid conflict.

This happy relationship did not last through the construction period of University Hospital. Modernizing in part for their new ties with academic medicine, Worcester hospitals have been acquiring ambitions of their own. Two, St. Vincent's and Memorial, now offer specialty services that duplicate those being installed at University Hospital. In addition, the fashion, if not the substance, in academic medicine has changed. The medical school has been under pressure from state officials to have its students and its teaching hospital involved in community medicine. The more the medical school moves in the direction of offering training in family practice, establishing outpatient clinics, and the like, and the more the larger Worcester hospitals discover the joys of medical technology, the greater the clash between University Hospital and the local medical community. What was once described as complementary by some now appears competitive to many.

There are, of course, those who would wish the problem away. A recent resolution of the local medical society called upon Worcester area physicians to refer all tertiary cases to University Hospital rather than to Boston while reserving all their secondary referrals for local hospitals other than University. But medical school officials are adamant in adhering to the plan to have 400 beds opened at University Hospital. The achievement of that goal will of necessity involve increased competition for secondary referrals and the treatment of uncomplicated as well as complicated cases. Apparently nothing short of closing a major hospital will eliminate Worcester's excess supply of hospital beds.

Worcester City is vulnerable for a number of reasons. Unlike St. Vincent's and Memorial, Worcester City has been slow to modernize. The belief is that it would require a multimillion dollar effort to repair the hospital's many physical defects and to add essential equipment. A renovation plan of that scale is said to have been prepared, but as yet has not been presented. In addition, Worcester City is the other public hospital in a city adjusting to the arrival of a new public facility. Worcester's only proprietary hospital, the 130-bed Doctor's Hospital, has already been driven out of the acute care business, having become primarily an alcoholic rehabilitation facility. The city's dominant non-profit hospitals naturally see any further bed shrinkage occurring in the public sector. So do the planners. In their view, St. Vincent's (600-plus beds) and Memorial (400 beds) are stable, effective institutions and Worcester's other nonprofit hospitals, Hahnemann (200 beds) and Fairlawn (100-plus), are too small to matter. Finally, Worcester City has not been able to expand or even protect its clientele. Several of Worcester's hospitals have built outlier clinics, but Worcester City has not. Within its own service area it competes for patients with a publicly supported neighborhood health center. And thanks to Medicare and Medicaid, Worcester City is losing even its traditional client base; Memorial now treats more poor patients than does Worcester City.

To be sure, City Hospital is not without supporters. The City Manager has been steadfast in backing the hospital's administration in its fight for survival. (For example, he is reported to have told the director of the city-supported neighborhood health center to stop referring patients to other hospitals and has made the center's financial assistance from local government contingent upon the approval of the director of City Hospital.) The City Manager's importance in local politics is legendary as is his interest in patronage such as is available at

City Hospital. (He holds the longest tenure of any city manager in the country and has recently been extended beyond the normal retirement age.) City Hospital's work force, heavily unionized and numbering over 1,000, is another source of support, as is its attending staff, many of whose members have no other hospital affiliations.

The merger proposal first surfaced in 1977 during a dispute the hospital was having with its residents. The residents had formed an association the year before and sought bargaining recognition. The association's often-repeated assertion was that its concern was with working conditions and the quality of care at the hospital and not with salaries. According to the residents the hospital was in desperate need of new equipment and increased levels of nursing services. Community groups claiming to represent the hospital's poverty clients supported these claims. The hospital's trustees and the city government, however, initially refused to bargain with residents, arguing that they were students not employees. A strike was threatened.

The hospital and the city sought a ruling on the status of residents from the Massachusetts Labor Relations Commission to settle the issue. Some thought this move strange since the Commission in a recent case involving Cambridge City Hospital had ruled in favor of the residents. Just before the Commission was to decide the Worcester City Hospital case, the president of the hospital's board of trustees stated publicly that the hospital would bargain with the residents. A few weeks later the hospital's trustees submitted an emergency request to the city for the appropriation of $1.45 million to upgrade the facility. Rumors circulated that a multi-million dollar building program was soon to follow. (Some of the residents feared that they were being used by the hospital to justify renovations at a time when the planning system opposed such major capital expenditures. Their fears may have been justified as within a year the hospital had terminated most of its residency programs, thus ridding itself of most of its vocal junior staff.)

Although taken aback by the size and emergency nature of the request, the City Council seemed willing to support the hospital. The City Manager was given permission to establish an equipment revolving fund for the hospital. To still employee fears that the hospital would close, the Council toured the institution and pledged in a 9 to 0 vote to keep it open. Some questions though were raised about the accuracy of the hospital's financial records. The suspicion was that the hospital's losses were greater than was being reported, largely due to the failure to recover third-party reimbursements. Few seemed to relish the idea of embarking on a major rebuilding program, especially at a time when the city voters were resisting a bond issue for a civic center. The new rumor, perhaps started by the hospital's nonprofit rivals, was that merger with University Hospital might be a better idea.

No one though knew what a merger would actually mean. To help clarify the impact, the local congressman obtained a grant from HEW to hire a consultant to study the outline of a merger. The consultant's much delayed report called for the joint siting of the institutions with independent managements within the physical plant of University Hospital (the consultant labeled this a "Condominium Arrangement") and the transfer of a city-run nursing home to the location of City Hospital, proposals which pleased neither potential partner. University Hospital wanted its full complement of beds and no involvement of City Hospital's management in the operation of the facility. City Hospital preferred no merger and its present site. The local health systems plan which was being developed at the same time picked up on the idea that there be a merger between the institutions, but specified only that the resulting bed complement be no greater than that originally planned for University Hospital. This plan gained state and HEW approval.

If a merger does occur, University Hospital is certain to be the surviving partner as it has the newest physical plant, the most prestigious staff, and the deepest pocket, facts well-known to City Hospital and its supporters. It also seems obvious that the longer City Hospital's physical renewal is postponed, the more likely that there will be a merger. Given the prospect of achieving a major planning goal by preventing the rehabilitation of City Hospital, the HSA, as presently structured and led, is strongly disinclined to recommend rehabilitation through the Determination of Need process. Without the endorsement of the HSA, the state is unlikely to approve the rehabilitation project even if the Worcester City Council continues to back the hospital. Thus the need for City Hospital to develop a counter strategy.

The counter strategy was revealed at the 1978 election meeting of the HSA when over a thousand City Hospital supporters, including staff allegedly released from work for the occasion, showed up to vote for a slate of board members favorable to the hospital. The election produced four new pro-City Hospital board members which, when previous board supporters are included, give City Hospital direct or indirect influence over seven of 30 board seats. If City Hospital supporters had been better organized, they could have gained full control of the board and the HSA at that session for they had the voting strength present to amend the bylaws of the agency.*

The HSA has sought to protect itself. Conveniently, the HEW

*Personal communication, HSA and Region I HEW staff.

Regional Office soon notified the HSA regarding the Office's concern about the agency bylaws that would allow the domination of policy by a single institution or group within the community. Election procedures were quickly altered to make it difficult for the politically isolated City Hospital to field candidates. Candidacy for board membership now requires nomination from constituency groups rather than being open to all who qualify by income, residency, or occupation. But the danger of a takeover remains. The 1979 elections have been postponed because of challenges to the new procedures by City Hospital supporters and others.

City Hospital's new found aggressiveness, however, may be its undoing. Recently it was discovered that City Hospital was renting a CAT scanner without previously obtaining the required Determination of Need approval. The HSA is mobilizing provider and consumer opposition to this violation of the rules. The state has threatened suit. And federal regulators are rallying to the cause of the local regulators. There is no better way to unite officials than to be contemptuous of their authority. City Hospital is not likely to be permitted to win this or any other of its battles.

Case 4

The New England Baptist Hospital:
An Upset Victory for Planning

On May 1, 1974, the New England Baptist Hospital (NEBH) submitted a Determination of Need application, documenting the rationale for constructing a 250-bed facility to replace the current hospital, as well as a 500-car garage, and a doctors' office building. This original application was withdrawn on December 16, 1974. A second application, cosponsored by NEBH and Cabot, Cabot & Forbes (a real estate firm), was submitted in September of 1975. This called for a 266-bed replacement facility, a 367-car garage, and proposed a unique financing scheme for the project. On June 10, 1976, the Massachusetts Public Health Council voted unanimously to deny permission for construction. Subsequently, two attempts by NEBH to win exemptive legislation in the state legislature failed. The route New England Baptist took and the reason for its failure thus far have important implications for Certificate of Need.

The Initial Proposal

To support the proposal to build a replacement facility at a new site on Parker Hill, the NEBH made several major arguments. The hospital presented data which showed increases in patient days and occupancy rates over the past two years, as well as expansion of the general medical staff associated with the NEBH. NEBH further claimed that an increase in the use of ancillary services over the past ten years and the adoption of new operating techniques were taxing the capacity of the existing physical plant. NEBH also used noncompliance with codes as a justification for the proposed replacement project, claiming that only 66 of its 250 beds, or 26 percent were "conforming" to Hill-Burton standards. The hospital emphasized that the design of the replacement facility would lead to economies of a more efficient layout, reducing staff requirements by 155 full-time equivalents, and resulting in annual operating cost savings of $1,770,000. Throughout the application ran the theme that NEBH was a specialty hospital, unique by virtue of the distribution of procedures performed there, and the national and international arena from which it attracted patients.

The application also cited traffic flow difficulties in the Mission Hill area, its current location, as a rationale for the proposed 500-car garage. The adjacent doctors' office building would provide greater accessibility to the hospital for the medical staff, and was considered an important component in the delivery of "quality" care.

The estimated capital cost of construction, assuming completion of the project by August, 1977, was $20.7 million for the replacement hospital plant, $4.6 million for the garage structure and land, and $3.15 million for the office building, a total expenditure of $28,450,000. It was assumed that costs would be covered in part by a federal grant and by guaranteed loans.

"a" Agency Review

On October 9, 1974, the Review Committee of the Advisory Council of the Office of Comprehensive Health Planning recommended denial of the NEBH proposal, but also suggested that NEBH submit a revised application. The revised version was to take into account four matters of concern to the "a" Agency:

1) It should suggest alternative methods of funding, should the Hill-Burton grant not materialize.
2) There were to be assurances that hospital revenues (31 percent of which were derived from Medicare) would not be used to subsidize possible cost overruns on nonpatient care facilities such as the garage and office building.
3) NEBH was to take a more analytical view of the effect of disaffiliation with the Lahey Clinic (which had recently been granted permission to build its own 200-bed facility in Burlington, Massachusetts) on occupancy and patient days. In fact, although the percentage of patient days attributable to the NEBH general medical staff had been increasing, actual total patient days had been decreasing by an average of 3 percent *per annum* between 1967 and 1973. The increase in the occupancy rate mentioned in the application was derived by dividing the number of patient days by

a reduced number of beds, and by using only winter month statistics for 1973 and 1974 to show an artificial increase in occupancy.

4) The "a" Agency also suggested that the revised application explore the possibility of sharing services with neighboring hospitals, and required evidence of a commitment on the part of the Baptist to work with the Affiliated and other hospitals, the community groups, and the "b" Agency on a compromise equitable to all.

"b" Agency Review

The Board of Directors of the Health Planning Council of Greater Boston (HPCGB) had already voted, in August, 1974, to recommend denial of the NEBH proposal. One major concern of the "b" Agency was the number of beds proposed for the replacement facility. Using various formulas, HPCGB found a need for only 160-190 beds in the service area of NEBH. These bed need formulas discounted the hospital's claim of being a national and international resource, since patient origin studies showed that 44 percent of NEBH admittees resided in the Greater Boston area. Another 22 percent lived in other parts of Massachusetts, while 17.4 percent came from neighboring New England states.

Determination of Need Staff Analysis

The Determination of Need staff voiced concern with the environmental effect of the project, especially the impact on traffic and parking congestion, and water pressure, a serious problem on Parker Hill. Their analysis of bed need led to a finding for 139-168 beds, instead of the 250 proposed. Lack of community involvement in the planning process, the effect of the loss of Lahey physicians, and the questionable specialty orientation of the Baptist (which had no emergency room facilities for community use) led to a negative recommendation on the part of the DON agency.

Ten Taxpayer Groups

Two community groups, the Mission Hill Health Movement, Inc., and the Mission Hill Planning Commission, requested and were granted a public hearing six weeks after the original application was submitted. By October of 1974, these groups had reached a consensus, and recommended denial of the NEBH proposal. Although they agreed with the construction of a replacement facility, they staunchly opposed the building of a garage at the top of their heavily congested hill, and proposed alternative sites for garage and office construction. The community groups had felt disenfranchised during the planning process, and wanted a say in how the vacated hospital facility would be used, and some guarantee of employment of community members in the new facility.

By November the Baptist agreed, in a letter to the DON agency, to withdraw the garage and office building from the application, but increased the anticipated capital expenditure to $33,653,155. This necessitated filing an official amendment to the application.

Environmental Impact

While the Baptist was taking steps to comply with the demands of the planning agencies and the community groups, another barrier to approval emerged. Along with the original proposal, NEBH had filed an environmental impact report, delineating the effect of construction on traffic flow, water pressure, and other matters of ecological concern. The DON office determined that the project would have no adverse environmental effects on the community. The DON recommendation was rejected by the Secretary of Environmental Affairs when it was noted that the environmental study had been done to support the federal grant application. NEBH would have to prepare a full environmental impact report in concordance with the standards of the Massachusetts Office of Environmental Affairs. In November of 1974, Envirovestment, Inc., was hired by NEBH to work with the DON staff in preparing such a report.

Withdrawal

A letter dated December 16, 1974, contained the news that the Executive Committee of the New England Baptist Hospital had voted to withdraw their application for a Determination of Need.

The Revised Application

On August 6, 1975, representatives from the NEBH, Cabot, Cabot & Forbes, and the Health Planning Council for Greater Boston, Inc., met to discuss issues related to the possible submission of a revised DON application. Discussion focused on the factors that had led to recommendations of denial for the initial proposal: bed need and length of stay, the definition of NEBH's service area, the effect of disaffiliation with the Lahey Clinic, the establishment of need for the office building and the parking garage, and especially the financial feasibility of the project, which NEBH felt had been the primary element leading to previous recommendations for denial. HPCGB representatives also elaborated on recent changes in the DON regulations, which required that the applicant involve the community in the planning process prior to submission of the application and show evidence of concern for "regionalization." This meant that the applicant must document its attempt to avoid duplication of services and must consider the possibility of sharing services with similar institutions. A joint application, co-sponsored by NEBM and CC&F, was submitted to the DON office on September 1, 1975. Despite previous DON and "b" Agency analysis which showed need for no more than 190 beds, the applicants requested permission to build a 266-bed facility. CC&F also intended to construct an 800-car garage on the site, of which 367 spaces were intended for NEBH use and were therefore included in the application. The doctors' office building, although still part of the hospital's long-range plan, was not included in this application. Unique to this application was the financing arrangement worked out between CC&F and NEBH. As stated in the HPCGB analysis

> NEBH proposes to lease land for a fixed annual rate to CC&F. On this land, CC&F will build a hospital facility and two levels (below ground) for parking . . . . CC&F will lease one level of the garage and the hospital facility to NEBH for a fixed annual rate for 35 years. At the end of 35 years, all improvements on NEBH's property will be given over to NEBH for no extra cost.

Under this arrangement capital project expenditures were estimated to range between $26,650,000 and $29,850,000.

Rate Setting Commission

The financing arrangement of the NEBH-CC&F proposal required a complex analysis of its effect on cash flow, reimbursement, and the handling of depreciation. After much deliberation, the Rate Setting Commission made the following assessments:

1) The arrangement would be treated as a purchase of assets, rather than a lease, under Medicare regulations.
2) Any return on equity or profit earned by CC&F and any cost overruns on the garage construction would not be reimbursable since the Baptist was a nonprofit voluntary hospital, and CC&F

was a joint applicant. (Had CC&F or any other company bid competitively to do the construction, it would have been allowed its usual profit margin).

3) Analysis of revenues showed that the coverage ratio for the lease payment would be less than 1.2 in the early years of operation of the new facility; this margin was too low to ensure financial feasibility of the project.

PSRO

During the August meeting, the staff of the HPCGB suggested that a PSRO audit of length of stay would be helpful in determining bed need and the appropriateness of bed use at NEBH. (Blue Cross had performed utilization review of NEBH cases in support of the initial DON application, and found no length-of-stay problems.) The Bay State Health Care Foundation accordingly reviewed a sample of 104 medical records that length of stay was excessive in 24 percent of the cases examined.

Environmental Impact

The report submitted to the Office of Environmental Affairs by Envirovestment, Inc., gave detailed analyses of the impact of the NEBH project on the local water supply and air quality, and considered problems associated with solid waste disposal, parking and CO emission, and fossil fuel burning. The Secretary of Environmental Affairs recommended approval of the project, pending the satisfactory solution of the problems with CO and fossil fuel emission.

Denial

The DON process for the revised application came to an end at the Public Health Council meeting of June 10, 1976. By this time the process had incorporated analysis, review, and recommendations of the Rate Setting Commission, the PSRO, the Health Systems Agency (HPCGB, the former "b" agency), the Area 620 Planning Group, the Office of Environmental Affairs, the DON staff, the architectural consultants Shepley, Bulfinch, Richardson and Abbott, and five "ten taxpayer" groups. The "a" Agency, the State Office of Comprehensive Health Planning, had waived the right to comment on this second application.

The members of the Public Health Council voted unanimously to deny approval to the NEBH-CC&F application. As their rationale for denial, they presented many of the arguments contained in the HSA analysis:

1) lack of bed need (finding for 157 beds, vs. 266 proposed)
2) adequacy of the current physical plant (according to the Shepley, Bulfinch, Richardson and Abbott analysis)
3) the proposal was not the least-cost alternative (per HSA analysis)
4) lack of adequate inhouse planning at NEBH, and lack of cooperative planning with the HSA and community groups
5) uncertain financial feasibility due to potential cash flow problems, and reimbursement uncertainty (Medicare)
6) environmental impact concerns which had not yet been completely resolved.

Exemptive Legislation

Faced with a denial from the Public Health Council, the New England Baptist took its case to the Massachusetts legislature. The Baptist's attempt at exemptive legislation was unsuccessful. It failed mainly because it had been filed very late in the legislative session in 1976. The Baptist's second attempt, filed in the next legislative session, was successful. However, Governor Dukakis, voicing concern both with health care costs and with the integrity of the DON process, vetoed the exemption. Attempts to override the Governor's veto in the State Senate were unsuccessful.

In failing to win exemptive legislation, the New England Baptist was unable to achieve what many other hospitals and nursing homes in Massachusetts had already accomplished. The Baptist's failure is particularly conspicuous since none of the successful petitioners for exemptive legislation were as prestigious or as well-connected politically as the New England Baptist Hospital. There are several special circumstances that contributed to the Baptist's failure.

Lobbying efforts for NEBH were led by ex-Massachusetts Attorney General Robert Quinn. Inside observers report that this was more a hindrance than a help; Quinn apparently had as many enemies in the legislature as he had friends. The same observers also report that Quinn made a series of tactical errors, including bypassing, and therefore alienating, State Senator Robert Bernashe, the prime supporter at the time of provider causes in the Massachusetts legislature. The Baptist project was also expensive; at $28 million it was considerably more expensive than any project that had been granted an exemption in the past. Perhaps most important, the Baptist was unable to offset these difficulties by mobilizing support in the Parker Hill community. Indeed, the community group that did mobilize opposed the Baptist project, citing the Baptist failure to involve the community in major decisions, the limited community services offered by the hospital, and the environmental impact of the Baptist's construction plans as the primary reasons for their opposition. In voting to deny the Baptist application, the Health Planning Council board was particularly concerned that the Baptist had not involved the community in the planning process and that community groups had organized in opposition to the hospital's project. Thus, for the Baptist, what is often a hospital's strongest asset, the ability to mobilize strong local support, became the hospital's chief liability.

The Baptist's petition for an exemption occurred at a time when a number of others were pending before the legislature. These, too, were approved by the legislature and vetoed by Governor Dukakis. The Baptist was the only case where the Governor's veto was not quickly overturned in the State Senate. A fairly unusual convergence of factors—the inability to mobilize community support, apparent tactical errors in the legislature, and the project's high price tag—resulted in a situation in which the Baptist became the victim in what amounted to a trade-off in the legislature between proponents and opponents of Determination of Need.

Following the defeat in the legislature, the Baptist sought to downgrade its modernization plans, hiring a management consultant to oversee the task. In 1978, however, Governor Dukakis was replaced by Edward King, a campaign critic of Determination of Need regulation. Many observers expected that the Baptist would once again petition for exemption, this time to a presumably more sympathetic administration. This was what *The Boston Globe* predicted when it ran a story reporting sizeable campaign contributions from Longwood Orthopedic Associates, Inc., a group of Baptist-affiliated physicians. To date, however, the Baptist has not made the predicted third attempt to win an exemption, despite the fact that a number of providers have already sought exemptions from the King Administration—some going directly to the legislature without applying for a Determination of Need in the first place. Determination of Need has once again become a hot political issue in Massachusetts, but the New England Baptist Hospital has not yet re-entered the controversy.

Case 5

Suburban Memorial Hospital: Hospital Bed Expansion in Spite of Strong State Opposition

Suburban Memorial Hospital (SMH)* is an acute care community hospital located in a relatively affluent suburban area within 10 miles of Providence. SMH opened in 1951 as a 200-bed acute care community hospital. As a result of experiencing high occupancy rates in the mid-1960s, an expansion program including an addition of 200 medical/surgical beds, was proposed in 1968. Although no Certificate of Need (CON) program was in effect at that time, the expansion program was reviewed by the private Health Planning Council (HPC) which was created in 1966 to serve as a voluntary health planning agency for Rhode Island. Based on their analysis of acute bed needs for the SMH area in 1968, the HPC recommended that only 96 beds be added. The hospital voluntarily complied with the HPC recommendation and the 96-bed addition was constructed, bringing the total licensed bed complement to 309.

During the mid-1970s SMH once again experienced high occupancy rates and proposed a second expansion program. By this time, Rhode Island had a stringent CON program which openly stated its opposition to any increase in hospital beds in the state. Both the applicant and the CON staff displayed a high level of sophistication with respect to the CON review process; the success of the applicant attests to the fact that a determined and sophisticated hospital staff can win a CON approval even in a tough regulatory environment.

*The name of this hospital is disguised in accordance with our agreement with SEARCH for access to Rhode Island hospital use data.

Before deciding on a bed expansion strategy, SMH formed a Community Advisory Committee composed of a cross section of citizens from the hospital's service area. In a one-year period the Committee developed an impressive description of the health care needs of the community and outlined a series of recommendations for SMH in its final report delivered in November, 1975. The Committee's recommendations, many of which focused on improving health education in the community, also included addition of 50 acute medical/surgical beds at SMH to relieve overcrowding.

Using a variety of approaches to determining bed need for the community (Hill-Burton, state and national bed ratios plus projections of future increases in patient days), the Committee concluded that a minimum of 50 additional medical/surgical beds would be required to meet current community needs. The SMH Certificate of Need application incorporated much of the description and analysis prepared by the Committee.

Ten months prior to submitting its CON application, SMH requested that the HPC suggest alternative mechanisms to bed expansion for relief of the hospital's utilization pressure. By involving the HPC in advance of the formal CON application, the hospital hoped that the 180-day review cycle could be reduced and that a short-term solution to overcrowding at SMH could be developed. In November, 1976, the Health Planning Council offered the following recommendations for short-term alternatives to bed expansion:

1) increased use of other nearby hospitals through such means as encouraging SMH staff physicians to obtain admitting privileges at other hospitals, limiting elective admissions to patients living in "Suburban" County, and educating community residents to use other hospitals
2) increased rigor of utilization review to further reduce average length of stay
3) transfer of some patients to skilled nursing facilities
4) implementation of a second opinion program for elective surgery
5) elimination of the obstetrics service at SMH and conversion of the 26 obstetrics beds to medical-surgical beds

The HPC suggested that these short-term alternatives to bed expansion be tried for at least six months before a final decision to add beds was made.

After considering the HPC's recommended alternatives to bed additions, SMH submitted its formal application for the 50-bed expansion project. The proposal cited many of the arguments developed by the

Community Advisory Committee and offered a rebuttal to the suggestions of the HPC for short-term relief of bed pressure.

The basic argument for more beds was based on the fact that
occupancy was high in all services, resulting in overcrowding, waiting
lists for elective admissions, and the use of corridor beds. Using analyses
developed by the Community Advisory Committee, the hospital
showed that, after applying a variety of formulas to determine the
appropriate number of acute beds for the community, a minimum of 50
additional beds were required at present.

The hospital stated that it had been trying to relieve bed pressure by
implementing a variety of innovative programs over the past several
years. For example, it reported that 5,000 patient days had been
eliminated in the past year through an ambulatory surgery program and
an additional 8,000 patient days were saved through a home care
program. In spite of these innovations, overcrowding continued.

SMH presented a specific rebuttal to each of the HPC's suggested
alternatives to bed expansion. The hospital rejected the concept of
diverting potential admissions to other nearby hospitals, citing both
inconvenience to patients and their families and interference with the
patient's choice of a SMH staff physician. The possibility of having staff
physicians divide their time among several hospitals was challenged as
an inefficient use of physician time. Moreover, it was stated that SMH
had recently attempted to use this approach with minimal success.

The hospital also indicated that it had been the first hospital in Rhode
Island to be delegated by the PSRO for concurrent review. The
overcrowding problem persisted in spite of this concurrent review.

In response to the HPC suggestion that consideration be given to
increased efforts to transfer appropriate patients to skilled nursing
homes, SMH cited its excellent record of discharging patients to sub-
acute facilities as noted in a current report from SEARCH, an independent health data collection and analysis agency in Rhode Island. As
constraints on nursing home transfers, the hospital pointed to a Rhode
Island Department of Health estimate of a shortage of skilled nursing
home beds in the local SMH area and to the Medicare regulations that
require a patient to stay in an acute care facility 72 hours before
nursing home costs can be covered.

SMH further dismissed the suggestion that its obstetrics service be
eliminated, indicating that the hospital had the second most active
obstetrics unit in the state and that diverting deliveries to Women and
Infants Hospital in Providence (as the HPC had proposed) would place
an unnecessary travel burden on community residents. Having thus

considered numerous alternative solutions to the problem of over-crowding, SMH concluded that expansion of beds was the only reason-able strategy.

State Agency Review

The SMH application was subjected to an intensive review process, incorporating volumes of statistical and other data. The analysis focused on three key issues: (1) The potential for expanding admitting privileges of SMH staff physicians at other hospitals; (2) utilization of hospital services in SMH area relative to the rest of the state; and (3) health status indicators in SMH area compared to the rest of the state. Bed need formulas were also examined.

The most effective alternative to construction of new acute beds was viewed by the Health Services Council* review committee to be the increased use of underutilized neighboring hospitals. Data indicated that SMH physicians admit their patients almost exclusively to SMH despite the fact that some 60 percent of these physicians have privileges at other hospitals. The problem did not seem to be one of negotiating with other hospitals to secure such privileges; rather it was one of making use of those already secured. This solution, the review com-mittee recognized, was short-term; during the interim period, however, it was hoped that longer run solutions to the problem of excess capacity throughout the state would be found.

Population-based data analysis indicated that aggregate measures of inpatient utilization—i.e., age-adjusted discharges and patient days per capita—were nearly the same for the SMH area as for the remainder of the state. The traditional indicators of health status, however (including mortality rates, prevalence of chronic conditions and activity limita-tions, and bed days of disability), were uniformly better for the SMH area than in the state as a whole. These comparisons, the committee concluded, did not argue for a pressing need for additional hospital beds.

Bed need projections were also analyzed. The committee questioned the projections prepared by or on behalf of the hospital, arguing against

---

*CON decisions in Rhode Island are made by the Director of the Department of Health based on advice given by a 19-member Health Services Council whose composition is determined by statute and which includes nominees of the legislature and the governor.

the assumption that past utilization patterns would persist in the face of current trends to substitute ambulatory care for inpatient services. The committee raised additional questions about the basis for the population projections as well as the definition of a hospital service area in an urbanized region.

The committee also noted the influx since 1972 of 35 additional physicians on the active medical staff. Population growth and other factors aside, this was considered to be the "single most important factor responsible for the overcrowded conditions . . . ."

The committee concluded, in short, that any benefits accruing from the addition of 50 new beds would not be worth the cost, which was estimated to be $2.8 million in capital costs and $2.2 million in annual operating costs. The burden of these costs, it was noted, would not fall exclusively on local residents but would be spread to all state residents, since nearly all SMH revenues come from third-party sources. The arguments presented in support of the project were seen by the committee as essentially ones of patient and physician convenience. Despite the fact that an adequate case for *institutional* need had been demonstrated, the committee determined that under its statutory authority its perspective had to be that of Rhode Island as a whole. Given the existence of statewide excess capacity, the presence of alternatives to new acute beds, and the lack of obvious health status deficiencies, the committee could not justify approving the application.

These conclusions were initially presented in a draft report to the full Health Services Council in early August, 1977. At that time, representatives of SMH appeared to address the conclusions expressed in the draft report as well as to argue the merits of their case. The delegation was headed by the President of the Board of Trustees and the administrator. In a prepared statement, the administrator contended that occupancy rates higher than 100 percent pointed to a shortage of acute beds for the surrounding community. The hospital's perspective must be the community it serves, he argued, and statewide need should be considered as a separate issue from Suburban County's need.

Subsequent presentations were made by the President of the Board, the head of the medical staff, and a local citizen who had been active in the Citizens Advisory Committee. The President described the heavy pressure received from administrators, hospital staff, and trustees about the overcrowding situation. If the decision is negative, he predicted, "other alternatives" will probably be pursued and the "will of the public" will prevail. The head of the medical staff pointed to the difficulties inherent in delivering patient care under current overcrowded conditions and alleged that, given current circumstances and the talk of sending patients elsewhere, not enough emphasis was being given to patient safety. Finally, the citizen representative argued that due to the constraints hampering its operations, SMH was unable to take the leadership role in the health affairs of the community that she believed it ought to have.

The next HSC meeting to consider the SMH application was held under very unusual circumstances. For the first time, members of the public were allowed to present their views before the Council; ordinarily, the public may attend HSC meetings, but may not participate. There was a sizeable citizen turnout for the meeting, and those present overwhelmingly supported the SMH application. However, in spite of the heated, often hostile debate, the HSC voted unanimously to deny the application. Justification for the denial rested mainly on the perceived excess capacity among Rhode Island hospitals, regardless of the particular needs of the SMH community, and on the state's inability under existing law to reallocate beds from underutilized hospitals to those experiencing excess demand. As is customary, the Director of the Department of Health followed the Council's recommendation and issued an official denial.

SMH immediately asked for an administrative hearing within the Department of Health. Concurrently, its attorneys filed suit against the Department in Superior Court, contending that the state had not complied with the administrative requirements under the CON statute. The point of contention related to the interpretation of language in the CON statute dealing with the procedure and timing of a public hearing:

> . . . If the licensing agency proposes to disapprove an application for construction, it shall afford the applicant an opportunity for a public hearing and it may, on its own motion, hold a public hearing on any application for construction. (From Rhode Island Statutes 23–16–12.)

The attorneys for the hospital contended that no bona fide public hearing was held within the six-month CON review period specified in this provision. CON staff argued that the HSC meeting which allowed public participation satisfied the requirements for a public hearing.

The case was never heard before the Superior Court. An administrative hearing was held during late 1977 and early 1978, during which extensive testimony was taken concerning the merits of the application and the basis for the state's decision. After considering the arguments, the adjudicative officer recommended that the denial be overturned on procedural grounds. In particular, he interpreted the CON statute as requiring that the application review as well as the administrative appeal should have taken place within the six-month review period. The Director of the Health Department, who could have appealed this decision to the court system, chose to accept the hearing officer's decision, and SMH's 50-bed expansion was therefore approved in March, 1978.

Throughout the process, the HSC had been sympathetic to the institutional need demonstrated by SMH, but stood firm to the belief that Rhode Island as a whole was overbedded. Under the circumstances, the HSC believed it could not approve a net addition of beds in Rhode Island. Even while the hearing was taking place, the CON staff were negotiating with other hospitals to voluntarily close empty beds so that a redistribution to SMH could be justified. One hospital had agreed to close 25 beds; it was hoped that an additional 25 beds could be located.

Up to the time the hearing officer's decision was announced, CON staff and the HSC had hoped to achieve a negotiated solution. If such a redistribution of beds could be achieved, both the hospital's and the state's purposes could have been served without damage to the credibility of the CON process. Both because this solution had not been achieved and because the denial had been overturned on procedural rather than substantive grounds, the final outcome of the case ' was extremely frustrating to HSC and CON staff members.

Analysis

An application for additional acute medical and surgical beds is a rare event in Rhode Island. In view of the state's position of discouraging new bed construction, SMH was wise to obtain support from a broad-based community group and to respond to a set of alternatives to bed expansion provided by the HPC in advance of the application. The hospital administration, in fact, stressed that the impetus for the bed expansion proposal came from the community, not the hospital itself.

A number of significant issues arise in this case and make it an instructive example of the problems inherent in regulation. The first is the conflict between the perceptions of need of the community and that of the planners and regulators. No one on either side questioned that need had been demonstrated for this institution, given prevailing patterns of medical practices. The issue became whether this need could be paramount when excess capacity existed in surrounding areas; the alternatives of either changing prevailing patterns of hospital use or redistributing beds from underused hospitals to SMH were far more palatable to the state than adding beds. A related issue is the definition of the community whose interests the law is to protect. The view of staff and the HSC is that the state is the relevant community, not a particular sub-region. The hospital, of course, sees as its community the local area in which most of its patients reside.

The second set of issues relates to the weights given particular factors during the decisionmaking process. How important should patient and physician preference be? How much should health status and utilization indicators be taken into account? Since widespread third-party coverage of hospital care means that consumers do not absorb directly the cost of the resources they use, true resource costs to the local community do not figure heavily in decisions to pursue capital projects. Regulators, on the other hand, are asked to make decisions based on social costs and benefits. Given the market distortion present, this usually means consumers will get less from the regulators than they desire. The process of making these choices and protecting the community's interest is inherently difficult and inevitably controversial.

The essence of the predicament this application presented to the Health Services Council is captured in the draft report of the committee assigned to review the SMH application:

> [This report] documents a classic dilemma which will inevitably face regulatory agencies with greater frequency in the near future—the case of a community hospital which has been innovative in its approach to alternatives to inpatient hospitalization, serving a growing population, in good conscience, proposing an increase in its bed complement in order to satisfy perceived consumer and physician demands placed upon it, denied by a governmental agency charged with a responsibility for controlling health care costs through the control of potential duplications of limited health care resources. The hospital's focus is the satisfaction of the needs or demands of its service population; the Council's focus is the optimal allocation of resources to derive maximum benefit for all of the citizens of the State of Rhode Island within the context of the fiscal constraints necessary to effectuate a cost-effective health care system. (Report of the Committee of the Health Services Council to Review the Proposal of the SMH to Construct 50 beds.)

Ultimately, the Council assigned its heaviest weight to its perceived charge to control the state's bed supply. This objective is the most long-standing and clear-cut within the Certificate of Need program, and despite the arguments presented by SMH, the Council ultimately felt it had to continue to enforce its "moratorium" on new beds if CON were to continue to be credible.

It is clear that the Department would have liked to approve the beds, but only under the condition that those beds would not constitute a net addition to the system. Although, the hearing officer's decision did not come as a surprise to many, the Health Department Director's refusal to take the case to court for a ruling surprised and disappointed key staff and Council members. His reason was thought to be that he believed the Department would lose in court and he wanted to avoid both the embarrassment and the potential damage it might cause to the overall CON process. Following the initial denial, hospital representatives met with both the Director and HSC members to discuss "alternatives." While it was actively pursuing the appeals route, SMH would have been willing to get the beds approved under almost any circumstances and was hopeful that a compromise solution—such as the redistribution plan proposed by the Department—could be worked out. The Director though apparently felt that a negotiated solution was not possible and that the matter best be dropped.

Conclusions

The SMH application put the Rhode Island CON program to its strongest test to date. At the time the application was filed, the program had matured considerably; most noticeably, the participants—particularly the HSC—had become knowledgeable and sophisticated with regard to health planning and regulation. It was this mature system that had the confidence to deny the SMH application, in public and in the face of considerable popular support.

For this reason, it is particularly unfortunate that the outcome was decided not on the substantive issues, which were significant and which could have been employed as the foundation for future CON decisions, but on a procedural technicality. The wording that led to that technicality has since been clarified.* While no applications for new beds have been submitted since the decision was made, and none are anticipated, the CON process was greatly damaged as a result of the resignation of key CON staff in part as a protest over the SMH decisions. During the year since the SMH decision, few CON applications have been submitted, providing little basis from which to conclude whether the Department's capacity to deny applications or negotiate solutions has been damaged. But SMH proved that a determined institution can gain CON approval even in the toughest regulatory environment.

*Chapter 269 of Rhode Island's Public Laws (May, 1978) eliminates the ambiguous wording of the previous CON statute (see page 9) and does not require a pubic hearing.

Case 6

"A" General Hospital:
The Use of Data in Health Planning

In the Spring of 1976, "A" General Hospital ("A"GH), a 72-bed acute care hospital in rural Maine, submitted an 1122 application for a $1,472,500 renovation and expansion program including the addition of 11 new acute care beds within a new patient care wing. The project encompassed the following: The replacement of 29 obsolete beds, the addition of 11 new acute general hospital beds, and remodeling to provide additional space for emergency care, an outpatient department, radiology, a laboratory, a pharmacy, mechanical services and an operating room.

The argument for the additional hospital resources at "A"GH was based on the fact that more physicians were coming to the area and that they would require increased hospital facilities. The following quote from the administrator of "A"GH summarizes the need argument:

> For many years, our area has experienced a shortage of physicians and only within the last two years has our physician population begun to increase with the addition of three new doctors to our Medical Staff. We are anticipating another doctor joining us in August of this year and are actively recruiting for other doctors and dentists. As you know, additional doctors have a great impact on the utilization of a hospital.

> We are experiencing definite overcrowding in our service areas and find the need to increase in order to accommodate our present workload and prepare for future growth. To find the needed space for the many new and increased activities in the hospital, an impact is made on the present nursing areas, one of which has small, dark patient rooms without toilets and bathing facilities.

By the addition of a new wing, we plan to solve many of the problems in ancillary services and improve the patient care areas. The past four years show a gradual but continued increase in the use of our services; it would appear shortsighted not to add a few beds at this time to prevent needed construction in the next five to ten years. This new wing would contain a special care unit, new pediatrics unit, solarium, and 40 patient beds. Twenty-nine of these would be replacing our present beds in the original hospital with 11 new beds in total, changing our total bed count to 83.

Background and Project Review

"A"GH is the major hospital serving a population of approximately 10,000 in an isolated area of Maine. The hospital was originally built in 1954. A 30-bed extended care facility was added in 1968, and these beds were subsequently converted to acute care in 1971. At the time of application the hospital was licensed for 71 acute care beds including 56 medical/surgical, 7 pediatric, and 8 obstetric beds. The community had been successful in recruiting several new physicians who accounted in large part for the observed increase in the annual number of hospital admissions. Tables C.3 and C.4, adapted from the "A"GH application, show the admission and occupancy statistics. Table C.3 shows that the number of admissions increased by 33 percent between 1971 and 1975 and that occupancy showed a concomitant increase from 60.5 percent in 1971 to 75 percent in 1976. Table C.4 shows that the net increase in the annual number of admissions could be accounted for by the fact that admissions of new physicians G, I, and N had more than compensated for the loss of admissions from physicians no longer on "A"GH staff.

The need for improvement in existing space was never disputed by the HSA or the SHPDA staff. The state did hire a consulting architect to assess the feasibility of a less costly renovation alternative to the construction of a new wing. The consultants agree with the hospital's plan to construct new space. The real issue in review of this 1122 application was the assessment of the need for additional beds.

Some Human Services staff members had been concerned for several years about reports of unjustified surgery performed at "A"GH. In 1972, as part of a licensing evaluation, the state had sent a consultant surgeon to study the quality of surgical services at "A"GH. After review of patient records and tissue, the consultant reported that, in his opinion, a significant number of surgical procedures were unjustified. This opinion was reinforced in the minds of the SHPDA staff when population-based analyses of the rate of surgery for residents of the

Table C.3

"A" General Hospital

Census	Number of Beds	Average Daily Census, Overall Occupancy Rates, and Number of Admissions from 1971 through 1976					
		1971*	1972*	1973*	1974*	1975*	1976**
Medical, Surgical	56	36.3	38.2	38.5	39.1	45.0	N/A
Pediatric	7	4.3	3.9	4.1	3.6	3.9	N/A
Obstetric	8	2.4	2.3	2.3	2.6	2.4	N/A
Total Hospital	71	43.0	44.4	44.9	45.3	51.3	53.2
Occupancy Rate		60.5%	62.5%	63.2%	63.9%	72.5%	75.0%
Number of Admissions		2,363	2,546	2,483	2,652	3,145	75.0%

*"A" General Hospital application, with appropriate adjustments.
**Additional information, received by the BHP&D 1/18/77.

Table C.4

"A" General Hospital

Staff Physicians	Number of Admissions Annually by Physician				
	1971	1972	1973	1974	1975
A	24	25	17	11	6
B	10	55	126	190	144
C	13	17	20	19	7
D	0	0	0	0	2
E	0	0	0	46	19
F	863	565	678	696	542
G	0	0	0	47	483
H	0	0	3	5	0
I	0	0	0	209	668
J	471	734	760	774	607
K	0	0	0	0	1
L	0	0	0	3	3
M	19	31	23	20	28
N	0	0	0	0	350
	1,400	1,427	1,627	2,020	2,860
Other physicians not presently on staff	963	1,119	856	632	285
TOTALS	2,363	2,546	2,483	2,652	3,145

"A"GH service area showed it to be among the highest rate areas in the state.

Population-based data covering all hospitalizations of Maine residents have been available in that state since 1974. Analyses of the utilization of hospital services of area residents were introduced into the 1122 review process by staff members of the Maine Health Data Service (MHDS), a private organization (administratively part of Maine Blue Cross) responsible for collecting hospital use data in Maine. Although no formal mechanisms existed for introducing these analyses into the 1122 process, MHDS staff presented their studies to both the HSA and SHPDA staffs. The following findings were reported:

1) The age-adjusted discharge rate for residents of the "A"GH area was the second highest in the state:* 248 discharges per 1,000 population compared to the state averages of 164.

2) The age-adjusted rate of surgery for residents of the "A"GH area was one-third higher than the state average.

3) The rates for appendectomy, hemorrhoidectomy, cholecystectomy, and hysterectomy were all over twice the state average.

Table C.5 presents a summary of the MHDS analyses.

The statistical analyses prepared by MHDS occasioned another site visit by the state's consultant surgeon. This review concentrated on hysterectomies, cholecystectomies, and appendectomies. Again, the consultant reported his belief that a significant amount of unneeded elective surgery was being performed. This opinion plus the statistical analysis of MHDS convinced some SHPDA staff that the application should be denied and that a new application, without an increase in the bed complement, might be entertained after the admissions and surgical policy at "A"GH were improved.

Anticipating the SHPDA's concern, the hospital sought to obtain an outside assessment of admission and surgical practice, and thus hired the PSRO to carry out an evaluation of more than 300 patient records with special attention to surgical patients. The PSRO review, the full report of which was never made public, was summarized to the HSA and SHPDA staff as showing that 89 percent of all admissions were clearly justified using the AMA admission criteria (See *Screening Criteria to Assist PSROs in Quality Assurance,* AMA, Chicago, June, 1976) and that the remaining 11 percent could not be termed unjustified.

The positions of the various institutions and agencies involved in this 1122 application can be summarized as follows.

*The highest area in the state is an isolated rural area with approximately 1,200 residents.

Table C.5

"A" General Hospital

Ratio of "A" General Hospital to Maine Discharge Rate			
Surgical Procedures	1973	1974	1975
T & A	1.17	0.91	0.63
Appendectomy	1.71	1.85	2.67
Hemorrhoidectomy	0.57	0.71	2.71
Hernia	1.36	1.30	1.23
Prostate	0.58	1.09	0.56
Cholecystectomy	1.17	1.94	2.31
Hysterectomy	2.37	2.14	2.43
Mastectomy	1.29	1.29	0.95
D & C	2.04	1.80	1.67
Varicose Veins	0.80	0.71	0.57
Total	1.33	1.34	1.55
Diagnosis Discharge By Group	1973	1974	1975
Infectious and Parasitic Diseases	1.87	1.00	1.22
Neoplasms	1.41	1.38	0.65
Endocrine	1.36	2.04	1.96
Mental	1.29	1.37	1.96
Nervous and Sense Organs	1.07	0.95	0.79
Circulatory	1.30	1.27	1.31
Respiratory	1.71	1.73	1.85
Digestive	1.99	2.22	1.92
Genito-Urinary	1.67	1.82	1.72
Pregnancy	1.20	1.48	1.41
Skin and Tissue	1.21	1.34	1.18
Congenital	1.11	1.09	0.23
Ill-Defined	1.64	1.82	2.21
Injuries	1.53	1.97	1.80
Total	1.51	1.63	1.54
Patient Days Ratio	1.44	1.56	N/A

Source: Maine Health Data Service Analysis.

The hospital staff could not understand why the SHPDA was concerned over the rates of admissions in the "A"GH area. They were convinced that the quality of care they provided was good and predicted that the PSRO would find the admission policy justified. The hospital staff indicated that the high rate of alcoholism in the area plus the medical needs of the local poor, largely American Indian community accounted for the high admission rate in the area. Privately, the hospital staff agreed that in the past some physicians might have been overly enthusiastic in offering surgical treatments, but that this was now checked by an active tissue committee.

The HSA project review group made a site visit to the hospital and was impressed by the need for the overall project. The HSA advised the hospital to reduce from 11 to 7 the number of new beds to be added to the hospital. After the application was modified to the lower number of additional beds, the HSA formally recommended that the SHPDA approve the application.

The PSRO staff, although publicly reporting no evidence of unnecessary admissions at "A"GH, privately indicated that the quality of surgical practice could be strengthened. The PSRO staff believed that a denial of the 1122 application would alienate the hospital staff and jeopardize the opportunity to improve the quality of care through a future, joint "A"GH-PSRO program. Seven additional beds were seen as a small price to pay for the potential improvement of the quality of care.

The SHPDA staff was generally opposed to increasing hospital bed capacity of any hospital without unusual justification. In this case, the high bed-use rates combined with the opinion of the state's surgical consultant that significant unneeded surgical procedures were being performed at "A"GH were seen by the SHPDA staff as irrefutable evidence for denial of the application. The fact that the hospital and the PSRO would not release the results of the patient record review strengthened the staff belief that unneeded admissions and surgery were the cause of the high rates of hospital use among area residents.*

In spite of staff opposition to the bed expansion portion of the project, the Deputy Commissioner for Health approved the project after several meetings with hospital staff. His decision was based on his belief that the state could not challenge the appropriateness of admissions at "A"GH in the face of the PSRO's public statements. Further, the Deputy Commissioner believed that the absence of a State Facilities Plan would, in combination with the PSRO's position, cause a reversal of a negative decision on appeal. (Both the hospital and the HSA had made it clear that a negative decision would be appealed.) The project was formally approved on April 29, 1979.

---

*After considerable negotiation, the Hospital did release the first portion of the PSRO report to the SHPDA—the portion dealing with the appropriateness of admission. Findings on the indications for surgery were not released.

Discussion

This case illustrates the limitations of an analytical approach to health planning and regulation. The kind of epidemiologic studies performed by MHDS in this case are only possible in a few other states and, in fact, had never been applied to CON or 1122 reviews outside Maine. While similar analyses and arguments had been made (also unsuccessfully) in opposition to one previous 1122 application for bed expansion in Maine, the "A"GH case is significant because of the extreme nature of the hospital use statistics for area residents. In fact, no more extreme epidemiologic analysis could be anticipated for any other area of Maine or any other New England state. (Among areas with greater than 10,000 population, the "A"GH area is the second highest hospital use area in New England). Yet the unusual hospital use patterns of area residents were effectively rebutted by the PSRO patient record review. This case illustrates the fact that hospital planning is not essentially an analytic undertaking, but rather a process of negotiation and political trade-off.

The hospital completed its construction project in June, 1978, and has subsequently experienced a reduction in occupancy. The cost per patient day has been increased to compensate for the lower use rates and the added cost of the capital project. Hospital staff attributed the lowered occupancy rates to the effectiveness of its delegated, concurrent review program which reviews all patient admissions. No special PSRO quality assurance program has been undertaken to date.

The 1122 review of the "A"GH application has had serious implications for the hospital data collection system in Maine. In the course of the review process, the hospital threatened to withdraw from the data system implying that other hospitals would follow suit. Why should a hospital voluntarily provide its data to MHDS, to have the data used in opposition to its capital projects?

The role of the MHDS in hospital planning and facilities review had always been ambiguous. Though not actually prohibited from participating in 1122 and CON reviews, MHDS was not developed to support hospital regulation and no formal mechanism existed (or exists) to introduce population-based analyses into the facilities review process. In fact, the MHDS data are not directly accessible by the HSA and SHPDA; their availability to planners is dependent on the philosophy of the current MHDS staff.

At this writing, health data collection in Maine is undergoing a major reorganization; the Maine Health Information Center (MHIC) will become a private superagency responsible for all health data collection in the state. A major issue still to be resolved is how the collection of the Uniform Hospital Discharge Data Set will administratively relate to the MHIC, and which agencies will have access to this data. The issue of data access raised by the "A"GH case has not yet been resolved—how can a voluntary hospital data collection system be utilized by a state regulatory program? Although this issue would have doubtless been raised without the "A"GH experience, that case did serve to focus debate on who controls the use of these data. The Maine Hospital Association would like to control use of the data; the state and HSA advocate an open data use policy. Whatever the outcome, it appears unlikely that the MHDS staff will be able to continue indefinitely their ad hoc participation in hospital planning and regulation.

Case 7

"The Leonard Morse Incident": Whose Consumers Have More Clout?

Section 1501 of the National Health Planning and Resources Development Act of 1974 directed the Department of Health, Education and Welfare to develop "National Guidelines" for state and local health planning agencies by mid-1976. The guidelines were to include quantitative standards for the "appropriate" supply and distribution of health resources.

On September 23, 1977, a notice of proposed rulemaking on National Guidelines for Health Planning was issued in the *Federal Register*. The proposed guidelines, which had been developed in hurried fashion during the previous summer by a high-level HEW work group, caused an immediate furor. In short order, HEW was deluged by a record number of written comments. Providers, mustering considerable local support, complained that the proposed guidelines were too stringent, that they were unsubstantiated by empirical evidence, and that they would have an especially severe impact on smaller and rural hospitals. Local planning agencies complained that the proposed guidelines violated the spirit of "bottom up" planning. And in December, the House of Representatives unanimously passed a resolution calling on Secretary Califano to clarify and soften the proposed guidelines. About half the Senate signed a letter with a similar message to the Secretary. Secretary Califano responded in a letter to Congress in which he stated that the guidelines, although stringent, did not include any federal authority to close hospitals or to eliminate services. Speaking on the floor of the House of Representatives, Congressman Paul Rogers, a prime supporter of the planning program, reassured the members that the guidelines were only advisory in nature.

Despite these apparent clarifications and disclaimers, locally the Health Systems Agencies felt obliged to develop their own standards. The HSAs believed that it was crucial to their organizational viability to maintain the semblance of "bottom up" planning and to avoid appearing to be the pawns of HEW policy. At the same time, however, the HSAs were also keenly aware of the need to maintain good standing with HEW.

In the summer of 1977, the Boston HSA struggled with this balancing problem for one of the most controversial areas addressed in the proposed National Guidelines, obstetrical beds and maternity services. The controversy in Boston, which centered around one particular suburban hospital, came to be known locally as "The Leonard Morse Incident." The Leonard Morse story contains any number of lessons about health planning. The emphasis here will be on the difficulties encountered by HSAs when planning issues move beyond the HSA board room to the community arena. The Leonard Morse Incident highlights a key dynamic of citizen participation in health planning, the differences in motivation and perspective of consumer representatives on HSA Boards and consumers in the local community.

In late September of 1977, the Boston HSA, the Health Planning Council for Greater Boston, Inc., circulated the draft of its Health Systems Plan (HSP). The draft HSP contained a series of goals and objectives for obstetric beds and maternity services. These became the focal point of the Leonard Morse controversy. The most relevant sections of the HSP were these:

Hospital maternity services that are performing fewer than 1,000 deliveries should be required immediately to close or consolidate with other maternity services, subject to geographic constraints.* Services performing fewer than 1,500 (but more than 1,000) deliveries should be closed or consolidated by 1985. . . .

The number of obstetric beds in HSA IV should be reduced through closure and consolidation of maternity units.

By 1985, the following numbers of obstetric beds should exist in each Metro area: 244 beds in Central Metro; 78 beds in Northwest Metro; 18 beds in Southwest Metro, 51 beds in South Metro and 69 beds in West Metro.

*An exception would be made where travel time exceeded 30 minutes.

The 1,000 delivery standard fell below the state's 1,500 delivery figure and fell well below the 2,000 delivery figure in the Proposed National Guidelines for Health Planning. Nevertheless, it was a figure that few hospitals in the state could meet. In the West Metro area, where Leonard Morse is located, one hospital was (barely) able to meet the 1,000 delivery requirement. The specification of obstetric bed targets by Metro area added to the apparent stringency of the delivery target. It meant that the HSA was prepared to do more than simply promulgate broad quantitative targets for the HSA region as a whole. Indeed, the HSA indicated that it planned to specify institutions failing to meet the standards by name when it undertook the "appropriateness review"* of the health services in its area.

The 1,000 births and obstetric bed targets contained in the draft HSP were the products of the HSA's Plan Development Committee, working closely with the plan development staff. The 1,000 delivery figure had been proposed initially by the Director of Plan Development. Although there was considerable discussion within the Committee regarding the paucity of evidence supporting the 1,000 delivery target, it was accepted by the committee as a reasonable alternative to the 1,500 and 2,000 figures being advanced by the state and HEW, respectively. Provider members of the Committee raised some questions regarding the wisdom of generating any HSA policy on deliveries in the absence of compelling cost/quality information, even if seemingly "more reasonable" than the Massachusetts and national targets. But consumers on the Committee persuaded that it was important to "do something" to protect "bottom up" planning in the face of the proposed federal guidelines. In fact, consumer members considered the 1,000 delivery target as an obvious and sensible choice and chose to direct the Committee's attention to the issue of alternative delivery settings, preempting an extensive discussion of the 1,000 delivery target.

The Plan Development Committee primarily responsible for developing the HSA's maternity policies had ten members. The makeup of the Committee is shown below:

Plan Development Committee

Chairperson	VA Hospital Director
Provider	Blue Cross Representative
Provider	Director, major Boston Teaching Hospital

*PL 93-641 requires that HSAs periodically review the "appropriateness" of "all institutional health services" in their areas.

Provider   Harvard Community Health Plan
                                     Representative
Provider   Hospital Representative
Consumer   Female with background in Mental
                                     Health Organizations and Issues
Consumer   Below median income female with
                                     background in League of Women Voters
Consumer   Black female involved in neighborhood health
                                     centers
Consumer   Suburban housewife
Consumer   Below median income female active
                                     in women's health-related organizations

Leonard Morse Hospital (LMH) is located in the western suburbs of Boston. The hospital had only recently undergone a major expansion, from 70 beds to its current capacity of 262 beds. When the draft HSP calling for the 1,000 delivery minimum was first released, LMH was doing just under 700 deliveries per year. The Director of LMH, not favorably predisposed towards health planning generally, regarded the standards contained in the draft HSP as a direct threat to the hospital's future. Indeed, he believed that the hospital had been named in an earlier version of the draft plan as one of the many hospitals failing to meet the maternity targets. Accordingly, in an attempt to protect the hospital's interests, the Director initiated an extensive campaign designed to mobilize local support and to place the Leonard Morse maternity issue at the top of the community agenda. The strategy was to come to a head on November 16, 1977, when a "cavalcade of buses" would descend on the West Metro Public Hearing on the draft HSP.

LMH's opposition plan began with a major internal organizational effort. Working with the hospital's Department of Community Relations, the Director enlisted the support of the medical staff, the administrative staff, the Hospital Aid Association and the Trustees.* The attached letter to the administrative staff characterizes the internal organization effort.

---

*In 1972, when the Director first came to LMH, he had organized the trustees into three local Trustee Councils with membership elected by the community, enabling him to claim later that, in a sense, the community "owned" the hospital.

Leonard Morse Hospital-Natick

November 2, 1977

TO: All Management Staff

FROM: John H. Luttrell, Sr.
         Director of Community Relations

General Director O. David West has asked me to remind you that not much time remains until the November 16 hearing at Newton City Hall on the Health Systems Agency recommendations to close our Maternity and Pediatric Units.

If you have simply postponed writing a letter to Mr. West in support of continuing these vital services at Leonard Morse, do it today! Preferably, this should not be done on hospital letterhead, but use your personal stationery instead. It might also convey to the HSA the erroneous impression that Leonard Morse is trying to "stack the deck," if you were to identify yourself as a member of our staff.

You may also wish to emphasize the short time limitations to other members of your respective departments. We have had some written responses but many, many more are needed to produce the desired effect upon those who may be judging the very future of Leonard Morse.

Won't you do it now?

The next step was to mobilize support in the community. Letters went out to some 2,000 mothers who had delivered babies at LMH over the past three years, to 70 expectant mothers in the community, to Senator Edward Brooke and Congressman Margaret Heckler, to all Natick Town Meeting members and members of the Board of Selectmen, to the South Middlesex Legislature Caucus, to the Mothers of Twins, the Newcomers Club, the Natick Jaycees, to the State Senators and Representatives in the western suburban area, to the local clergymen, and to the local fire chiefs, among others. Special luncheons and coffee hours were held for some of these groups and those who attended were encouraged to drum up further support. The letter to Senator Brooke is an interesting example of the campaign to seek outside support:

Leonard Morse Hospital-Natick

October 24, 1977

U. S. Senator Edward W. Brooke
2003F John F. Kennedy Building
Boston, MA   02203

Dear Ed:

Although we have not corresponded since your apologetic inability to participate in the dedication of our totally new community hospital back in June of 1969, I can remember you expressed desire to be of any tangible help to Leonard Morse Hospital if or when the occasion ever arose.

On Wednesday, November 16, beginning at 7:30 p.m., in War Memorial Auditorium, Newton City Hall, spokesmen for this hospital and all of the eleven communities it serves, must show cause at a hearing conducted by Health Systems Agency (Area IV, West Metro) why our Maternity Unit, then Pediatrics should not be closed and consolidated into a regional hospital approach. By using arbitrary figures, that not even the HSA can authenticate, they are advancing the theory that "bigger is better" and that Leonard Morse cannot offer the same high quality patient care available at strictly maternity and newborn care centers.

We have all of the documents to prove that they are grossly in error but we are also realistic enough to know that we need strong political clout. Peg Heckler is hoping to testify, or, at least, to send one of her staff aides with a strongly worded objection to any maternity closure here. I honestly hope that you can do the same.

Although we do not wish to create a circus atmosphere, please rest assured that our supporters, overwhelmingly consumers, will be arriving at Newton City Hall in a stream of chartered buses. We shall have all top local legislators of both parties and selectmen from every town in our service area, together with uncounted numbers of mothers who have delivered here and expectant mothers planning to have their babies at Leonard Morse Hospital. Full newspaper, radio and television coverage is guaranteed.

Ed, if you can help bail us out, especially bearing in mind your ranking posture on the HEW Committee in Washington, we would be eternally grateful. If another commitment precludes a personal appearance by you, we would vastly appreciate a letter expressing your opposition to be read into the record, but addressed to either me or our General Director O. David West.

Ending on a more personal note, I have totally lost track of our mutual friend Cheako Ciarlone of Revere and I've wondered whether you have had further chance to encounter him during your return visits to Boston.

Willya try to give our request some priority in sufficient time for us to make plans for the November 16 presentation? With every kind personal regard, and with vivid memories dating back to your days on the Boston Fin Com, I remain

Warmly,

John H. Luttrell, Sr.
Director of Community Relations

The letter writing effort to mobilize community support was augmented by a media campaign. Advertisements were purchased in local newspapers to recruit support at the public hearing. (See Figure C.)

Editorials were written for both local and citywide print and electronic media. Reporters were invited to Leonard Morse to learn of the hospital's opposition to the draft plan. Much of the media response was favorable. This selection from a local newspaper article is typical:

> In an unprecedented saturation campaign involving the use of news and broadcast media, mass mailings, and the support of State senators, representatives, area selectmen, and selectmen, and Congressional aides, Leonard Morse has served strong notice that it plans to fight HSA tooth and nail. But, the hospital cannot possibly do it alone.
>
> If the HSA should only 'half-listen' to what hospitals are normally expected to say in justification of maintaining their services, it most certainly will perk up if the hearing chamber is packed with angry consumers who have instinctively turned to full-service Leonard Morse for the past 78 years.

Figure C

From *The Natick Bulletin*, Wednesday, November 2, 1977, pp. 1 and 6

AN ESSENTIAL NOTICE!

TO THE CONSUMERS
OF THE COMMUNITIES SERVED BY
LEONARD MORSE HOSPITAL:

Natick - Sherborn - Dover - Medfield - Millis - Medway - Framingham
Wellesley - Wayland - Needham - Holliston - Milford - Norfolk - Ashland
Franklin -Bellingham - Hopkinton

The Massachusetts Health Systems Agency (Area IV, West Metro), a consumer-dominated advisory board to the State Public Health Council, is recommending the immediate closing of all Maternity Units which have less than 1,000 deliveries per year. Pediatrics clearly will be next!

THIS MEANS LEONARD MORSE

Do you want YOUR children, YOUR grandchildren, YOUR nieces and nephews or YOUR BABY delivered in a distant impersonal regional setting . . . "Beating the clock", fighting traffic, unable to find parking?

OF COURSE NOT! SO HELP DO SOMETHING ABOUT IT

Consumers will listen to consumers. Attend the HSA hearing at Newton City Hall's War Memorial Auditorium, 1000 Commonwealth Avenue, on

Wednesday, November 16

beginning at 7:30 p.m. Let your voices be heard! Make your presence felt in overwhelming numbers!

FREE CHARTERED BUSES

Leaving Leonard Morse Hospital Main Entrance at 7 p.m.

Write to Your State Senators, Your Representatives, and Your Selectmen. Insist that they help us preserve and protect the Family-Oriented Health Care Needs furnished by LEONARD MORSE HOSPITAL for the past 78 years.

And, write your supportive letters to me, too. I will hand-deliver them at the Health Systems Agency Hearing on Wednesday, November 16. Remember, the ultra-modern Leonard Morse Hospital WAS BUILT for today's children and tomorrow's generations still unborn.

To Reserve Free Bus Reservations,
Call the LMH Office of Community
Relations, 654–3400, Extension 606,
No Later Than Monday, Nov. 14 by 4 p.m.

O. DAVID WEST, FACHA,
General Director,
Leonard Morse Hospital

Things don't just 'happen.' What a calamity and an irretrievable loss if Leonard Morse were forced to eliminate that newborn and sick young child from its patient population by default. And that is what could happen unless the 'inhabitants of Natick,' who literally own their fine community hospital, join hands with their neighboring townspeople in a massive outpouring at the November 16 hearing.

There's a tinge of bitter irony here, because the Health Systems Agency has absolutely no control over hospitals in Massachusetts, It can only recommend' its findings to the State Public Health Council, which has the muscle to make recommendations a reality. The names and numbers may have changed, but the 'game' remains the same.

Regretfully, the HSA appears to be playing a numbers game. Maternity-Pediatrics occupancy and cost figures seem to be its primary concern, with little or no thought given to the humanitarian and social aspects of patient care.

Leonard Morse, instead, prefers to concentrate exclusively on fulfilling total patient needs in its family-oriented hospital.

We also believe that an overwhelming majority of consumers served by Leonard Morse must be and should be appalled at this 'backdoor' approach to eroding the capabilities of one of the Commonwealth's superior hospitals.

But becoming angry and resentful simply isn't good enough. Action and personal involvement are inescapable, if the unspoken 'silent majority' apathetically sits on its hands while the vocal minority grabs all of the marbles. By then, it's too late.

In all of these enterprises, the internal organizational effort, the community campaign and the media campaign, the hospital stressed not only ideological and theoretical objectives to the draft plan, but presented the substantive merits of its case as well. The key points in the hospital's arguments were these:

1) Utilization of the LMH maternity facility had increased over the previous year from 675 to 692 births.
2) Rate-setting cost figures showed that costs at LMH were $100 less "per weighted delivery" than the region's average cost and, in any case, considerably less than the average cost in Boston.
3) Stillbirth rates, neonatal mortality rates, and premature infant rates at LMH were comparable to the West Surburban Hospital Association member hospitals and superior to state figures.
4) Concerns about travel time to larger regional centers and about the impersonal quality of care are legitimate.

As might be expected, given the size and scope of their organizational effort, Leonard Morse was able to have its case heard at the public hearing. About 500 supporters attended, including the recent and expecting mothers, local politicians, and representatives from Senator Brooke and Congresswoman Heckler's offices. Boston television and newspapers also gave the hearing wide coverage. "We had 500, but the problem was to keep the number down. We could have had 5,000," said the LMH Director.

In January 1978, the HSA published its final Health Systems Plan. The maternal and pediatric components of the plan softened the policies advanced earlier in the draft. The changes in policy reflected the intensity of the Leonard Morse opposition. They also reflected the results of public hearings held in other Metro areas, and the nationwide criticism that had been directed at the draft national guidelines. In December, in response to the proposed guidelines, Congress passed its resolution designed to protect smaller and rural hospitals. In Massachusetts, the state had served notice that it intended to qualify its 1,500 delivery and other targets. In a November letter to Congress, Secretary Califano allowed that "the currently proposed standard (2,000 delivery) for obstetrical units may be too strict." Indeed, on March 28, 1978, HEW issued final guidelines that, among other changes, considerably softened the delivery standard.*

The changes in policy in the Boston HSA's final HSP reflected this broader reappraisal. Moreover, the fact that an overall reappraisal was occurring allowed the HSA greater flexibility in deviating from federal and state standards and greater leeway to avoid taking immediate policy positions that would be difficult to substantiate. The final HSA plan could openly reflect the fact "that there is no unanimity of opinion, professional or other, on what the minimum size of hospital maternity units should be." Consistent with this, the policy in the final plan was, in fact, both more flexible and more tentative. It was not, however, really a major change. In the words of the HSA Plan Development Director, it was "two steps forward, one step back."

The relevant differences with the draft HSP were these:

1) Where the draft plans called for immediate closure or consolidation where a standard of 1,000 deliveries was not met, the final plan rolled back the time period to 1981, and to 1985 for services below 1,500.

2) The final plan allows that "exceptions may be justified on the basis of quality, location, cost and aggregate system cost criteria."

---

*In fact, the new standard of 1,500 births annually applied only to hospitals providing care for complicated obstetrical problems, see *Federal Register*, March 28, 1978, p. 13046.

3) The final plan abandoned the effort to specify pediatric levels by each Metro area, saying only that between 650 and 824 pediatric beds should exist in the entire HSA region.

This change in overall policy, of course, represented a victory of sorts for Leonard Morse. In addition, the hospital gained private assurance from both the HSA Executive Director and the Director of the State Health Planning and Resources Development Agency. These assurances, in the words of the LMH Director, amounted to a bargain—"you leave us alone, we'll leave you alone."

In fact, of course, neither the HSA nor the state had made any specific concessions to Leonard Morse. The HSA plan had never specifically targeted Leonard Morse or any other hospital. The "Leonard Morse Incident," after all, had involved broad planning policy and not specific regulatory decisions. In reality, neither the HSA nor the state had any real authority to close Leonard Morse or any of its services. And privately, the planners at the HSA acknowledged that on a cost and quality basis, the maternity services at Leonard Morse were up to par, perhaps better than most.

Postscript

The Leonard Morse Incident did not end with the publication of the HSA's final plan. In October of 1978, the HSA completed the First Annual Update of its Health Systems Plan. In the areas of maternity services and pediatric beds, the update reiterated the policies established in the plan. Nevertheless, Leonard Morse again primed to oppose the HSA Update, once again pointing its strategy towards a public hearing, this one scheduled for December of 1978. In a letter to the LMH General Director, the Director of Community Relations explained the hospital's interest in further opposition:

> Although the threat of closure of our maternity unit no longer appears as immediate, it exists nonetheless; and we would be well advised to conduct an update of our own to indicate what positive steps we have taken since last November 16 in the important areas of total deliveries, cost factors and the quality of health care.

In addition, the Community Relations Director expressed specific concern with two proposed HSA-wide task forces, one to look at low-volume maternity services and a second to initiate a pediatric regionalization project.

Hearing of the hospital's plans, the Executive Director of the HSA decided to visit the LMH trustees. Her visit allayed some of the trustees' fears if only inasmuch as it provided some perspective on the plan, pointing out that the HSA neither would nor could take any immediate action affecting Leonard Morse. At about the same time other hospitals began withdrawing some of their support for the LMH project. They felt that the basic objectives of the planned second protest had already been accomplished and, along with many community groups, felt that other issues deserved attention at the public hearing.

As a result, Leonard Morse re-evaluated its plan to stage a repeat of its earlier public protest. According to the LMH Director:

> This time prompting a massive turnout would be both inappropriate and unnecessary . . . last year Leonard Morse supporters astonished and impressed the HSA, and we made our point.

Planners at the HSA speculated that Leonard Morse had played down its protest because the hospital's image had begun to suffer, damaging both its substantive case and whatever positive fund-raising effort the earlier protest had caused.

Conclusion

A number of lessons can be learned from the "Leonard Morse Incident." This narrative, for example, might have emphasized the substantive and technical aspects of the disagreement regarding maternity and obstetric policy. It might have paid close attention to the reaction of other local providers. Or it might have focused more directly on interaction between federal, state, and local planning agencies and its impact on planning process and policy. Instead, this rendition of the Leonard Morse story has emphasized the role of citizen participation when planning issues reach the community agenda, paying close attention to the differences between consumer representatives on HSA boards and consumers in the community, and to the processes by which community consumers are mobilized.

At the HSA Board and Committee level, many of the ingredients of consumer support for planning are present in the LMH example. Most important were the size of the HSA area and the internalization by HSA consumers of broader organizational goals. None of the members of the HSA's Plan Development Committee, consumers or providers, came from the west suburban area. As a result, the members of the Committee could advance a policy aimed at regionalizing maternity and obstetrical services, although expressing some uncertainty as to the exact parameters of the policy, without involving any material interests of their own. In practice, given the size of many HSA areas, local and "public" interests are not always in conflict. In addition, the members of the Committee, especially the consumer members, regarded the interests of the HSA as a top priority. While there was some disagreement over the exact contour of the maternity and obstetric policy and a general uneasiness that data were not available to determine a "best" policy, there was a consensus that the HSA had to "do something" to protect the concept of local planning and to distinguish its policy from that of the state and federal agencies.

Since it was less stringent than the originally proposed federal (2,000) or state (1,500) delivery standards, the 1,000 target adopted seemed a reasonable compromise, one that would allow the HSA to walk the fence between federal and state approval and provide cooperation. One can only speculate whether the other major determinants of HSA consumer support for planning, ideological predisposition of consumer representatives, previous encounters with the expansionist tendencies of medical institutions, and on-the-job learning, played an important role.

The community support for Leonard Morse, on the other hand, demonstrates the difficulties planning encounters in the broader community arena. Although it required a substantial organization effort, it was a relatively straightforward matter for Leonard Morse to mobilize local support and place its case at the top of the community agenda. As interest and attention snowballed, so did the scope of the issues involved. A conflict that began over the possible impact of numbers in a plan on a local hospital came to involve a series of broader issues, including big government, the city versus the suburbs, and statistics versus human values.

Communities provide a ready pool of groups which can be mobilized around the bread-and-butter aspects of health planning, including jobs, local availability of services, tradition and civic pride, and so forth. The extent to which the supporters of Leonard Morse are representative of their communities is, of course, unclear. But the breadth of the support and the numbers involved do support the suggestion that the residents mobilized were more rather than less representative.

In the Leonard Morse example, local support was strengthened by the relative merits of the hospital's case and by a general sense that the interests of the west suburban area have been of little concern in the big city politics. Indeed, when PL 93–641 was first passed, the west suburban area had lobbied hard to have its own HSAs, and conflicts regarding the representation of suburban interests still play a major role in HSA politics. Neither of these factors is atypical. Few planning decisions are "clear choices," and identification with regional interests within an HSA area is common. In contrast to the HSA board room, in the community arena perceptions of local and public interest are often in conflict.

The Leonard Morse Incident also raises a question that cannot be resolved here: whether or not the residents of a community are always accurately represented by the demographic ambassadors who surface as consumer representatives on HSA boards and committees. Even where the demographics are the same, the interests may differ. Critics of planning would argue that in the Leonard Morse case, residents of the West Metro Area were neither accurately nor well represented on the HSA Board and the Plan Development Committee. Proponents would argue that the "Public" interest was served; they were "well" represented, irrespective of whether the demographic fit was exact. In his own way, the Director of Leonard Morse presented as a certainty what is, in fact, the central question in the Leonard Morse case:

> The HSA is comprised of consumers; we are certain they will not turn a deaf ear to the plans of other consumers who have been served so well by our fine hospital.

Case 8

Body Scanners in Boston: Protecting the Integrity of the Planning Process

On February 24, 1976, the Massachusetts Public Health Council, acting on the advice of the Director of the Office of Radiation Control and the Office of State Health Planning, authorized the installation of a single full body scanner in Massachusetts on condition that the institution acquiring it develop a sophisticated research program for evaluating the efficacy of CBT (Computerized Body Tomography) scanning. In his advice to the Council the Director of the Office of Radiation Control had said:

> The Council should consider an application for one, third generation body scanner within the state provided that such a machine is located in a research institution and is installed under rigid research protocols to determine the efficiency of the whole body CAT Scanner on patient outcome.

The Director's choice of words was significant. They implied that the DPH would apply the full range of criteria in evaluating CBT scanning; efficacy would depend not just on CBT producing better diagnostic information or a change in patient treatment, but on CBT's ultimate impact on patient outcome as well. In the context of the time, the Director's choice of language signaled the intention of DPH planners to take a hard line on CBT scanners limiting distribution until efficacy, which was expected to be great, had been more fully documented.

As far back as September of 1975, the Peter Bent Brigham Hospital, one of Boston's major teaching hospitals and a major referral center for

complicated medical cases of all kinds, had made an application for a
CBT scanner, and had worked closely with planners to establish
satisfactory research protocols. The planners were particularly encouraged by the Brigham's willingness to accept patients from Children's
Hospital, Beth Israel Hospital, Boston Hospital for Women, Sidney
Farber Cancer Institute, New England Deaconess, and a number of
community clinics. Five years of experience conducting utilization
studies of radiological diagnostic procedures for the National Institutes
of Health counted in the Brigham's favor as well. Capital costs for the
scanner ($570,000 later increased in a revised DON application to
$625,000) were at the low end of the spectrum for CBT scanners. The
Brigham's projected utilization of 2,500 patient procedures per year and
projected total charges of $260 per procedure ($200 technical component, $60 professional component) were also acceptable to the
planners in early 1976. The Brigham was expected to win approval for
its CBT scanner.

The Massachusetts General Hospital

While the Brigham's DON request was pending before the Public
Health Council, the Massachusetts General Hospital (MGH) moved to
acquire a CBT scanner of its own. MGH, however, was able to acquire
its scanner without going through the DON process. It did so by
entering into an arrangement with the manufacturer, EMI Ltd., of
England, whereby EMI would install a scanner at MGH for demonstration purposes for one year only. Massachusetts law requires a
Determination of Need only where a facility makes a "major capital
expenditure."* EMI classified the costs associated with the scanner as
"inventory costs chargeable against current operations," and therefore,
not as capital costs. Thus, neither MGH nor EMI had made a capital
expenditure in excess of $100,000 (the Massachusetts DON threshold
at the time). Technically, a Determination of Need was not required.

This turn of events posed problems for HSA and state planners.

---

*G.L. ch. 111 § 25 (c) reads: "no person . . . may make a substantial capital
expenditure for construction of a health care facility or a substantial change in
service unless the Department has determined that there is a need for such
substantial capital expenditure or change in service." In Section 5 (3) of the
Massachusetts Determination of Need regulations, "capital expenditure" is
defined as: "any expenditure, past, present, or future, which under generally
accepted accounting principles, is not properly chargeable as a cost of operation
and maintenance."

Although the EMI loan was for a one-year period, planners regarded the MGH scanner as more permanent. They expected MGH, with a sophisticated research program already well underway, to file for a DON at the end of the one-year period. Indeed, MGH had worked just this strategy successfully some years earlier when acquiring a head scanner. But both state and HSA planners had determined that only a *single* body scanner could be justified for research purposes in Massachusetts. They had urged strongly that proliferation of the new technology should await further investigation of its merits and they had worked closely with the Brigham to develop a research plan. To deny the Brigham application, they believed, would be to reward MHG for circumventing the DON processes and to disregard the Brigham's efforts to work within the planning process.

The DON staff phrased the dilemma clearly in their report to the Public Health Council:

> Staff has recommended that only one scanner is necessary to determine the efficacy of the procedure . . . but . . . staff notes that it may not be fair to deny an applicant who has, in good faith, undergone the rigors of the DON process because another institution has been successful in bypassing the very same process without violating the statute. In addition, would a denial encourage other institutes to follow the path MGH took? Staff is very concerned that a denial would be a clear incentive to all other institutions to exhaust all possibilities of bypassing the DON process.

Thus, what the planners had initially regarded as a clear and reasonable planning decision, to grant a single DON to the Brigham to evaluate full body scanning, had become a much more complicated problem. Rational planning principles had to be balanced against concern for the question of equity, and for the integrity of the planning process. On June 29, 1976, in an effort to uphold the credibility and integrity of the planning process, the Public Health Council approved the acquisition of a whole body scanner by the Peter Bent Brigham. In October of 1977, the CBT scanner was delivered to the Brigham and operation began a month later.

On January 1, 1977, the Massachusetts General Hospital formally requested a DON for the CBT scanner it had been operating on loan from EMI. When informed by both HSA and DON staff that the application would not be approved, MGH arranged to table its application. MGH continued to operate the scanner for the remainder of 1977 and 1978, building a comprehensive record of the efficacy of CBT scanning in the process.

In January of 1979, MGH again filed a DON for its scanner. The

DON request, however, was not for the body scanner it had "bor-rowed" from EMI. That scanner had experienced mechanical diffi-culties. Rather than apply to recondition the scanner, at an estimated cost of $500,000, MGH submitted a DON application for a new, state-of-the-art, $800,000 body scanner. It is anticipated that the MGH DON will be approved. One indication of this is the fact that HSA planners have decided to regard it as a "replacement scanner" rather than as a new machine being introduced to the hospital for the first time. This is explained, in part, by the fact that the new MGH application occurs in a context very different from 1976, the chief difference being that the efficacy of body scanning has been much more fully established. In addition, the MGH scanner is no longer the high-priority body scanning issue it once was. With CBT scanning now accepted as a routine diagnostic procedure, planners are directing their attention to CBT application from 14 other hospitals attempting to acquire scanners for the first time.

Conclusion

The Peter Bent Brigham-MGH case is short and straightforward. First, it illustrates the resourcefulness of hospitals attempting to evade regulatory programs. MGH was able to "borrow" a body scanner and eventually will parlay it into a new, state-of-the-art, CON-approved CBT scanner. Second, the Brigham-MGH case underscores the impor-tance of nontechnical factors in the review process. The Peter Bent Brigham scanner was ultimately approved in order to safeguard the integrity and the credibility of the planning process. It was approved in spite of the fact that, as a result of the MGH maneuver, the quota for CBT scanners then deemed acceptable by planners had already been met.

Case 9

Lewiston, Maine:
Hospital Ambitions Frustrated

On November 6, 1979, the voters of Lewiston had the opportunity to end the rivalry that existed between Lewiston's two hospitals, St. Mary's and Central Maine Medical Center. The hospitals' rivalry, of course, was not the issue on the ballot. Rather, it was the apparently mundane question of whether or not St. Mary's would be permitted to close a public street, Campus Avenue, in order to build a replacement hospital. As it turned out the election was close, with the proposal to close Campus Avenue losing by 149 votes out of the 14,000 plus cast. If the proposal had passed, St. Mary's ambitious $26 million rebuilding project, its "Health Care Campus Plan," would have taken an important step forward, gaining a clear indication of public support. The defeat, narrow though it was, places the rebuilding project in severe jeopardy.

The rivalry between the hospitals is an intense one, with deep roots in ethnic and class conflict. St. Mary's ties are to Lewiston's French-Canadian population which is said to constitute a majority of the city's 41,500 residents. The hospital is owned and operated by the Sisters of Charity (the Gray Nuns) who came to Lewiston a hundred years ago from Quebec to teach French to the children of the city's immigrant mill workers and who founded the hospital in 1888. The sign near the hospital's main entrance still reads Hôpital Général Sainte-Marie, reflecting the institution's ethnic heritage.

Central Maine Medical Center traces its origins to the hospital that the mill owners founded in 1891. While St. Mary's draws its patients mainly from Lewiston proper, Central Maine's prime service area is the surrounding communities, predominantly Yankee in composition, and especially the adjacent smaller, but wealthier, city of Auburn (see Table C.6).

Until recently, Central Maine was known as Lewiston General

Table C.6

Towns in Lewiston Service Area (1975)

	Percentage Distribution of Towns' Hospital Admissions			
Town	% To C.M.M.C.	% To St. Mary's	% To Lewiston	% To Other
Auburn	61.0	32.4	93.5	6.5
Durham	72.2	0.0	72.2	27.8
Greene	51.0	41.7	92.8	7.2
Leeds	55.9	19.1	75.0	25.0
Lewiston	34.3	61.7	96.1	3.9
Lisbon	37.9	27.2	65.1	34.9
Livermore	44.3	1.6	45.9	54.1
Livermore Falls	23.6	11.7	35.3	64.7
Mechanic Falls	63.4	19.4	82.8	17.2
Minot	72.1	14.0	86.0	14.0
Poland	49.2	19.4	68.7	31.3
Turner	70.2	15.6	85.8	14.2
Wales	50.0	40.9	90.9	9.1
Sabattus	43.1	51.2	94.3	5.7
Buckfield	48.6	14.1	62.7	37.3
Hebron	47.4	11.5	59.0	41.0
New Gloucester	53.6	16.8	70.4	29.6

Hospital. It acquired its new title in 1975 when the hospital was applying for permission from the state to purchase a CT scanner. The three other hospitals in Maine that were candidates to purchase scanners at the same time all claimed to be regional referral hospitals and had medical center as part of their name—Maine Medical Center (Portland), Eastern Maine Medical Center (Bangor), and Mid-Maine Medical Center (Waterville). By becoming Central Maine Medical Center, Lewiston General was seemingly proclaiming its ambition to be the referral hospital for the Lewiston-Auburn area, Maine's second largest population concentration.

Central Maine's ambition is frustrated by the existence of St. Mary's. The hospitals are nearly identical in size. Central Maine has 239 beds; St. Mary's had 233 beds. As might be expected, they have similar budgets and numbers of personnel. In the communities where Maine's other referral hospitals are located, the facility with medical center in its title clearly dominates (see Table C.7).

The competition between St. Mary's and Central Maine has intensified in recent years. Both have moved aggressively to add services and to attract physicians. St. Mary's has a cobalt unit, but so does Central Maine. St. Mary's has a new doctors' office building and subsidizes the

Table C.7

Hospital Statistics for Areas with
Competing Hospitals in Maine, 1978

		Beds	Admissions
Lewiston	Central Maine	239	9,000
	St. Mary's	233	7,600
Portland	Maine MC	525	20,950
	Mercy	176	7,000
	Osteopathic	180	6,850
Waterville	Mid-Maine	309	12,350
	Osteopathic	78	3,000
Bangor	Eastern MC	379	13,650
	St. Joseph	130	4,550
	Taylor Osteopathic	98	1,420

Source: American Hospital Association, *Hospital Statistics 1979*.

relocation of physicians to Lewiston, but so does Central Maine. When Central Maine applied for the scanner, St. Mary's reported that it intended to continue to refer patients in need of that service to Portland.

The height of competition has been the hospitals' duplication in emergency care. Lewiston is the core of a tri-county Emergency Medical Service region that requires the designation of a single hospital as the region's coordinator. Because emergencies constitute about 20 percent of local hospital admissions, potentially much was at stake. Both hospitals began to augment their EMS capacity. When the tri-county region decided to designate Central Maine as the coordinator and purchase an ambulance service and dispatch, St. Mary's withdrew from the regional groups and purchased its own ambulance company and dispatch. Lewiston is now blessed with two well-trained and highly rivalrous emergency units.

Perhaps because of the interhospital conflict, but more likely because of the closeness of Lewiston to Portland (only 30 minutes down the Maine Turnpike), the state's hospital regulators have always not been receptive to Central Maine's efforts to become a regional referral center. They delayed approval of the scanner for two years, permitting its purchase only after Portland's had reached capacity. Central Maine's requests for an argon laser and an eight-bed neonatal care unit also met regulator opposition. Fortunately, from Central Maine's perspective, the hospital's major renewal effort was completed in 1975 before facility regulation became a developed art in Maine.

St. Mary's is in a more difficult position. Although it has a relatively new wing, a building completed in 1960, its main unit is nearly eighty years old and no longer meets accreditation standards. Moreover, St. Mary's sister institution, the Marcotte Home, a 350-plus-bed nursing facility also run by the Gray Nuns, operates on a waiver from the state's Life/Safety Code that will soon expire and is unlikely to be renewed. The Health Care Campus Project, which involves the construction of a hospital addition and a new Marcotte Home and the conversion of existing buildings to service spaces, thus represents the hope of survival for St. Mary's and its affiliated activities.

Survival of St. Mary's is important to the Sisters of Charity. It is the last of several hospitals the order has operated in the United States and Canada, the others having been sold or closed becuase of financial difficulties and the pressure of government regulation. The Sisters are deeply committed to the practice of Catholic medical care and the preservation of French-Canadian culture, as are many of the older French-Canadian physicians and community members in Lewiston. Although members of the St. Mary's staff scoff at Central Maine's goal of becoming a teaching hospital in an area that has a service population of only 100,000 people, they take pride in the fact that their institution is the fifth largest in Maine and the only Catholic hospital in the state that can provide, independently, a near full range of medical services.

The cultural gap though between the hospitals may be fading. Half of Central Maine's clientele is Catholic. Despite the fact that it performs abortions and sterilizations, Central Maine now has the greatest share of Lewiston births. Occupancy is a perpetual problem at St. Mary's. Fading also may be strong ethnic ties. The French language daily in Lewiston ceased publication 20 years ago. The local radio stations offer two or three hours of French language broadcasting on Sunday mornings and have trouble finding announcers for the programs.

Central Maine did not provoke the opposition to the closure of Campus Avenue. Neighbors worried about expansion of St. Mary's and Bates College (the original campus on Campus Avenue) and the loss of a convenient public way initiated the referendum after the Lewiston City Council on a 4 to 3 vote approved its closure. But Central Maine makes clear its opposition to new facilities for St. Mary's that were not jointly planned. Dozens of times it has offered merger or other combinations in order to end the rivalry, not unmindful of Mid-Maine Medical Center's successful amalgamation with a competing Catholic hospital. Continually rebuffed, it now plans expansion of its own, an action certain to bring additional regulatory attention to the duplication of facilities in overbedded Lewiston. A source close to Central Maine said that St.

Mary's is now in "Box Canyon." He believes St. Mary's failure to accept merger or joint planning with Central Maine dooms its renewal plan to destructive regulatory harassment and will eventually force the very combination it seeks to avoid.

St. Mary's certainly expects problems with the regulators. It believed though that the referendum call on the street closure would be a potential blessing in disguise. A big victory for St. Mary's, certainly a possibility in predominantly French-Canadian Lewiston, would have meant that community support had been documented in a way regulators and state politicians could not ignore. Thus St. Mary's openly contributed funds to the supposedly independent Citizens to Close Campus Avenue Committee and helped select the committee's advertising agency for the referendum. Perhaps it was too blatant about its ambitions.

The defeat was crushing for St. Mary's, but it has not yet surrendered to Central Maine. St. Mary's announced subsequent to the election that it would proceed with the construction of a replacement building for the Marcotte Home. The plan to construct a new acute care facility was deferred, but not canceled. Opinions differ on the likelihood of a revised Campus Plan ever being presented. It is clear though that St. Mary's will now have to consider more seriously than it had in the past the option of reaching some sort of accommodation with Central Maine.

For Central Maine the election means that its frustrated plans to become a major referral center have new life. Any combination with St. Mary's would give it equal standing at the regulation table with centers in Portland, Bangor, and Waterville. Soon instead of having three of every medical innovation, Maine may have four. The voters in Lewiston may have kept Campus Avenue open, but in so doing they may have closed the opportunity for regulators to play one Lewiston hospital against the other in the effort to control the diffusion of medical technologies and services.

Index

About the Authors

DREW ALTMAN is currently Special Assistant to the Deputy Administrator of the Health Care Financing Administration. Prior to going to the government, Mr. Altman was a Research Fellow in the Interdisciplinary Programs in Health at the Harvard School of Public Health, a lecturer in the Department of Political Science at MIT, and a Principal Research Associate with the Codman Research Group. A Ph.D. candidate in Political Science from MIT, he received his M.A. in Political Science from Brown University. He has published several articles on health planning and the social sciences.

RICHARD GREENE, M.D., is Acting Director of Medical Research, Acting Director of Rehabilitative Engineering Research and Development Services, and Director of Health Services Research for the Veterans Administration. He was principal investigator in the Codman Research Group in Washington, D.C., and before that on the staff of the Harvard University School of Public Health. Dr. Greene has a Ph.D. in biology from Massachusetts Institute of Technology and an M.D. from Johns Hopkins University. He is author of *Assuring Quality in Medical Care* published in 1976.

HARVEY SAPOLSKY, currently Professor of Public Policy and Organization at the Massachusetts Institute of Technology, is the author of *The Polaris System Development: Bureaucratic and Programmatic Success in Government* and co-author of the forthcoming text *Blood Policy*. He has published a wide variety of articles on science, defense, and health issues and has contributed to *The Handbook of Political Science*. Dr. Sapolsky received his Ph.D. in Political Economy from Harvard University.

...micians — for example, the chief compiler of the *Ssu-ku ch* ... s... — would have it, might have been widely accepted by the ... ...rs. But the scholarly concerns of Li Kuang-ti 李光地 (1... ...ly one of the most influential court scholar-officials during t... ...gn, had by then already fallen into dispute.[86] This partly expla... ...e of Sung Learning: Li's effort to promote Chu Hsi's teaching ...ial sponsorship actually prompted a powerful yet subtle reaction ag... ...ficial line of interpreting the classics, or "official learning" (*kuan-h*... ...[87] It is thus important to note that the concept of learning was as mu... ...tical notion as an intellectual ideal. And Li Kung's uneasiness in h... ...rly endeavours, viewed from this perspective, may have been reflectec... ...umber of sensitive minds in the Ch'ien-Chia reign.

...e of the most intriguing problems in the study of early Ch'ing thought ...eral and the Ch'ien-Chia tradition in particular is the issue of "literary ...tion".[88] The attempt to establish the claim that the practice of *wen-tzu* ...字獄 ("literary cases") featured prominently in early Ch'ing politics is, ...r, not a fruitful way of approaching it. The issue involved is not one ...ermining how the system of ideological control actually worked in ...of the precise number of people directly affected. Rather, it has to ...h the "felt reality" of a highly oppressive atmosphere created by a ...us imperial policy of bringing the articulate minority in line with ...l" and thus "orthodox" learning. The difficulty of understanding this ...ex phenomenon partly lies in a subtle and fundamental metamorphosis ...self-image as well as the prescribed role of the Confucian scholar in ...ien-Chia era. This metamorphosis resulted in no small measure from ...erate imposition of political standards on scholarship and ingenious ...riation of intellectual ideas for the purpose of ideological control. ...ly the Confucian scholar, as a full participating member of society, ...s the responsibility of not only cultivating his personal self but also ...ng the human community as a whole. Although in practice he may ...a minor official in a local government, his spiritual self-identification ...cated on a comprehensive vision of self, society, world, and cosmos. ...ue scholar is thus a keeper of the Way as well as the master of his ...use. His consciousness of duty and his loyalty come from a morality ...in broad humanist terms rather than from a commitment to an

...*hung-kuo tsao-ch'i ch'i-meng ssu-hsiang*, 411–12.

...12.

...of examining this complex issue is to ascertain the nature of the books not included in the ...Although the methodological problems are by no means simple, the possibility is perhaps ...xploring. See William Hung's article mentioned in n. 68.

his teacher as a theorist of statecraft, he himself, as a result of the trips, significantly departed from his teacher in both methodology of study and epistemology.[75] Li's sense of guilt toward Yen, recorded in his chronological biography and expressed in his own writings, made the trips dramatic in terms of both his life history and the magnetic power of "erudition".

It is commonly assumed that Mao Ch'i-ling 毛奇齡 (1623–1716), the prolific author who was notorious for his questionable moral integrity, was mainly responsible for Li's involvement in a mode of scholarship fundamentally different from "real learning". Li's decision to study the classics, especially the *Book of Change*, under Mao in 1698 is considered the crucial event in this connection.[76] It seems, however, that Li's fascination with the kind of learning characterised by Mao's work was symptomatic of a much more complex process. Mao may have been the principle tempter, but Li had been already exposed to what may be called the "philological studies of the south" through his friend Wang Fu-li 王復禮 during his first journey to the south in 1695. According to Li's chronological biography, his encounter with Yen Jo-chü, Hu Wei, and Wan Ssu-t'ung in Peking in 1700, two years after his meeting with Mao, was particularly significant for his intellectual development.[77] But since Jo-chü died in 1704 and Wan in 1702, Li could not have studied with them for very long. Nor does he seem to have maintained a close relationship with Mao for an extended period of time. Perhaps it was not the influences of single individuals but the atmosphere of scholarly centres such as Yang-chou 揚州 and Ch'ang-chou 常州 in the south and Peking in the north that can really account for Li's "conversion".

Nevertheless, it is quite misleading to take the idea of conversion literally. Li's personal loyalty to Yen Yüan remained strong throughout his life, lasting for almost two decades after Yen's death in 1704. Furthermore, it was because of Li that the single-minded scholar Wang Yüan 王源 visited Yen and pledged his total dedication to Yen's teaching when he himself was approaching sixty years of age.[78] And it was because of Wang's introduction that Li befriended the T'ung-ch'eng scholar Fang Pao 方苞 (1668–1749).[79] The controversy of Fang's interpretation of Li's departure from Yen in an

---

[75] Ch'ien, *Chung-kuo chin san-pai nien hsüeh-shu shih*, 203; Hou, *Chung-kuo tsao-ch'i ch'i-meng ssu-hsiang*, 386–90.

[76] Ch'ien, *Chung-kuo chin san-pai nien hsüeh-shu shih*, 206–9.

[77] *Li Shu-ku nien-p'u*, under 42 *sui*, 3:8a–14a.

[78] Ibid. 3:2b.

[79] Ibid., under 45 *sui*, 3:21a.

unsolicited epitaph should not concern us here.[80] Yet the very fact that a committed Sung scholar could claim the example of Li as support for his philosophical position is worth noticing. It should also be noticed that after Li's first trip to the south, his exposure to Lu Shih-i's *Ssu-pien lu* prompted him in 1698 to compose a treatise on the *Great Learning*.[81] The treatise fully demonstrates that Li subscribed to a version of the Chu Hsi view that knowledge and action are in principle separable and that the acquisition of knowledge should precede its transformation into action.[82]

Neither the cause nor the effect of Li Kung's newly assumed cast of mind allows an easy explanation. But the form in which his scholarship was constructed clearly symbolises the social prestige of erudition. The ability to conduct purely scholarly inquiry, specifically the capacity to acquire professional skills in philological studies and textual analyses, became an unquestioned standard of excellence in intellectual circles. No matter what other competences one happened to possess, this was the required "rite of passage" in the Ch'ien-Chia scholarly world. Was it, then, social prestige that motivated Li Kung to change his mind?

It is beyond question that erudition as a mode of scholarship was a social as well as an intellectual ethos. The case of Tai Chen is instructive. Tai's entrance into the Peking coteries of learning was mainly the result of his sound knowledge of the classics. But without the proper introduction of well-established authorities such as Ch'ien Ta-hsin, Tai could not have gained an easy access to "establish friendship" with Wang An-kuo 王安國 (1694–1757), Chi Yün 紀昀 (1724–1805), and Wang Ming-sheng 王鳴盛.[83] His ability to develop an impressive network of social relations was certainly a major reason for his success in the high-powered group clustered around Wang and a few other senior scholars. In the light of examples of this kind, it is possible that the combined force of personal push and communal pull accounted for much of Li Kung's significantly altered scholarly orientation. Li's dilemma is quite understandable: his credibility as a serious scholar was necessary for transmitting the way of his teacher to the centres of learning; yet the only way for him to earn that credibility was to take up a mode of

---

[80] Hou, *Chung-kuo tsao-ch'i ch'i-meng ssu-hsiang*, 383–84.

[81] See Li's acknowledgment in his *Ta-hsüeh pien-yeh* 大學辨業 (A critical exercise on the *Great Learning*), in *Yen-Li ts'ung-shu*, vol. 25, *t'i-tz'u*, 3a.

[82] Ibid. 3:2a–b.

[83] See Tai's *Nien-p'u* in *Tai Chen wen-chi*, under 33 *sui*, p. 221. The *Nien-p'u* notes in fact that the other outstanding members of the class of 1854 of *chin-shih* 進士, such as Chi Yün, Wang Ming-sheng, Wang Ch'ang 王昶 and Chu Yün 朱昀, knew about Tai at the same time as Ch'ien did.

...holarship defined in terms fundamentally different ...ught to appreciate as the practical and the real w...

Li Kung's ambivalence toward what his teacher, ...as the learning of the "students of books" and of t... probably not an isolated phenomenon. The very ... scholars preferred to characterise their learning as ... Learning) and that the students of Ch'ien Ta-hsin oft... as *P'u-hsüeh* 樸學 (Plain Learning) indicates that t... themselves by no means saw erudition merely as a f... sense, I suppose, Chang Hsüeh-ch'eng's insistence o... "singularity" (*chuan* 專) was really meant to be a c... narrowly defined as *K'ao-cheng* 考證 (philology).[84] ... among Confucian scholars of all persuasions was t... words" (*k'ung-yen* 空言). For the study of the cla... exercise in words, it would have to be linked up w... ing greater than philology. Li Kung's feeling of gu... old age that only after he had failed to establish ... meritorious service did he take up the task of wri... the efficacy of his words was more than simply a ... famous "three immortalities". With a sense of tra... poor health and frustrated ambitions compelled ... texts as a commentator and, by implication, to ...

One wonders if Li's sentiments were not als... contemporaries, including both those who gained a... tutors and those who received imperial recognitio... Intellectual giants such as Tai Chen and Ch'ier... seriously doubted the supreme value of their sch... of a new tradition, they considered scholarship a... concern". Even among the less-known Ch'ien-C... Ch'ang 王昶 (1724–1806), Chu Yün 朱昀 (1729–81)... (1717–95), there is no evidence to show that they... committed to their studies. The problem was n... researchers and teachers. The available documen... was a great deal of that in virtually all of the e...

However, it is an entirely different matter t... value of their intellectual pursuits. The idea of ...

---

[84] For example, see Chang Hsüeh-ch'eng's critical reflection on Tai ...篇後 ("Further thought on the essay on Chu Hsi and Lu Hsi...

[85] See Li Kung, "*Shih Ching chuan-chu* t'i-tz'u 詩經傳注題辭" (Pref... Book of Poetry), in *Yen-Li ts'ung-shu*, vol. 31, 11:7b.

---

acade... Yün ... maste... certai... hsi re... declin... imper... the of... 官學)... a poli... schola... in a n...

On... in gen... inquis... *yü* 文... howev... of det... terms ... do wi... consci... "officia... comple... in the ... the Ch... a delib... approp...

Idea... 'assume... regulat... serve a... is predi... The tr... own h... defined...

[86] Hou, ...

[87] Ibid., ...

[88] A way ... Ssu-k'u... worth ...

existing polity. For example, Ch'eng Hao 程顥 (1032–85) took his assignments as a low-level bureaucrat (such as keeper of records or assistant prefect) no less seriously than his role as a teacher. His younger brother, Ch'eng I 程頤 (1033–1107), maintained that only through a detailed description of what Hao did as a bureaucrat could the meaning of his exemplary teaching be fully appreciated.[89] Yet it is evident in Ch'eng Hao's case that the dignity of serving as a minor official was linked to a structure of meaning not at all reducible to the political realm. In other words, it was precisely the morality that transcended politics that informed Master Ch'eng's role as both a bureaucrat and a teacher, for he never doubted that he, as well as anyone else, had a legitimate claim to speak for the Way.

In a highly politicised culture, the emperor tried to monopolise access to and claims on the Way: he alone was the keeper of the Way. The role of the scholar, by contrast, was reduced to little more than an echo of the "sageliness" of the king. The Ch'ing emperors were in fact more deserving to assume such a privilege than, say, the Ming emperors. K'ang-hsi, for one, actually worked very hard to achieve it. But by the Ch'ien-Chia period, when such an assumption had been defended with absolute authority, the intellectual atmosphere was extremely oppressive. Tai Chen's attack on the philosophy of "principle" (*li*) may not have been motivated by political considerations. Yet his appeal to human feelings as a repudiation of the imposition of rigid moral standards on the people had political implications.[90]

There were seemingly self-contented Ch'ien-Chia scholars who pursued learning for its own sake, for the eighteenth century was generally peaceful and prosperous and highly conducive to uninterrupted scholarly endeavours. Ch'en Ho 陳鱣 (1757–1811), whose diary provides us with a rare glimpse of the daily life of a well-known erudite over a period of fifty years, is a case in point.[91] A dedicated disciple of Ch'ien Ta-hsin, Chi Yün, and other masters, his whole life can be summarised as *tu-shu* 讀書 (book reading). Underlying his apparently uneventful career and vocation as a student-teacher, numerous anecdotes vividly depict his social relations, familial ties, intellectual encounters, personal feelings, and political concerns. His "book reading", an

---

[89] For Ch'eng I's biography of Ch'eng Hao, see *I-ch'uan wen-chi* 伊川文集 (Collected literary works of Ch'eng I), in *Erh-Ch'eng ch'üan-shu* 二程全書 (The complete works of the two Ch'engs; Ssu-pu Pei-yao ed.), 7:1a–7a.

[90] See Tai, Chen, *Meng Tzu tzu-i shu-cheng*, 4–5.

[91] See Ch'en Ho, *Tu-shu kai-kuo chai ts'ung-lu* 讀書改過齋叢錄 (Miscellaneous records of the *Study of Reading Books and Correcting Mistakes*; photocopy of the original manuscript in the National Central Library, Taipei: Cheng-chung 正中 Book Co., 1969).

intense and unceasing effort at intellectual and moral self-development, was perhaps the norm of pure scholarship in his age.

From the perspective of intellectuals in the nineteenth century, the single-minded commitment of the Ch'ien-Chia masters to pure scholarship must have evoked a sense of nonreality. Even the great phonologist and classicist, Ch'en Li 陳澧 (1810–82), whose scholarly interests were very close to theirs, predicted that as Han Learning declined it was inevitable that Sung Learning would again emerge as a dominant intellectual force.[92] This is particularly remarkable because Ch'en was so much overwhelmed by the erudites that he confessed, as he turned fifty, that he could never reach the standards of excellence set by Chiang Yung 江永 (1691–1762) and Tai Chen and that all he could hope for was a level somewhere between the Chu Hsi study of Wang Mou-hung 王懋竑 (1668–1741) and the Han Learning of Ch'eng Yao-t'ien 程瑤田 (1725–1814).[93] Despite Ch'en's awe-inspiring list of scholarly accomplishments, however, he was deeply concerned about the fate of the dynasty and the future of the Confucian Way at the time of the Opium War of 1842.[94] Like his learned friend Wei Yüan 魏源 (1794–1857), Ch'en symbolised by his extensive involvement in geographical studies the emergence of a new perception of learning, which expectedly reopened many fundamental issues in Neo-Confucian thought.[95] By contrast, Ch'ien-Chia scholarship was "pure", "plain", and remotely "ancient".

---

[92] See Wang Tsung-yen 汪宗衍, *Ch'en Tung-shu hsien-sheng nien-p'u* 陳東塾先生年譜 (Chronological biography of Ch'en Li; Hong Kong: Commercial Press, 1964), 47–48.

[93] Ibid., 79.

[94] Ibid., 26–27.

[95] Ibid., 43–44.

8

Towards a Third Epoch of Confucian Humanism

In his "Values of Confucianism", Vitaly A. Rubin observes that "the last decades have witnessed an extremely significant phenomenon in Chinese cultural and intellectual life outside Communist China: the revival of Confucianism. This movement, which is about thirty years old, has been called 'New Confucianism'".[1] For those of us actively involved in the movement, Rubin's encouraging words are most precious. It is gratifying to hear such sympathetic words in the wilderness where perpetual silence has been taken for granted. Although I never had the opportunity to speak with Rubin face to face, I have heard his inner voice in his writings and felt this intelligence and his searching mind. Rubin thought not only with his head but also with his heart, indeed with his entire body and soul.

In this essay I intend to discuss the possibility of a third epoch of Confucian humanism, an issue that fascinated Rubin. I will first take the Levensonian interpretive stance as a point of departure in order to identify the question. After a brief survey of the historical background, I will try to assess the contemporary situation in the perspective of the modern transformation of Confucian China. The essay ends with a look toward the future.

The Question

The question of whether a third epoch of Confucian humanism is possible has intrigued students of Chinese intellectual history for decades. Joseph Levenson's monumental attempt to understand the dilemma of the modern

---

[1] Vitaly Rubin, "Values of Confucianism", *Numen* 38, no. 1 (1981): 72. For a comparable interpretive position, see Rubin, "The End of Confucianism?" *T'oung Pao* 49 (1973): 68–78.

Chinese thinker responding to the impact of the West answers this question in the negative.[2] For those who were privileged to know Levenson personally, however, the statement that the "Mozartian historian"[3] makes about Confucian China and its modern fate is not only the verdict of a disinterested judge but also the lamentation of a poet-philosopher. Levenson is said to have been anguished over the demise of the Confucian amateur ideal. Yet, despite his admiration for the Confucian literatus, he concluded that, in an increasingly specialised and professionalised modern society, the scholar-official ideal was outdated. As the feudal society that nourished Confucians degenerates, Levenson observed, Confucian humanism inevitably fades into the background.[4]

An important assumption in the Levensonian interpretation is Max Weber's characterisation of the modern West as the triumph of rationality. An obvious implication of Weber's thesis is that traditional forms of life will all be destroyed as the modernising process that originated in the Calvinist spirit of capitalism in Western Europe engulfs the whole world. The levelling power of science and technology will eventually render major historical religions inoperative as differentiating cultural factors. The technocrat, rather than the literatus, will rule the universe. Confucian humanism, in the Levensonian perspective, can only remain a faint memory in the minds of those who still cherish the ideal of the amateur who writes poetry and thinks great thoughts for pleasure.[5] The Confucian heritage may still have a place in the "museum without walls",[6] dominated though it is by what Weber refers to as "bureaucratic authority".[7] This remaining place contains little hope, however, that Confucianism can reemerge as a dynamic intellectual force in the twentieth century.

Levenson's interpretation of the fate of Confucian China may be arbitrary. But the argument that Confucianism has only historical significance for contemporary China is widely accepted as self-evident and thus as true. A clear

---

[2] Joseph R. Levenson, *Confucian China and Its Modern Fate: A Trilogy* (Berkeley and Los Angeles: University of California Press, 1968).

[3] The term is borrowed from the title of a collection of essays in memory of Levenson, *The Mozartian Historian: Essays on the Works of Joseph R. Levenson*, Maurice Meisner and Rhoads Murphey, eds. (Berkeley and Los Angeles: University of California Press, 1976).

[4] Levenson, *Confucian China*, general preface, x.

[5] Ibid.

[6] Ibid.

[7] From *Max Weber: Essays in Sociology*, H. H. Gerth and C. Wright Mills, trans. and eds. (New York: Oxford University Press, 1958), 196.

indication of the influence of the Levensonian interpretation is the common practice among Western students of modern China to label post-May Fourth (1919) Confucians as traditional, conservative, or reactionary. They take it for granted that the incongruity between Confucian traditionalism and rational, scientific modernism is so clear-cut that the rise of modernity in China entails the demise of the Confucian tradition.[8]

A number of scholars have tried to develop alternative explanatory models. A fruitful approach has been to explore the lives and thoughts of the "traditionalists", "conservatives", and "reactionaries" in order to see how they wrestled with "modern" Western questions. In the collection of essays *The Limits of Change*, the perimeters of Confucian conservatism are extended to include spiritual values.[9] These essays serve as a corrective to the stereotypical image that Confucianism caused traditional Chinese political culture to be dominated by an authoritarian, gerontocratic, and male-chauvinist orientation. Guy Alitto's study of Liang Shu-ming 梁漱溟 vividly attempts to apply Confucian ideas to village governance in the twentieth century.[10] Liang may very well have been "the last Confucian", but the Confucianism that he advocated may outlast such influential modern ideologies as socialism, liberalism, democratism, and scientism in both theory and practice in China.

Thomas Metzger, in his thought-provoking reflection on the "predicament" of the Neo-Confucian personality, seriously challenges the Weberian explanation of the Confucian ethic as one of making "adjustment to the world".[11] Instead Metzger demonstrates that the dilemma of a typical Confucian, caught between self-cultivation and social service, is likely to generate an internal psychic dynamism comparable in intensity to that generated in the Calvinist under the influence of the Puritan inner asceticism. The Confucians, in this view, shape the world according to their cultural ideal; they do not simply submit themselves to the status quo. It is debatable whether the Neo-Confucians were inescapably constricted by what Metzger describes as the unpleasant state of affairs, given their ontological assumptions and existential conditions. Metzger's claim that the impact of the West actually provided an outlet by which the Neo-Confucians escaped their unbearable

---

[8] Levenson, *Confucian China* 3:110–25.

[9] *The Limits of Change: Essays on Conservative Alternatives in Republican China*, Charlotte Furth, ed. (Cambridge, Mass.: Harvard University Press, 1976); see articles by Chang Hao 張灝, Lin Yü-sheng 林毓生, and Tu Wei-ming 杜維明.

[10] Guy S. Alitto, *The Last Confucian: Liang Shu-ming and the Chinese Dilemma of Modernity* (Berkeley and Los Angeles: University of California Press, 1979).

[11] Max Weber, *The Religion of China*, Hans H. Gerth, trans. and ed. (New York: The Free Press, 1964), 235.

predicament is also debatable. However, his assertion that Confucian ethics is transformative in the Weberian sense is well founded.[12]

A concerted effort to investigate the inner logic as well as the internal dynamics of the Neo-Confucian tradition began in the United States in the early 1960s. Led by Wm. Theodore de Bary, a series of research conferences was held in America and Europe to encourage scholars from both the East and the West in the study of the second epoch of Confucian humanism. The four collections of essays subsequently published represent an attempt to probe the meanings embodied in the lives and philosophies of Neo-Confucian thinkers.[13] This attempt would have been impossible without the active participation of contemporary exemplars of the Confucian heritage, notably Wing-tsit Chan 陳榮捷 of the United States, T'ang Chün-i 唐君毅 of Hong Kong, and Okada Takehiko 岡田武彦 of Japan. By their exemplary teaching, they inspired a whole generation of American scholars to undertake the difficult task of understanding and interpreting Confucian "codes" in terms of contemporary Western conceptual apparatuses.

On the surface, Levenson's assessment of the fate of Confucian China is diametrically opposed to de Bary's faith in the relevance of the Confucian project to the concerns of our times. Political events since the untimely death of Levenson in 1969 suggest that the fate of Confucianism in China remains an open question. Few people doubt the relevance of the Confucian tradition to the emerging political culture in the People's Republic of China. Industrial East Asia's success in the last two decades in competing with the United States and Western Europe in manufacturing enterprises and high technology presents another situation. Its ingenious employment of culturally specific development strategies raise challenging questions about the relationship between Confucian ethics and the East Asian entrepreneurial spirit.[14] Some sociologists, fascinated by the economic performance of the "post-Confucian states" (Japan, South Korea, Hong Kong, Taiwan, and Singapore), have even proposed new concepts such as "modern capitalism"

---

[12] Thomas A. Metzger, *Escape from Predicament: Neo-Confucianism and China's Evolving Political Culture* (New York: Columbia University Press, 1977).

[13] *Self and Society in Ming Thought*, Wm. T. de Bary, ed. (New York: Columbia University Press, 1970); *The Unfolding of Neo-Confucianism*, Wm. T. de Bary, ed. (New York: Columbia University Press, 1975); *Principle and Practicality: Essays in Neo-Confucianism and Practical Learning*, Wm. T. de Bary and Irene Bloom, eds. (New York: Columbia University Press, 1979); and *Yüan Thought: Chinese Thought and Religion Under the Mongols*, Hok-lam Chan 陳學霖 and Wm. T. de Bary, eds. (New York: Columbia University Press, 1982).

[14] Tu Wei-ming, "Confucian Ethics and the Entrepreneurial Spirit in East Asia", seminar presentation in Business Administration, National University of Singapore, August 31, 1982. Included as chapter 3 in Tu Wei-ming, *Confucian Ethics Today: The Singapore Challenge* (Singapore: Federal Publications, 1984).

and "second modernity" to describe the new phenomenon.[15] If Levenson were alive today, would he fundamentally revise his interpretive stance?

Levenson, as an intellectual historian dedicated to probing the thinking person in his total context, was particularly sensitive to the ability of the Confucian in contemporary China to produce original and creative perspectives. This he felt to be painfully deficient. He did not find the influential intellectuals who shaped the currents of thought in modern China to be creative or original. In fact, he found virtually no evidence of the originality and creativity required for Confucianism to become a living tradition either in the active participation of articulate Westernisers or in the contemplative reflection of erudite classicists. One wonders, however, whether he would have changed his perception had he encountered the writings of an unusual metaphysician such as Hsiung Shih-li 熊十力, or a philosopher of culture such as T'ang Chün-i, or a concerned intellectual such as Hsü Fu-kuan 徐復觀, or an idealist thinker such as Mou Tsung-san 牟宗三.

As our knowledge of the lives and thoughts of the Sung–Ming Confucian masters increases, thanks to de Bary and his colleagues, the Levensonian outlook becomes even more poignant. The days of Chu Hsi 朱熹 (1130–1200) and Wang Yang-ming 王陽明 (1472–1529) are gone forever. Even the glory of Tai Chen 戴震 (1723–77) is hardly visible in the philosophical writings of modern Confucians. Many of the alleged followers of the Confucian Way are more reminiscent of the characters in Wu Ching-tzu's 吳敬梓 *Ju-lin wai-shih* 儒林外史 (The scholars): petty, superficial, selfish, and irrelevant. Lu Hsün's 魯迅 (1881–1936) apparent cynicism about Confucian ritualism realistically identifies much in the Confucian practice that is callous, insensitive, and outmoded. The more we learn about the Confucian tradition, the more we are convinced that its modern expression is not what it is supposed to be.

A comparison of the *t'i-yung* 體用 (substance–function) dichotomy in Chu Hsi's thought with Chang Chih-tung's 張之洞 (1837–1909) formula ("Chinese learning as substance and Western learning as function") clearly shows how the subtlety of a dynamic category can become an excuse for nonthinking. This, of course, does not mean that Chang's effort to bring such categories in traditional Chinese philosophy as *t'i-yung* to bear upon the modern situation is not significant. Indeed, his formula may have been an ingenious way of softening the Western impact. Nevertheless, in regard to creative thought, Chang's dichotomy is indicative of the paucity of the Confucian response to the intellectual challenge presented by the West. Levenson was right in characterising much of the wishful thinking among

---

[15] See Peter Berger's "An East Asian Development Model?" in *In Search of An East Asian Development Model*, edited by Peter L. Berger and Hsin Huang Hsiao (New Brunswick, USA and Oxford, UK: Transaction Books, 1988), pp. 3–11.

contemporary Chinese literati as an index to the identity crisis of the modern mind of China.[16]

In a deeper sense, Levenson's negative response to the question of whether there is a possibility for the development of a third epoch of Confucian humanism serves as an excellent point of departure for exploring the narrow ridge where a positive response might be found. To put it differently, the concrete procedure by which this possibility might be realised must begin with the recognition that the Confucian world studied by de Bary and his colleagues is no more. De Bary himself and some of his colleagues are aware of the intellectual challenge. This realisation does not imply, however, that the only hope for a Confucian revival in modern China is resurrection. Reanimating the old to attain the new is surely still possible in Confucian symbolism, but to do so the modern Confucian must again be original and creative, no matter how difficult the task and how strenuous the effort.

To retrieve the meaning of a tradition after the naive certainty of its universal truth has been thoroughly criticised is no easy task. The effort required to overcome the sense of estrangement and to bridge the gap between classical texts as dead letters and as living messages is no simple effort. The systematic inquiry into the lives and thoughts of the Sung–Ming Confucian masters is only the first step. Scholarly endeavour alone may not bring about an intellectual renaissance. Egyptologists, or for that matter Buddhologists, cannot by themselves breathe vitality into ancient scripts. Nor can Sinologists alone bring about a new epoch in Confucian learning. Numerous political, social, and cultural factors are involved. The upsurge of interest in Confucian ethics in the 1980s, sharply contrasted with the anti-Confucian sentiments of the 1960s, was not predicted. Nor has there been a sophisticated explanatory model to help us appraise its seemingly far-reaching implications. The veil of ignorance is so extensive that we are at the mercy of external forces that are often beyond our comprehension.

This sense of uncertainty, verging on perplexity, is not at all alien to the Confucian experience. Confucius himself is said to have constantly worried about the fate of his teachings, although he was not particularly worried about his own lot.[17] His concern for the well-being of the cultural tradition, for a form of life that was thought to have been inherited from King Wen 文王 and the Duke of Chou 周公, was shared by Mencius 孟子, Hsün Tzu 荀子, and virtually all subsequent Confucian masters. The idea that the line of transmission has been broken and that extraordinary measures must be

---

[16] See Joseph R. Levenson's argument in his *Liang Ch'i-ch'ao and the Mind of Modern China* (Cambridge, Mass.: Harvard University Press, 1953).

[17] *Analects* 7:3.

taken to ensure the proper transmission of the Way (*tao-t'ung* 道統) began long before Han Yü's 韓愈 (768–824) famous essay on the subject. Han Yü's unique contribution lies in his definition of the *tao-t'ung* as the human way, in contradistinction to the Buddhist dharma.[18] Neo-Confucians since Chang Tsai 張載 (1020–77) have taken this identity of the Confucian Tao as their ultimate concern. A fear that "this culture" (*ssu-wen* 斯文)[19] would perish if they did not continue to embody the Tao in their ordinary daily existence was pervasive among the Neo-Confucian thinkers.

Historical Background

Han Yü's claim that the transmission of the Confucian Way had been broken since Mencius was widely accepted by Confucians of the Sung–Ming 宋明 period, but historically it is a gross exaggeration. The claim overlooked the fact that it was in the Han 漢 dynasty (206 B.C.–A.D. 220) that the Confucian polity become firmly established. The interplay between the Confucianisation of the Legalist bureaucracy and the politicisation of Confucian moral values characterised much of the dynamics of the Han governing mechanism.[20] It is true that the following Wei 魏 (220–65) and Chin 晉 (265–420) periods are commonly known in intellectual history as the age of Neo-Taoism, and it is often assumed that after the fall of the Han empire, the Confucian method (*ju-shu* 儒術) was also eclipsed. Yet, as Yü Ying-shih 余英時 and others have pointed out, the Confucian form of life at the societal level not only continued but even flourished. The emergence of lineage organisations, clan cooperatives, and family rules in this period, all defined in Confucian terms, clearly indicates that, despite the disintegration of the Confucian polity, Confucian norms played an important role in society.[21]

Even during the Sui 隋 (581–618) and T'ang 唐 (618–907) dynasties, when Buddhism was the predominant spiritual force in Chinese society, Confucian classics, history, and ritual studies developed further. The completion of the

---

[18] Han Yü, "Yüan Tao 原道" (The origin of the Way), in *Ch'ang-li ch'üan-chi* 昌黎全集 (Complete works of Han Yü), 5 vols. (Shanghai: Commercial Press, 1918), 2: 11/6b.

[19] *Analects* 9:5.

[20] For an example of the conflict between Confucians and Legalists, see *Chung-kuo ssu-hsiang shih* 中國思想史 (History of Chinese thought), Hou Wai-lu 侯外廬 et al., eds. 5 vols. (Beijing: Jen-min 人民, 1957), 2:172–80.

[21] See Yü Ying-shih, "Han-Chin chih chi shih chih hsin-chih-chüeh yü hsin-ssu-ch'ao" 漢晉之際士之新自覺與新思潮 (The new awakening of the literatus and new currents of thought in the transition between Han and Chin), *Hsin-ya hsüeh-pao* 新亞學報 (New Asia journal), 5, no. 1 (1959): 25–144.

commentaries, and subcommentaries of the Thirteen Classics, the compilation of the T'ang codes, the composition of great works in historiography
and in instituional history, and the elaborate effort to analyse Confucian
rituals signify the high level of T'ang scholarship in Confucian studies.[22]

What we see from Mencius to Han Yü, then, is a broadening of the
Confucian project to include political and social practices in its overall
concern. Ironically, it was the Confucian institutionalisation of polity and
the Confucian ritualisation of society that enabled Han Yü to lament that
the true message of Confucian humanism had been lost for more than a
thousand years. What Han Yü and the defenders of the Confucian Tao
wanted was not the minimum survival of Confucian ethics but the maximum
expression of Confucian truth; they wanted the most authentic manifestation
of the Confucian way of life. This quest for a holistic vision grounded in
Confucian spirituality led to a redefinition of the Confucian project. The
defenders of the Confucian Tao were no longer satisfied with Confucianism
as a political ideology and a social norm. They wanted to make the teachings
of the sages the centre of their form of life. To be sure, they were deeply
concerned about politics and society, but they took Confucian self-realisation
as their ultimate concern. They clearly set a new priority: political and
social practicality had to radiate from self-cultivation. The classical Confucian
ideal, "inner sageliness and outer kingliness",[23] became a defining characteristic of their rediscovered "learning of nature and destiny" (*hsing-ming chih
hsüeh* 性命之學).

Undoubtedly, without the rise of Buddhism in China and the Chinese
transformation of Buddhism,[24] the second epoch of Confucian humanism
could not have come about. Despite the broadening of the Confucian project, the Chinese intellectual scene from the third to the tenth century was
dominated by the introduction, growth, maturation, and transformation of
Buddhism.[25] Viewed from a comparative perspective, it is one of the most
significant chapters of intercultural communication in human history. The
scope, depth, and lasting effect of the Indian influence on China represent

[22] Edwin G. Pulleyblank, "Neo-Confucianism and Neo-Legalism in T'ang Intellectual Life, 755–805",
in *The Confucian Persuasion*, Arthur F. Wright, ed. (Stanford: Stanford University Press, 1960), 77–114.

[23] The *locus classicus* for this expression is found in *Chuang Tzu* 莊子, chap. 32. See *Chuang Tzu yin-te*
莊子引得 (Index to *Chuang Tzu*; Cambridge, Mass.: Harvard-Yenching Institute, 1947), 91/33/15.

[24] The following monographs are pertinent to this issue: Erik Zürcher, *The Buddhist Conquest of China:
The Spread and Adaptation of Buddhism in Early Medieval China* (Leiden: Brill, 1959); and Kenneth
K. S. Ch'en 陳觀勝, *The Chinese Transformation of Buddhism* (Princeton: Princeton University Press, 1973).

[25] Arthur Wright, *Buddhism in Chinese History* (Stanford: Stanford University Press, 1959).

a phenomenon laden with far-reaching implications.[26] It signifies, for one thing, the universality of the Buddhist message and the receptivity of the Chinese mind.

The emergence of Neo-Confucian thought in response to the challenge of Buddhism has often been portrayed as a departure from the cosmopolitan spirit of the T'ang. The rise of narrowly defined official orthodoxy may give the impression that Neo-Confucianism as a political ideology was inextricably linked with a form of xenophobic culturalism. The history of China from Sung to Ch'ing 清 is a story of conquest dynasties. Neo-Confucianism, with its emphasis on legitimacy in historiography and authenticity in culture, aroused interest in ethnicity and proto-national sentiments. However, it is ill-advised to associate Neo-Confucianism with exclusivistic Chineseness, let alone with a particular Chinese dynasty, be it Sung 宋 or Ming 明 (1368–1644). The historical record speaks for itself. As the story of Neo-Confucianism unfolds, we see that the term is a generic one covering not only Sung–Ming Confucianism but Chin 金 (Jurchin, 1115–1234) Confucianism, Yüan 元 (1271–1368) Confucianism, and Ch'ing (1644–1912) Confucianism. By stretching the term, we may also include Chosŏn 朝鮮 dynasty (1392–1910) Confucianism in Korea, Tokugawa 德川 (1600–1867) Confucianism in Japan, and Later-Le 李 dynasty (1428–1789) Confucianism in Vietnam. As our awareness of the complexity sharpens, we may even find the term "Neo-Confucianism" misleading.

A distinctive feature of the second epoch of Confucian humanism is the spread of Confucianism to Korea, Japan, and Vietnam. As Shimada Kenji 島田虔次 implies, it is parochial to describe Confucianism as Chinese; it is Korean, Japanese, and Vietnamese as well.[27] Confucianism has never extended beyond East Asia; unlike Buddhism, Christianity, or Islam, it is not a world religion. It has not yet transcended the linguistic boundary. Even though Confucian classics are now available in English translation, the Confucian message still seems inextricably entwined with written Chinese. However, it is at least conceivable that, if there is a possibility for the development of a third epoch of Confucian humanism, its message will be communicable in languages other than Chinese.

Levenson's analogy of the relationship between vocabulary and language is particularly pertinent in this connection.[28] The revival of Confucianism

---

[26] Kenneth K. S. Ch'en, *Buddhism in China: A Historical Survey* (Princeton: Princeton University Press, 1964), 471–86.

[27] This is what I interpret as the implicit message in Shimada's article, "Chan-hou Jih-pen Sung-Ming li-hsüeh yen-chiu te kai-k'uang" 戰後日本宋明理學研究的概況(A survey of Sung-Ming Confucian studies in postwar Japan), *Chung-kuo che-hsüeh* 中國哲學 (Chinese philosophy; Beijing) 7(1983): 146–58.

[28] Levenson, *Confucian China* 1:156–63.

in the tenth century ushered in a new epistemic era partly because it created a new language, indeed, a new grammar of action. The Sung Confucians absorbed much from Taoism and Buddhism. Their vocabulary of self-cultivation was greatly enriched by Taoist and Buddhist ideas. A strong and yet open sense of identity enabled them to take advantage of symbolic resources in other ethicoreligious traditions without losing the main thrust of their own spiritual direction. Since they advocated an all-inclusive human way that neither denies nor belittles nature and heaven, they tried to incorporate a wide range of experience as a constitutive part of their ultimate concern. They firmly believed that their thoughts engaged reality and characterised what they taught as "real learning" (*shih-hsüeh* 實學).[29] To them, "nature and destiny", "body and mind" (*shen-hsin* 身心), and "principle and vital force" (*li-ch'i* 理氣) were all real. The moral metaphysics[30] that they constructed as a collective enterprise provided the final justification for their teaching. Prior to the impact of the West, East Asian polity, society, and, to a great extent, psychology were shaped by Confucian values. The language and, indeed, the grammar of action of the East Asian people was distinctively Confucian.

Modern Transformation

Since the middle of the nineteenth century, Confucian China has undergone unprecedented transformation. The Opium War of the 1840s and the Taiping Rebellion of the 1850s signalled a perpetual pattern of "domestic trouble and foreign invasion" in modern Chinese history. The abortive Self-Strengthening Movement that followed was symptomatic of the impotence of the Chinese leadership in dealing with Western aggression. The encroachment of the Western powers from the coast to the interior and the total collapse of the Chinese defense occurred in one generation. By the time of the Reform Movement in 1898, Wei Yüan's 魏源 (1794–1857) recommendation, "Learn their superior technology in order to control them",[31] made more than half

---

[29] It should be noted that, although the term *shih-hsüeh* has often been rendered as "practical learning", its occurrence in Ch'eng I's 程頤 writings, cited by Chu Hsi in his preface to the *Great Learning*, clearly shows that *shih-hsüeh* is opposed to *hsü-wen* 虛文 ("ephemeral literature", referring to the literary studies required for the examinations) and to *k'ung-li* 空理 ("empty principle", referring to the Buddhist doctrine of *śūnyatā*), and that the term is also used by Sung masters to define what Confucian learning really entails.

[30] The expression is used by Mou Tsung-san to characterise the Sung-Ming Confucian approach to questions about ontology and cosmology. See Mou Tsung-san, *Hsin-t'i yü hsing-t'i* 心體與性體 (The substance of mind and the substance of nature), 3 vols. (Taipei: Cheng-chung 正中, 1968), 1:115–89.

[31] *China's Response to the West: A Documentary Survey, 1839–1923*, Ssu-yü Teng 鄧嗣禹 and John K. Fairbank, eds. (Cambridge, Mass.: Harvard University Press, 1954).

a century previously, had been tried, it was thought, and had failed. The T'ung-chih Restoration 同治中興 (1862–74), depicted by Mary Wright as the last stand of Chinese conservatism, was not sufficient to turn the tide.[32] K'ang Yu-wei's 康有為 (1858–1927) radical attempt in 1898 to reform all the institutions — military, economic, political, and educational — lasted for only one hundred days. His vision for the Age of the Great Unity was truly utopian, for it was "nowhere" and, for all practical purposes, irrelevant.[33]

Liang Ch'i-ch'ao 梁啟超 (1873–1929), K'ang Yu-wei's disciple, described his teacher's "New Text" interpretations of the Confucian tradition as "a cyclone, a mighty volcanic eruption, and a huge earthquake".[34] The furor that K'ang created among conservative scholars marked an important change in Confucian rhetoric. We may not accept Liang's glorification of K'ang Yu-wei as the Confucian Martin Luther, but K'ang was revolutionary in his action as well as in his vision. K'ang's speculations about the ideal state significantly changed Confucian discourse. If Confucius was a reformer in K'ang's sense, Confucianism was not only a reformist ideology but also a comprehensive utopia. For K'ang, Confucianism had little to do with differentiation and hierarchy. It was thoroughly universalistic. In order to modernise Confucianism, K'ang felt free to draw inspiration from many sources — Taoist, Buddhist, Christian, social Darwinian, and scientific sources, as well as common sense. His eclecticism supplied a significant new context for Confucian scholarship. His attempt to undermine the scholasticism of the Ch'ien-Chia 乾嘉 (1736–1820) period aroused much resentment among the "Old Text" scholars, notably Chang Ping-lin 章炳麟 (T'ai-yen 太炎, 1868–1936). Thanks to K'ang's unrestrained imagination, the shape of the Confucian tradition became indeterminate and thus susceptible to a wide range of interpretations.[35] As the Confucian repertoire expanded, however, its core curriculum became problematic.

This becomes apparent in the case of Liang Ch'i-ch'ao. Levenson defines Liang's intellectual predicament as one of emotional attachment to Chinese

---

[32] Mary Wright, *The Last Stand of Chinese Conservatism: The T'ung-chih Restoration, 1862-1874* (Stanford: Stanford University Press, 1957).

[33] For a comprehensive study of K'ang, see Kung-ch'üan Hsiao 蕭公權, *A Modern China and a New World: K'ang Yu-wei, Reformer and Utopian, 1858-1927* (Seattle: University of Washington Press, 1975). See also Jonathan Spence, *The Gate of Heavenly Peace: The Chinese and Their Revolution, 1895-1980* (New York: The Viking Press, 1981), 1–60.

[34] Quoted from Wing-tsit Chan, *Source Book in Chinese Philosophy* (Princeton: Princeton University Press, 1969), 724. For the original statement, see Liang Ch'i-ch'ao, *Intellectual Trends in the Ch'ing Period*, Immanuel C. Y. Hsü 徐中約, trans. (Cambridge, Mass: Harvard University Press, 1959), 94.

[35] Wolfgang Bauer, *China and the Search for Happiness*, Michael Shaw, trans. (New York: The Seabury Press, 1976), 300–29.

history and intellectual commitment to Western values.[36] This is a controversial judgment. As Benjamin Schwartz's subtle analysis of Yen Fu 嚴復
(1854–1921) shows, the dichotomy of China and the West, or the dichotomy
of history and value, is too simplistic a scheme to account for how an
intellectual mind like Liang Ch'i-ch'ao's actually works. Often the truth lies
somewhere in between. Its elusiveness can only be overcome by nuanced
investigation.[37] Nevertheless, Liang's seemingly unlimited selection of sources
may well have been a reflection of his inability to find a niche for his intellectual enterprise. This sense of spiritual homelessness must have been acute
for the sensitive minds of his generation.

The effort of some of the most influential intellectuals during the May
Fourth period (1917–21) to criticise Confucianism was on the surface the
result of an existential choice by progressive Chinese youth to make a clear
break with China's feudal past: familialism, authoritarianism, antiquarianism,
passivity, submission, and stagnation were their targets. However, underlying
their elated sense of liberation was an extremely persistent and destructive
cynicism. The slogan "wholesale Westernisation" was probably embraced
by only a small minority of the iconoclasts, but it was symptomatic of a
widespread attitude. The demand for radical change was so overwhelming and
the inability of the political structure to make any adjustment so obvious
that the level of frustration among concerned intellectuals became unbearable.
The situation was not at all conducive to quiet reflection and deep thinking.
The tendency toward action was so strong that the very act of writing was
transformed into a weapon for effecting concrete changes in society. Escapism
became rampant merely as a reaction to this collective impulse to be engagé.
The political question dominated the intellectual scene.[38] When Wei Yüan
offered his advice on how to deal with urgent matters on the coast in the
1840s, the issue of cultural identity was not even raised. Chang Chih-tung's
wishful thinking in the 1890s was at least a compromise between identity
and adaptation. The May Fourth Westernisers accepted the survival of the
Chinese race and nation as the supreme goal; for them, cultural identity
consisted of its instrumental value in helping China to adapt to a new order
defined in Western terms.

[36] Levenson, *Confucian China* 1:107–8, 2:37. For a critique of Levenson's position, see Hao Chang,
Liang Ch'i-ch'ao and Intellectual Transition in China, 1890–1907 (Cambridge, Mass.: Harvard University
Press, 1971), 224–37.

[37] For an example of this nuanced approach to modern Chinese intellectual history, see Benjamin I.
Schwartz, *In Search of Wealth and Power: Yen Fu and the West* (Cambridge, Mass.: Harvard University,
1964).

[38] Tse-tsung Chow 周策縱, *The May Fourth Movement: Intellectual Revolution in Modern China* (Cambridge,
Mass.: Harvard University Press, 1960), 19–40.

Ironically, at the time that Chinese youth, especially students, were demonstrating great patriotism and nationalism, Confucianism was being thoroughly criticised as a defining characteristic of Chineseness. What had made China and, indeed, East Asia a society of ritual and music was now blamed as the cause of backwardness in the Chinese economy, polity, society, and culture. Hu Shih 胡適 was not entirely serious when he announced that the Chinese cultural essence was foot binding and opium smoking.[39] Lu Hsün 魯迅, however, was absolutely serious in his scathing attack on "Confucius and Sons".[40] Ch'en Tu-hsiu's 陳獨秀 (1879–1942) short-lived magazine *New Youth* was not particularly informative in its promulgation of science and democracy, but its comments on Confucianism were devastating.[41] Mao Tse-tung's 毛澤東 depiction of the "three bonds" (*san-kang* 三綱) as the authoritarianism of the ruler, the father, and the husband was in perfect accord with the May Fourth appraisal of the Confucian heritage.[42]

The writers of *New Youth* believed that the introduction of Western ideas to China was predicated on a fundamental turnabout of Chinese attitudes toward Western currents of thought and that the rejection of the Confucian mode of thinking was a precondition for China's modernisation. For the brief period when virtually all major intellectual trends in vogue in America and Europe found a sympathetic audience in China, the sense that China was on the verge of an enlightenment was truly contagious. John Dewey and Bertrand Russell felt the excitement during their sojourns in China.[43] Liberalism, pragmatism, vitalism, idealism, socialism, anarchism, evolutionism, positivism, and scientism all seemed to have a brilliant future in

[39] For Hu Shih's strategy to present the dark side of Chinese culture as a way of undermining the complacency of the traditionalists, see his three essays on faith and reflection (*hsin-hsin yü fan-hsing* 信心與反省) in *Hu Shih lun-hsüeh chin-chu* 胡適論學近著 (Recent scholarly writings of Hu Shih; Shanghai: Commercial Press, 1935), 479–99.

[40] Chow, *The May Fourth Movement*, 308–12.

[41] Ibid., 58–61.

[42] Mao Tse-tung, "Hunan nung-min yün-tung k'ao-ch'a pao-kao" 湖南農民運動考察報告 (Report on the investigation of the peasant movements in Hunan), in *Mao Tse-tung hsüan-chi* 毛澤東選集 (Selected works of Mao Tse-tung), 4 vols (Peking: Jen-min, 1951), 1:32–35.

[43] For Dewey, see *Tu-wei wu-ta yen-chiang* 杜威五大演講 (Five major lectures by Dewey), recorded by Mu-wang 毋忘 et al. (Peking: Ch'en-pao she ts'ung-shu 晨報社叢書, 1920); *John Dewey's Lectures in China, 1919-1920*, Robert W. Clopton and Tsuin-chen Ou, trans. and eds. (Honolulu: University Press of Hawaii, 1973); Barry Keenan, *The Dewey Experiment in China* (Cambridge, Mass.: Harvard University Press, 1977). For Russell, see *Lo-su chi Po-la-k'o chiang-yen chi* 羅素及勃拉克講演集 (Collection of lectures by Russell and Dora Black), recorded by Li Hsiao-feng 李小峯 et al. (Peking: Wei-i jih-pao she ts'ung-shu, 1921); Suzanne P. Ogden, "The Sage in the Inkpot: Bertrand Russell and China's Social Reconstruction in the 1920s", *Modern Asian Studies* 16, no. 4 (1982): 529–600.

the thirsty minds of Chinese youths. In retrospect, it seems extraordinary that Marxism-Leninism emerged as the predominant ideological force less than two decades after the founding of the Chinese Communist Party in 1921. Li Ta-chao 李大釗 (1888–1927), the nationalist who saw the Leninist theory of imperialism as a way for China to become independent, was for years a lone voice hailing "The Victory of Bolshevism!"[44]

This description of the May Fourth intellectual ethos may give the impression that the Westernisers failed to make any positive contribution to a fair-minded appraisal of Confucian tradition. This is not the case, for by formulating an all-out attack on Confucius and his followers, the Westernisers rendered it virtually impossible for any reflective literatus to embrace the Confucian heritage uncritically. They forced the small coterie of thinkers who were committed to a living tradition of Confucianism to introduce fresh perspectives on their chosen tradition. Thus the Westernisers of the May Fourth generation paradoxically performed a great service: by their effort to prove the incompatibility of the Confucian value orientation and the spirit of modernisation, they helped purify Confucian symbolism.

The most serious damage to the public image of Confucianism did not come from the frontal attack organised by the liberals, anarchists, socialists, and other Westernisers. It came from the extreme right, specifically from the warlords and collaborating traditionalists who used Confucian ethics to stabilise their control. The notorious attempt of Yüan Shih-k'ai 袁世凱 (1858–1916) to revive the state cult of Confucius for the purpose of realising his own imperial ambitions must have provoked much anti-Confucian sentiment among the revolutionaries. Yüan's monarchical fiasco of 1915, as J. K. Fairbank calls it,[45] was most detrimental to the Confucian cause. Those who saw a gleam of a Confucian revival in Yüan's monarchical movement were totally disillusioned. Those who were directly involved were shown to have been either fools or knaves. Unfortunately, this corruption of Confucian symbols from within was continued by other warlords for at least another generation. Lu Hsün, for example, was repeatedly surprised by the haunting power of Confucian ghosts throughout China.[46] The vicious circle of frontal

---

[44] Maurice Meisner, *Li Ta-chao and the Origins of Chinese Marxism* (Cambridge, Mass.: Harvard University Press, 1967), 60–70.

[45] J. K. Fairbank, E. D. Reischauer, and A. M. Craig, *East Asia: Tradition and Transformation* (Boston: Houghton Mifflin Company, 1973), 756.

[46] Lu Hsün, "Sui-kan lu san-shih-pa" 隨感錄三十八 (Random Thoughts, no. 38), *Hsin ch'ing-nien* 新青年 (New youth) 5, no. 5 (November 15, 1918): 515–18. For a thought-provoking analysis of Lu Hsün's "complex consciousness", see Yü-sheng Lin, *The Crisis of Chinese Consciousness: Radical Antitraditionalism in the May Fourth Era* (Madison: University of Wisconsin Press, 1979), 142–51.

attack and internal corruption made Confucianism either a scapegoat for China's sins or a sinister ideology for beguiling the innocent.

Contemporary Situation

Needless to say, circumstances made it painful for a conscientious intellectual to philosophise in the true spirit of Confucian humanism. The few Confucian thinkers who managed to do so, often with originality and brilliance, deserve our particular attention. Methodologically, two sources of inspiration contributed to the revival of creative thinking in the Confucian tradition in the post-May Fourth era. One was the critical spirit of the West. In 1921 Chang Chün-mai 張君勱 (Carsun Chang, 1886–1969), who had accompanied Liang Ch'i-ch'ao to the Paris Peace Conference after World War I, proposed a new way of reexamining the national heritage in the perspective of a philosophy of life.[47] He later devoted himself to forming the Democratic Socialist Party as a way of integrating Western liberal democracy with Confucian socialism.[48] Although his "third force" made little impact on the Chinese political scene, he was a pioneer in using comparative philosophical methods to analyse Neo-Confucian thought.[49] Carsun Chang turned his attention to scholarship in the 1940s, but by then Fung Yu-lan 馮友蘭 and Ho Lin 賀麟 had reinterpreted the Confucian project in the light of Western philosophy. Whereas Fung reformulated Chu Hsi's system in the light of New Realism, Ho interpreted Wang Yang-ming's philosophy of mind from the viewpoint of German Idealism.[50]

Another source of inspiration came from Buddhism, specifically from Yogācāra (or the Consciousness Only) school. The revival of this tradition, under the leadership of Ou-yang Ching-wu 歐陽竟无 (1871–1943) and Abbot T'ai-hsü 太虛 (1889–1947), stimulated a great deal of original thinking among

---

[47] Charlotte Furth, *Ting Wen-chiang: Science and China's New Culture* (Cambridge, Mass.: Harvard University Press, 1970), 99–135. See also *Sources of Chinese Tradition*, Wm. T. de Bary, Wing-tsit Chan, and Chester Tan, comps., 2 vols. (New York: Columbia University Press, 1960), 2:172–81.

[48] Carsun Chang, *The Third Force in China* (New York: Bookman Associates, 1952).

[49] Carsun Chang, *the Development of Neo-Confucian Thought*, 2 vols. (New York: Bookman Associates, 1957–62).

[50] For Fung, see his *Hsin li-hsüeh* 新理學 (New learning of the principle; Ch'ang-sha 長沙: Commercial Press, 1939); *Hsin yüan-jen* 新原人 (New origins of man; Chungking 重慶: Commercial Press, 1943); *Hsin yüan-tao* 新原道 (New origins of the Way; Shanghai 上海: Commercial Press, 1945). For Ho, see his *Tang-tai Chung-kuo che-hsüeh* 當代中國哲學 (Contemporary Chinese philosophy; Nanking: Sheng-li, 1947).

Chinese intellectuals.[51] The analytical method of the Yogācāra, particularly its psychoanalytical technique, helped scholars in China to study human life and the world holistically. Although there is no clear evidence that Liang Shu-ming, Alitto's "last Confucian", directly benefited from the Yogācāra methodology, he was deeply influenced by Buddhism. His *Eastern and Western Cultures and Their Philosophies*, published in 1921, "championed Confucian moral values and aroused the Chinese to a degree seldom seen in the contemporary world"[52] by comparing the Sinitic worldview with the Indian view on the one hand and with the Western on the other. Hsiung Shih-li, who also drew inspiration from Buddhism, received his analytical training in a Buddhist institute under the tutelage of Master Ou-yang. Considered one of the most profound and original thinkers in contemporary China, Hsiung reconstructed Confucian metaphysics on the basis of a critique of Yogācāra presuppositions.[53]

It has been argued that Hu Shih's pragmatic approach to the issues of contemporary China failed partly because of his strong stand against "isms".[54] The triumph of Marxism in filling the ideological vacuum left by "bourgeois" scholars preoccupied with academic pursuits and a problem-solving mentality seemed inevitable. Yet the Chinese Communist movement, significantly shaped by nationalist sentiments, undertook the task of sinicising Marxism from the beginning. As a result, Confucianism figures prominently in this supposedly materialist interpretation of Chinese history and society. The shape of Confucian thought in Chinese Marxism is, however, one-sided. Because of Marxism's insistence on a simplistic and highly partisan view of history as a struggle between materialism and idealism, it relegates to the background such great architects of the Confucian project as Mencius, Tung Chung-shu 董仲舒 (ca. 179–ca. 104 B.C.), Chu Hsi, and Wang Yang-ming. Confucian thinkers with a perceived materialist predilection, such as Hsün Tzu, Wang Ch'ung 王充 (27–100?), Chang Tsai, and Wang Fu-chih 王夫之 (1619–92), receive much attention. Nevertheless, the Confucian question, whether concerned with evaluating the historical role of Confucius or determining the proper line of cultural inheritance for socialist China,

---

[51] Holmes Welch, *The Buddhist Revival in China* (Cambridge, Mass.: Harvard University Press, 1968), 51–71, 117–20.

[52] Chan, *Source Book*, 743.

[53] Hsiung Shi-li, *Hsin wei-shih lun* 新唯識論 (New exposition of the Consciousness-Only doctrine), 3 vols. (Beijing: Peking University Press, 1933).

[54] Jerome B. Grieder, *Hu Shih and the Chinese Renaissance: Liberalism in the Chinese Revolution, 1917–1937* (Cambridge, Mass.: Harvard University Press, 1970), 173–216.

continues to occupy the centre stage in intellectual debates.[55] As the Cultural Revolution unfolded, Levenson began to wonder how his earlier thesis that the Confucian heritage had been relegated to a museum of the past could be compatible with the fanfare of anti-Confucian campaigns. He had to accept that, beyond a doubt, Confucian symbolism was relevant to contemporary Chinese political culture.[56]

During the last thirty years Confucian humanism has developed significantly in Taiwan and Hong Kong. The New Asia College in Hong Kong, founded on the principle of revitalising the true spirit of Confucian education, played a key role in coordinating individual efforts to promulgate Confucian learning. Under the leadership of Ch'ien Mu 錢穆 and the aforementioned T'ang Chün-i, the college trained a generation of scholars in the study of various dimensions of Confucian culture. Especially noteworthy in their scholarship is their philosophical focus. Ch'ien and T'ang, later assisted by two intellectual luminaries from Taiwan, Mou Tsung-san and Hsü Fu-kuan, provided the most comprehensive curriculum for the study of Confucian thought in recent memory.[57] Even though the college has been incorporated into the Chinese University of Hong Kong, its position as a centre of Confucian studies has remained strong.

The situation in Taiwan is less focused. Since the most prestigious institute of higher learning on the island was dominated in the 1950s and 1960s by refugee scholars from Peking University, the intellectual atmosphere was not congenial to Confucian learning. Mou Tsung-san, first at Taiwan Normal University and later at Tunghai University, and Hsü Fu-kuan at Tunghai University were involved in a lonely struggle to deliver the Confucian message. The situation in the 1970s, however, was considerably different. Fang Tung-mei's 方東美 (Thomé Fang) impassioned lectures on Chinese philosophy at Taiwan and Fu-jen 輔仁 universities aroused a generation of young scholars to enthusiasm for investigating the spirit of Confucian

[55] Tu Wei-ming, "Confucianism: Symbol and Substance in Recent Times", *Asian Thought and Society: An International Review* no. 1 (April 1976): 42–66; also in Tu Wei-ming, *Humanity and Self-Cultivation* (Berkeley: Asian Humanities Press, 1979), 257–96. For an example of the surge in Confucian studies in the People's Republic of China, see *Lun Sung-Ming li-hsüeh* 論宋明理學 (On Sung-Ming Confucianism; Hangchou 杭州: Chekiang jen-min 浙江人民, 1983). This collection includes more than thirty essays originally contributed to the international conference on Sung-ming Confucian thought held in Hangchou, October 15–21, 1981.

[56] Joseph Levenson, "Communist China in Time and Space: Roots and Rootlessness", *The China Quarterly*, no. 39 (July–September 1969): 1–11.

[57] Briefly mentioned in Chang, *Development of Neo-Confucian Thought*, preface.

culture.[58] The surge of interest in Confucian studies in Taiwan in recent years, however, has been complicated by a lack of differentiation between official ideology, which promotes Confucianism as an anti-Communist weapon, and genuine scholarly pursuit. Surely, Confucian learning, by definition, is more than a genuine scholarly pursuit. Yet the distinction between the Confucian intention to moralise politics and the politicisation of Confucian values for ideological control is not only meaningful intellectually but also significant politically.

The question of a third epoch of Confucian humanism has been addressed by scholars such as T'ang Chün-i, Hsü Fu-kuan, and Mou Tsung-san. Indeed, their lifelong work has been to demonstrate that the possibility not only exists in their own minds and in the minds of those who share their vision but has also been realised in the acts of philosophising, the practices of writing, and the exemplary teachings of numerous like-minded intellectuals around the world. The real challenge to them is how a revived Confucian humanism might answer questions that science and democracy have raised. Even though these questions are alien to traditional Confucianism, they are absolutely necessary for China today. In a deeper sense, these scholars perceive the challenge to be the formulation of a Confucian approach to the perennial human problems of the world: the creation of a new philosophical anthropology, a common creed, for humanity as a whole. They are aware that concern for the survival of the Confucian tradition and for the continuity of traditional Chinese culture must be subsumed under a broader concern for the future of humankind. To them, what is at stake is not the relevance of the popular idea of the Confucian literatus to a functionally differentiated modern society but a much larger issue — the well-being of humanity — which can provide a locus for meaningful existence in our world, present and future.[59]

The Future

There is no way to predict the future direction of the Confucian humanism envisioned by T'ang, Hsü, and Mou. Given the fruitful indications to date, however, we can suggest the steps by which such a project can be further developed. If the well-being of humanity is its central concern, Confucian

---

[58] For a succinct account of Fang's philosophy, see Thomé H. Fang, *Creativity in Man and Nature* (Taipei: Linking Publishing Co., 1980).

[59] See "A Manifesto for a Reappraisal of Sinology and Reconstruction of Chinese Culture", signed by Carsun Chang, T'ang Chün-i, Mou Tsung-san, and Hsü Fu-kuan, in Chang, *Development of Neo-Confucianism Thought* 2:455–83.

humanism in the third epoch cannot afford to be confined to East Asian cultures. A global perspective is needed to universalise its concerns. Confucians can benefit from dialogue with Jewish, Christian, and Islamic theologians, with Buddhists, with Marxists, and with Freudian and post-Freudian psychologists. The attempt to analyse Confucian ideas in terms of Kantian and Hegelian categories, an attempt that has yielded impressive results, will have to be broadened to accommodate new philosophical insights in the twentieth century.

The Confucian response to the West must not weaken its roots in East Asian cultures. Interregional communication among Confucian scholars in Japan, South Korea, Taiwan, Hong Kong, and Singapore may lead to a genuine intellectual exchange with scholars in the People's Republic of China. The internal dynamics of China in the post-Cultural Revolutionary era are likely to generate unprecedented creativity in Confucian studies. Confucian scholars in North America and in Europe can take an active role in bringing all these dialogues into a continuing conversation.[60] Such conversation may bring about a communal critical self-consciousness among concerned Confucian intellectuals throughout the world. Original thinking from Confucian roots, the kind that Levenson felt no longer possible, may very well reemerge to inspire productive scholarship. Vitaly Rubin's prophetic insight, in the Levensonian sense, is historically significant.

---

[60] For two recent attempts to address this issue, see Wm. T. de Bary, *The Liberal Tradition in China* (Hong Kong: The Chinese University Press; New York: Columbia University Press, 1983), 91–108, and Tu, *Confucian Ethics Today: The Singapore Challenge*.

9
Iconoclasm, Holistic Vision, and Patient Watchfulness: A Personal Reflection on the Modern Chinese Intellectual Quest

Joseph R. Levenson, in his thought-provoking interpretation of Confucian China and its modern fate, lamented that "there has been so much forgetting in modern Chinese history" and that "the current urge to preserve, the historical mood, does not belie it." To underscore "the forgetting", he thought fit to conclude a story of China with a tale of the Hasidim:

> When the Baal Shem had a difficult task before him, he would go to a certain place in the woods, light a fire and meditate in prayer – and what he had set out to perform was done. When a generation later the "Maggid" of the Meseritz was faced with the same task he would go to the same place in the woods and say: We can no longer light the fire, but we can still speak the prayers – and what he wanted done became reality. Again a generation later Rabbi Moshe Leib of Sassov had to perform this task. And he, too, went into the woods and said: We can no longer light a fire, nor do we know the secret meditations belonging to the prayer, but we do know the place in the woods to which it all belongs – and that must be sufficient; and sufficient it was. And when another generation had passed and Rabbi Israel of Rishin was called upon to perform the task he sat down on his golden chair in his castle and said: We cannot light the fire, we cannot speak the prayers, we do not know the place, but we can tell the story of how it was done.[1]

Notwithstanding the suggestiveness of the Hasidic parable for our appreciation of the perennial problem of the gradual erosion of a cherished tradition –

---

[1] Joseph R. Levenson, *Confucian China and Its Modern Fate: A Trilogy* (Berkeley: University of California Press, 1968), vol. 3, pp. 124–125.

especially of a prophetic one with its sacred place, its religious ritual, and its esoteric meditation signifying an intimate "I–Thou" relationship with the transcendent – its relevance to the Chinese situation is ambiguous. For one thing, as Lin Yü-sheng 林毓生 notes, " one of the most striking and peculiar features of the intellectual history of twentieth-century China has been the emergence and persistence of profoundly iconoclastic attitudes toward the cultural heritage of the Chinese past."[2] If we must employ the theme of "forgetting" to depict the antitraditional mentality of the modern Chinese intellectual, we may have to imagine a sort of voluntary and active forgetting, in fact an outright rejection of and a frontal attack on tradition. As Benjamin Schwartz points out in his foreword to Lin's seminal study on modern Chinese "totalistic iconoclasm", China, "often regarded in the West as the very paradigm of traditionalism" during the nineteenth century, "had become for many the land of revolution – a society which had effected a total, fundamental break with the entire cultural and social order of the past" by the mid-twentieth century.[3]

Paradoxically, even iconoclastic intellectuals inadvertently subscribed to certain of the enduring "Confucian" presuppositions: "the notion of the integrated wholeness of culture, the notion that every aspect of society and culture could somehow be controlled through the political order, and the notion that conscious ideas could play a decisive role in transforming human life."[4] Indeed, these notions that "formed a powerful, widely shared syndrome of ideas within the cultural tradition"[5] contribute to the ambivalences and complexities of modern Chinese intellectual discourse.

When Lin Tse-hsü 林則徐 (1785–1850), judged by the distinguished British diplomat and Sinologist, H. A. Giles, to be "a fine scholar, a just and merciful official, and a true patriot",[6] sent his celebrated letter to Queen Victoria in 1839, his argument against the opium trade – expressing all the moral indignation characteristic of the Confucian scholar-official – showed that he had good reasons for taking an uncompromising attitude toward "those who smuggle opium to seduce the Chinese people and so cause the spread of the poison to all provinces". He was absolutely certain that "such persons

---

[2] Lin Yü-sheng, *The Crisis of Chinese Consciousness: Radical Antitraditionalism in the May Fourth Era* (Madison: The University of Wisconsin Press, 1979), p. 3.

[3] Ibid., p. ix.

[4] Ibid., pp. x–xi.

[5] Ibid., p. xi.

[6] William Theodore de Bary, et. al., comp., *Sources of Chinese Tradition*, 2 vols. (New York: Columbia University Press, 1964), vol. 2, p. 6.

who only care to profit themselves, and disregard their harm to others, are not tolerated by the laws of Heaven and are unanimously hated by human beings".[7]

While Lin's moral tone may sound naive and unrealistic to us, with our advantage of hindsight and knowledge of China's mighty fall from the Middle Kingdom to a semicolonial state in a few decades, he in fact spoke from the perspective of "a totally integrated social-cultural-political order presided over by a class which managed to embody within itself both the spiritual and political authority of the society".[8] Though such a perception was much more myth than reality, "the endurance of tradition seemed to be a function of its all-encompassing wholeness"[9] in imperial China.

A generation later, when Tseng Kuo-fan 曾國藩 (1811–1872) decided to send young men in their teens abroad to study superior Western technology as an integral part of the "self-strengthening" movement in 1871, he proposed that there be "interpreters and instructors to teach them Chinese literature from time to time, so that they will learn the great principles for the establishment of character, in the hope of becoming men with abilities of use to us".[10] Prepared to take bold measures to learn from the West, to make compromises in Sinic education to achieve practical ends, he was clearly willing to reorder his sense of priority, no longer certain that the world would long be governed by the principles that seemed so reasonable to him.

Yet, in Tseng's mind, the price exacted for some measure of Westernisation was not only affordable but painless. While he raised the issue of cultural identity in response to the challenge of the T'aiping Rebellion under the leadership of a Christian convert, the danger of a radical rejection of the Confucian tradition – not only by feeble minds corrupted by Western influences but by some of the most brilliant shapers of the Chinese intellectual landscape – was almost beyond his imagination. Tseng, an exemplar of the scholar-official, a distinguished literatus, an accomplished calligrapher, a sophisticated interpreter of Sung 宋 (960–1279) learning, an able administrator, and an effective military commander, had no doubt (as is evidenced in his copious writings) that the transformative potential of the Confucian tradition was great.

---

[7] Ibid.

[8] Benjamin Schwartz attributed this perception to China as the symbol of unchanging tradition; see Lin Yü-sheng, *The Crisis of Chinese Consciousness*, p. ix.

[9] Ibid.

[10] De Bary, *Sources*, vol. 2, p. 51.

When K'ang Yu-wei 康有為 (1858–1927) used his reinterpreted Confucianism as an ideological basis for reforming imperial institutions in 1898, the Confucian moral order was significantly compromised. To accommodate the Western impact as both a cultural challenge and as a military threat, the grammar of action, defined in terms of wealth and power, gained ascendency on the intellectual scene. A sense of urgency, prompted by the belief that the survival not only of the imperial polity but also of the Chinese form of life depended on the success of basic institutional changes, led him to undertake a comprehensive examination of all the available symbolic and spiritual resources for social reconstruction in the Confucian tradition.[11]

Chang Chih-tung's 張之洞 (1837–1909) catchphrase, "Chinese learning as substance (*t'i* 體) and Western learning as function (*yung* 用)",[12] coined in the same period, shows how an eclectic blending of indigenous cultural values and imported Western ideas was deemed necessary to provide an ideological formula for coping with the Western tide.

The "difficult task" of the Chinese intellectual, defined by the charismatic Liang Ch'i-ch'ao 梁啓超 (1873–1929) was fourfold. Liang wrote:

> I therefore hope that our dear young people will, first of all, have
> a sincere purpose of respecting and protecting our civilisation;
> secondly, that they will apply Western methods to study our civilisation
> and discover its true character; thirdly, that they will put our
> civilisation in order and supplement it with others' so that it will
> be transformed and become a new civilisation; and fourthly, that
> they will extend this new civilisation to the outside world so that
> it can benefit the whole human race.[13]

Levenson perceived in Liang's wishful thinking the dilemma common to the mind of modern China: an emotional attachment to China's past and an intellectual commitment to Western values.[14] Yet underlying all such intellectual efforts to come to grips with Confucian China and its modern transformation was the strong faith in the ability of human consciousness

---

[11] Hao Chang 張灝, *Chinese Intellectuals in Crisis: Search for Order and Meaning, 1890–1911* (Berkeley: University of California Press, 1987), pp. 21–65. Professor Chang's focused investigation of the ethico-religious world views of four of the major intellectual figures of this transitional era is most illuminating for understanding the breakdown of the Confucian moral-spiritual order and Chinese intellectuals' struggle to recreate a new holistic vision to fill the vacuum.

[12] De Bary, *Sources*, vol. 2, p. 82.

[13] Ibid., p. 187.

[14] Levenson first formulated this interpretive thesis in his *Liang Ch'i-ch'ao and the Mind of Modern China* (Cambridge, MA: Harvard University Press, 1953). For a summary of his argument, see his *Confucian China*, pp. ix–x.

to understand and to shape historical reality. While the undifferentiated masses might not have the vision or the persuasive power to effect fundamental changes in society, it was both the duty and the responsibility of the intelligentsia to do so.

The generation of the May Fourth Movement (1919), witnessing the abortive attempt by the Nationalist Revolution to bring about an integrated polity after the collapse of the imperial dynasty, resorted to a wide-ranging iconoclastic attack on the Confucian tradition. This was seen as a strategic move intended to prepare the ground for "wholesale Westernisation". For a brief time, China was hospitable to virtually all brands of Western thought: liberalism, pragmatism, vitalism, anarchism, socialism, romanticism, idealism, and nihilism each found a sympathetic and indeed enthusiastic audience.

In less than four generations after the Opium War, many of the most articulate members of the Chinese intelligentsia, notably those who had studied abroad, deliberately relegated their cultural identity to the background, taking it for granted that China's survival depended on her ability to adapt to the brave new world now defined in Western terms. It was perhaps no accident that Sun Yat-sen 孫逸仙 (1866–1925), the paradigmatic revolutionary, emerged as a political leader and national hero from the periphery of traditional Confucian culture.

Yet, without exception, Chinese intellectuals remained obsessed with Chinese culture, past and present. Nowhere in China is there a counterpart to the radical Fukuzawa Yukichi 福澤諭吉 (1835–1901), who, despite his solid Confucian education, openly advocated the policy of "cutting loose from Asia" to allow Japan successfully to play the Social Darwinian game. Ironically, the great scholarly accomplishments of the Chinese westernisers were principally in traditional Chinese studies. The lifelong work of Yen Fu 嚴復 (1853–1921), who singlehandedly translated the works of Thomas Huxley, John Stuart Mill, Herbert Spencer, Adam Smith, and others into classical Chinese, was an exception.[15] Yet, even in the case of Yen Fu, as the recent publication of his completed works in the People's Republic of China shows, his primary concern was with Chinese studies.

This combination of cultural iconoclasm and cultural obsession made the relationship of the post–May Fourth intellectuals to their Confucian tradition both ambivalent and complex. The deliberate effort to forget was never fully realised; conscious rejection and unconscious identification with traditional symbols and values were pervasive among the most influential figures in Chinese intellectual life. Levenson speculated as to whether the

[15] For a thought-provoking study of Yen Fu, see Benjamin I. Schwartz, *In Search of Wealth and Power: Yen Fu and the West* (Cambridge, MA: Harvard University Press, 1964).

modern fate of Chinese culture, so unlike the museumisation of ancient Egyptian culture by foreign curators, was not also a sort of museumisation. He wrote:

> By making their own museum-approach to traditional Chinese culture, the Chinese kept their continuity without precluding change. Their modern revolution — against the world to join the world, against their past to keep it theirs, but past — was a long striving to make their museums themselves. They had to make their own accounting with history, throwing back a new line, and holding fast to it, while heading in quite the opposite direction.[16]

This reading of the ability of Chinese intellectuals to detach themselves from the past by externalising and objectifying it so that it may be safely packaged for display is too optimistic, if not simple-minded. The truth of the matter is that the Chinese intelligentsia — including many who were consistently iconolastic — maintained unacknowledged, often unconscious, continuities with the culture of the past on every level of life: behaviour, attitude, belief, and commitment.[17]

The gradual erosion of the Chinese intellectual's faith in the viability of Confucian culture to sustain the fundamental restructuring of the Chinese polity (an inevitable consequence of Westernisation) may be witnessed in Lin Tse-hsü's moralism, by way of Tseng Kuo-fan's pragmatism, K'ang Yu-wei's reformism, and Chang Chih-tung's eclecticism, which eventually led to the iconoclasm of the May Fourth generation. Lin believed in the power and authority of the Celestial Court and the place of the Middle Kingdom under Heaven; he thought that he knew the proper ritual for dealing with uncivilised foreigners, and was confident that he possessed the spiritual resources to expiate sins against humanity. Tseng believed also that China was the centre of the world, that she had the spiritual resources to strengthen her national defence, but he was willing to learn the formula, the know-how, from the West. Although K'ang continued to believe in the supremacy of the imperial system and Confucian culture, he recommended drastic measures to revitalise both. For him, China's place in the world, her methods of governance, and the spiritual resources she could command in coping with the unprecedented crisis in her history had all become problematic.

Chang Chih-tung's eclecticism, rightfully dismissed by Levenson as a

---

[16] Levenson, *Confucian China*, vol. 3, p. 124.

[17] Schwartz notes in his aforementioned "Foreword": "The unconscious and unacknowledged continuities with the culture of the past on every level of life in contemporary China are being thoroughly examined." See Lin Yü-sheng, *The Crisis of Chinese Consciousness*, p. x.

fallacious rationalisation, was a desperate attempt "to consolidate Chinese devotion to Chinese culture in the modern world of western techniques":

> Chinese learning, which was to be the *t'i* [substance] in the new syncretic culture, was the learning of a society which had always used it for *yung* [function], as the necessary passport to the best of all careers. Western learning, when sought as *yung*, did not supplement Chinese learning – as the neat formula would have it do – but began to supplant it. For in reality, Chinese learning had come to be prised as substance because of its function, and when its function was usurped, the learning withered. The more western learning came to be accepted as the practical instrument of life and power, the more Confucianism ceased to be *t'i*, essence, the naturally believed-in value of a civilisation without a rival, and became instead an historical inheritance, preserved, if at all, as a romantic token of no-surrender to a foreign rival which had changed the essence of Chinese life.[18]

The sense of crisis experienced by the Chinese intellectual after 1895, when Japan, having successfully transformed herself into a Western-style power, threatened China militarily as a full-fledged imperialist, cannot be adequately appreciated in a traditional–modern/China–West dichotomy.[19] The psychocultural dynamics of the Chinese intellectual community, informed by a profound historical consciousness, added layers of complexity to the public debates, which, on the surface, seemed to follow neatly the two-line struggle between the traditionalists and the westernisers.

Wang Kuo-wei's 王國維 (1877–1927) agony was symptomatic. Caught between idealism and pragmatism, he, an aspirant philosopher, ruefully remarked that what he really loved (idealistic claims of the life of the Spirit) was no longer believable; what he believed to be true (empirical proofs in natural sciences) was utterly unlovable.[20] The painful recognition that the culture of the past, with its richly textured history, philosophical insight,

---

[18] Levenson, *Confucian China*, vol. 1, p. 61.

[19] For an informed critique of this sort of dichotomous methodology, see Paul A. Cohen, *Discovering History in China: American Historial Writing on the Recent Chinese Past* (New York: Columbia University Press, 1984).

[20] Wang's autobiographic account of how he gradually lost interest in philosophy is worth noting:
> In general those philosophical theories that can be loved cannot be believed, and those that can be believed cannot be loved. I seek truth and yet I love mistaken forms of it. Great metaphysics, rigourist ethics, and pure aesthetics – of these we are inordinately fond. However, in searching for what is believable, we turn instead to the positivistic theory of truth, the hedonistic theory of ethics, and the empiricist theory of aesthetics. I know the latter are believable but I cannot love them, and I know the former are lovable but I cannot believe. This has caused me great distress during the last two or three years.

See Joey Bonner, *Wang Kuo-wei: An Intellectual Biography* (Cambridge, MA: Harvard University Press, 1986), p. 95.

aesthetic sensibility, and literary taste could not be entrusted with the urgent task of "saving the nation", that Western ideas of science and democracy, functionally necessary for making China wealthy and powerful, did not in fact move the heart or inspire the soul, made many a Chinese intellectual both emotionally frustrated and intellectually unfulfilled.

The story of the life of the mind of the modern Chinese intellectual has yet to be told. The sense of urgency with which he or she has been impelled to deal with personal, familial, communal, or national crisis has not so far been congenial to long-term scholarship or deep thinking. The psychology of uncertainty, caused by continuous wars, hunger, and famine, not to mention political persecution, social unrest, and economic chaos, has constantly haunted the intelligentsia. It is understandable that for the overwhelming majority the political questions have loomed large. For them, the contemplative life was never a real option; at best, it was a dispensable luxury. The demand for relevance, participation, and activism was so overwhelming at times that those who opted for teaching or writing almost always developed a profound sense of guilt. The historical allusion to Pan Ch'ao 班超, who, fired by a strong patriotic impulse, threw his writing brush on the ground and joined the army, became a pervasive theme in the profile of the modern Chinese intellectual.

Ironically, as the intelligentsia accepted the rhetoric of relevance, with participation and activism appearing as the authentic way to engage in the struggle to save the nation, the rationale that the intellectual community was a centre of critical reflection and long-term deliberation was relegated to the background. As a consequence, the politicisation of culture became inevitable. The unreflective patriotism of the Chinese intellectual undermined the power of the pen as a prime weapon of social and political criticism in modern China. The spirit of self-sacrifice, with its attendant willingness to subordinate all personal concerns to the well-being of the group, motivated by an idealism to involve one's body and soul actively in the revolution to save China, served to weaken the intelligentsia in a way unprecedented in Chinese history.

The triumph of Marxism-Leninism as a political ideology demonstrates this point. When the Chinese Communist Party was founded in 1921, the philosophies of Kant, Schopenhauer, Nietzsche, Bergson, James, Dewey, and Russell were all more important than that of Marx. Although Li Ta-chao 李大釗 (1888–1927) enthusiastically hailed the victory of Bolshevism in an article published in the influential *New Youth* 新青年 in 1918, his Marxist study club, with its messianic hope for the future, attracted very few recruits. The intellectual debates that centred around scientism and the philosophy of life in the early 1920s were dominated by pragmatists and idealists.

The upsurge of interest in Marxism-Leninism politically may be attributed to the increasing popularity of the Soviet Union as a revolutionary model. Ideologically, however, the fact that Marxism-Leninism was Western to the core, while thoroughly critical of imperialism, made its persuasive power overwhelming to many totally iconoclastic and fiercely nationalistic intellectuals. Also, the breakdown of the traditional order in the economic, political, and social realms did much to generate a powerful ferment among Chinese intellectuals:

> Nothing is untouched: the self, the idea of nature, the relation to
> the other person, to the family, the group, the State. Love, ambition,
> respect, friendship, all are challenged at such intimate depths that
> anger becomes a protective reaction, pride a defence, hatred a strategy
> and contempt a reflex.[21]

The demand for a holistic vision — a worldview that would situate the Chinese problem in a global context, in a broad historical perspective — was urgent. Hu Shih 胡適 (1891–1962), inspired by Dewey's pragmatic instrumentalism and frightened by Marxist-Leninist ideology, urged his followers to avoid "isms" and to concentrate all their efforts on solvable problems. His plea for reason, liberty, and independent-mindedness was widely interpreted as being both unrealistic and irrelevant, if not positively selfish. After all, Dewey's instrumentalism grew out of the safe academic environment of the United States; it was never intended to address the burning issues of the kind that confronted the Chinese intellectual. A totalistic ideological turn was almost inevitable.

While the timeliness of the Marxist-Leninist ideology, as embodied in the Soviet revolutionary model, may have captured the imagination of the Chinese intelligentsia, it was the participation of the peasantry, the perpetual carriers of traditionalism, that fundamentally changed the political dynamics of the country and eventually brought about a revolution. The principal beneficiary of the rise of communism in China was not the intelligentsia, however instrumental it may have been in providing the symbolic resources that helped form a broad consensus, thereby preparing the whole nation for it. Though the Chinese Communist Party explicitly demanded a total iconoclastic break with the feudal past, it was in fact nativist to the core. Mao Tse-tung 毛澤東 (1893–1976) may have been a creative interpreter of Marxism-Leninism, but he was by no means a westerniser. Even discounting what has been revealed of Mao's style of leadership during the Cultural Revolutionary period (1966–1976), Mao Tse-tung's thought was

---

[21] François Geoffroy-Dechaume, *China Looks at the World* (New York: Pantheon, 1967), p. 131.

a deliberate attempt to bring Marxist-Leninist modes of analysis to bear upon the concrete situation in China; as such, it functioned primarily in a Chinese linguistic universe.

However, the Chinese linguistic universe that produced the thought of Mao Tse-tung and that was subsequently influenced by it cannot be seen as traditional. One does not prove Mao's traditionalism by pointing to his frequent use of historical allusions, conventional expressions, and classic literary styles; the message Mao tried to convey was iconoclastic; the utopia he envisioned was communist. Still, by and large, he was a traditionalist; his aesthetic sensibility, life-style, political skills, self-image, and conceptual apparatus were reflected in his familiarity with Chinese poetry, fiction, history and thought.

While the Chinese communists may have emerged from peasant movements and guerrilla warfare — and while the Long March and the Yenan Spirit certainly evoke sensations of earthiness, symbolically explaining why the Red Star over China is inherently rural rather than urban, nativistic rather than foreign — and while there is much truth in all such characterisation — the other side of the coin must also be considered. Chinese communists, as nationalists, returned students, intellectuals, and ideologists, are also the self-assigned inheritors of May Fourth iconoclasm. The Chinese Communist Party, Leninist in its conception and organisation, assumed the role of "saving the nation" as its manifest destiny. The belief that Marxism smashed the two great mountains — feudalism and imperialism — that had blocked China's way toward modernity for decades led to the self-righteous claim that the wave of the future was neither Western nor Chinese but socialist, combining the most "progressive" elements of both.

The intelligentsia's active participation in this, or at least its tacit acceptance of the communist agenda for "saving the nation", was crucial for developing an ideology with broad popular appeal. If Mao's investigation of peasant conditions in the heartland of Chinese agriculture in the 1920s helped him design a strategy for reordering China's power relationships (which involved the development of tactics of class struggle and brainwashing), his constant wrestling with intellectuals also taught him the complex art of symbolic control.

Symbolic control, in this sense, refers to a governing mechanism that gains its coercive, persuasive power through its appeal to cultural values and social norms. While legal sanctions are also applied, these are used only as a last resort. Social order is maintained not by law but by ritual. Members of the community, with varying degrees of sophistication, all have personal knowledge of the boundaries within which they interact as centres of specific relationships, not as isolated individuals. Underlying all overt behaviour and revealed attitudes, but also in subtle and inarticulate signs of human interaction, is a tacit understanding of what is acceptable, what is expected of each member. A seasoned member knows precisely the operational rules that derive from such understanding. This is not to say that individual members tend to think and act alike according to standards imposed from above; it does suggest, however, that the governing mechanism relies heavily on shared values and norms. Leaders cannot afford to take lightly a society's value orientation as a political force that is capable of enhancing or undermining their authority and power in consensus formation.

Mao and other founding members of the Chinese communist movement in the Party, but also in the government and in the army, were absolutely serious about ideology. The slogan "politics is in command" means more than that the civilian is in control of the military; it implies that every aspect of society, civilian as well as military, has to be guided by principles that emanate from the power centre, where a holistic vision of China's destiny resides.

The intellectuals, especially well-known professors and prominent writers, are not in this sense "rootless cosmopolitans"; they are dangerous shapers of public opinion. Having privileged access to the holistic vision because they have helped formulate it as the core of the sinicised socialist ideology, at least in principle, they have the authority to suggest an alternative vision, formulating such a new vision when occasion demands it. Theoretically, and occasionally in practice, Chinese intellectuals have exercised their right to criticise the state and the symbolic resources used by the state to legitimise both its *modus operandi* and its very existence. The thoroughness and incisiveness with which political, social, and cultural criticism was directed against the Party and its legitimising ideology during the Hundred Flowers campaign in 1957 clearly demonstrates that when intellectuals are given the opportunity, they are not unwilling to be outspoken critics. However, it is one thing to be thoroughly and incisively critical of a regime, and quite another to become an active dissident as a declaration of conscience.

The authentic possibility of becoming a dissident in Chinese political culture is very limited. Neither the political push nor the ideological pull has ever been strong enough. Historically, the Chinese intelligentsia was an integral part of the governing mechanism of the body politic. Although tension existed between the ruling minority and the cultural elite, the examination system (a Confucian contribution to social mobility in traditional China) enabled the literati to staff the higher echelons of the bureaucracy. As a result, politics was seen not only as a power game but also as an exercise of symbolic control. The intellectuals' role, as the most articulate members of society, was crucial to the success of any such governing mechanism. It is difficult to imagine that the imperial court in traditional China actually imposed Confucian ideology on the literati; rather, the literati, as carriers of the Confucian Way, initiated, implemented, and judged the whole process of symbolic control from the political and bureaucratic centre. Marxism-Leninism, as an implanted young ideology in the historical landscape of China, was imposed on the intelligentsia by the central government. However, given the fact that the rise of Marxism-Leninism in China was neither the result of an international conspiracy nor a domestic misunderstanding, but was a deliberate ideological choice made by the intellectuals (instrumental in creating the agenda intended to save the nation), it is entirely conceivable that they see themselves as the carriers of the socialist message. If they remain the government's collaborators, despite wave after wave of anti-intellectual campaigns, it is in large measure due to their perception that they have actually participated in the formation of the holistic vision of nation building. Chinese intellectuals may well be economically disadvantaged and politically oppressed; they are not ideologically alienated.

The collective memory of China's modern fate is so vividly implanted in the mind of every educated Chinese that — despite significant differences among historians' interpretations and evaluations of each major event — the chronology illustrated by Lin's abortive attempt to stop the British, Tseng's self-strengthening effort to catch up with the West, K'ang's reform inspired by the Meiji Restoration, and Sun Yat-sen's revolution, later guided or misguided by the Russians, shows that saving the nation is of great historical significance: that nothing else deserves more focused attention. By comparison, the fate of any single individual, however painfully unfair, can never match the cumulative injustice and humiliation that China, as a civilisation-state, has endured in modern times.

The personification of China's woes in literature, history and philosophy — in textbooks and the mass media — has done much to heighten the awareness of the young. Each generation relives and reexperiences the century-long tragedy of China, sharing a poignant sense that new painful realities will have to be endured as well. No one in the Chinese cultural universe is spared this historical and existential weight. While the Chinese have never known the Holocaust, they have suffered collectively a series of holocausts, a few self-inflicted by the people of the "land of ritual and rites", as the traditional Confucian scholar would choose to characterise the Middle Kingdom.

The Chinese intellectuals' desire for a strong centre, dictated by the modern conception of wealth and power as the essential imperatives for national survival, has been so pervasive that weakness, backwardness, and poverty have seemed even more heinous than dictatorship. Ting Wen-chiang 丁文江 (1888–1936), the champion of scientism, is alleged to have told his liberal friends that if Chiang Kai-shek 蔣介石, could defeat the Japanese by becoming a dictator, there was nothing wrong with dictatorship. It is well to recall that the communists, as well as anarchists and liberals, joined the Nationalist government in its fight against Japanese aggression. If Chiang had faded from the scene in the early 1940s, he would be honoured today as a national hero in China. The prestige that Sun Yat-sen now enjoys on both sides of the Taiwan Strait seems to have come from the perception that he was single-mindedly committed to the Nationalist cause. The deification of Mao in the Cultural Revolutionary period (1966–1976) may have been an aberration in this long and strenuous effort to find an incorruptible centre from which a holistic vision of national reconstruction could be persuasively articulated and effectively implemented. Mao's strength in mobilising a nationwide revolution came not from the power centres of the bureaucracy but from the authority of ideology. His ability to shape profoundly the direction of national sentiment may be attributed to his strategic choice not to exercise power directly through the Party apparatus. Had he, for example, been closely associated with implementing the Party's educational policies, he would have lacked the leverage to deal with the student demonstrations in the summer of 1968.

The reasons why ideology is still vitally important in China are many. To begin with, the mass mobilisation of energy from various echelons of the society to achieve national goals depends on the ability of the leadership to set the course of collective action in terms understandable and persuasive to the country as a whole. Because the agenda for saving the nation since the late nineteenth century has demanded a concerted effort to involve every Chinese (including those overseas), the art of persuasion, with emphasis on credibility, public-spiritedness, and goodwill, is not so much moralising propaganda as an essential ingredient that defines Chinese society.

Lurking behind the scene, however, is the dilemma of the May Fourth Chinese intellectual – caught between the necessity to learn from abroad and the urgency of consensus formation based on a shared cultural identity at home – which continues to haunt the communists. The vicious circle of wholesale Westernisation, together with the Boxer mentality, which generates both strong admiration for and rejection of foreignism, continues to aggravate all the highly charged ideological debates. Moreover, the imposition of a superficially domesticated ideology on a bureaucracy that is deeply rooted in peasant traditionalism has made the political culture in the People's Republic a pattern of domination that combines feudalist traditionalism with Leninist collectivism.

Unfortunately, the intellectuals who wholeheartedly support the communist agenda have found themselves targets of attack in wave after wave of political campaigns since 1958. The Chinese Communist Party, thought to embody the messianic hope for "saving the nation", consists mainly of peasants, workers, and soldiers; the majority have little more than a primary education. Vigorous recruitment of college graduates in recent years notwithstanding, illiterates still greatly outnumber those with any experience of higher education. The confrontation between the brightest but marginalised intelligentsia and the least educated but most powerful cadres seems almost unavoidable.

Still, the intelligentsia's willing participation in this most recent joint effort to make China both strong and wealthy remains the norm. Despite the activity of highly publicised dissidents, the Chinese intellectual community as a whole has never challenged the leadership of the Party. The phenomenon of *refusenik*, a familiar and common one in the political and social landscape of the Soviet Union, is not likely to have its counterpart in China in the near future. The idea that a member of the intelligentsia, influenced by the Enlightenment ideas of the West, would deliberately alienate himself from the ideological claims of the state to live a meaningful life guided by an alternative sense of truth and reality, has never been even a rejected possibility – though, given the intellectual effervescence of recent years, it may become an authentic existential option for an increasing number of writers-as-prophets in Chinese life.

I would suggest that two new mountains have emerged after the Cultural Revolutionary earthquake: Confucian humanism and democratic liberalism. It is too early to tell whether they will block China's predetermined course toward socialism. However, the articulated goal of China's reform effort, "to build China into a great socialist modern civilisation-state with a Chinese character", suggests that the iconoclastic attack on Chinese culture as poisonous feudalism together with the total rejection of Western civilisation as bourgeois imperialism, is no longer tenable. The antispiritual pollution campaign of 1983 and the more recent criticism of bourgeois liberalism do not appear to have the support of the intelligentsia. The upsurge in comparative cultural studies, evident in the systematic annotation of major traditional Chinese works in literature, history, and philosophy but also in the comprehensive translation and interpretation of Western classics, past and present, has fundamentally restructured the ideological landscape. The relevance of Confucian humanism and democratic liberalism to the viability of Marxism, if not of Leninism, as a continuous socialist ideology in China has been imaginatively and creatively explored by some of the most seminal minds in China today. Even if we choose to believe that the power struggle in China is more a political game than an ideological debate, it is worth noting that the widely accepted way to exercise power in this political game is through ideological debate.

It appears that the ideological debate, centred on the proper way of realising the Chinese dream of building a "socialist modern civilisation-state with a Chinese character", has taken a pluralistic turn. With the influx of Western ideas and practices and the exodus of Chinese officials, scholars, and students, the intellectual discourse has become more subtle and nuanced. It must sound positively cacophonous to those who assume that the intelligentsia automatically subscribe to the Party line. The days when the Party elders could actually "set the tone" for any ideological debate are gone. In their attempt to redefine socialism, they must now confront the challenge of both Western and Chinese humanism espoused by some of the most sophisticated journalists, columnists, and Marxist theoreticians. Teng Hsiao-p'ing's 鄧小平 reformers may want to confine the current ideological discussion to the Four Modernisations of agriculture, industry, military, and technology with only limited attention to institutional adjustment, but university students have called for participatory democracy, constitutionally guaranteed liberties, and legally protected human rights as essential features of modernity. The question of how a socialist modern society with a Chinese character should evolve is particularly intriguing: Who should have the authority to interpret and judge the rightness of such a concept for the nation as a whole — intellectuals or cadres? A communal critical self-awareness of the Chinese intellectuals is taking shape. Whether or not a civic society will emerge that significantly changes the conventional pattern of symbolic control in which the state is not only omnipresent but also virtually omnipotent, the conscience of the intelligentsia has already been voiced and heard.

In the spring of 1985, I had the good fortune to offer a lecture course on Confucian philosophy in Chinese at Peking University. About 150 people attended the class, mainly graduate and undergraduate students at Peking, Beijing Normal, and People's Universities, but also members of the Chinese Academy of Sciences, visiting college teachers from other provinces, and foreign students. I was struck first by the iconoclasm on the campus. There was nothing there to evoke a feeling of a traditional Chinese academy. The campus itself, the original site of the now discontinued missionary Yenching University, is charming. Though the University is blessed with more than eighty years of history, the collective memory is remarkably short. As a response to strong student campaigns, new bronze statues of Li Ta-chao and Ts'ai Yüan-p'ei 蔡元培 (1867–1940), the famous president of the University in the May Fourth era, added a little variety to the otherwise monotonous domination of the two gigantic stone figures of Mao.

Indeed, since the founding of the People's Republic in 1949, Peking University has undergone such dramatic change that many find it traumatic to recollect what it was like even a decade ago. The idea that an academic institution such as Harvard University, founded in the Ming dynasty (1368–1644), could survive the Manchu conquest, the T'aiping Rebellion, the collapse of the Ch'ing dynasty, the Warlords, the Sino-Japanese War, and the Cultural Revolution (as I tried to suggest in conveying a sense of continuity in the history of Harvard, which was celebrating its 350th anniversary) produced only incredulous looks among my Chinese students. They found it revealing that the United States, supposedly youthful, has enjoyed an uninterrupted history with impressive traditions for more than three centuries, while the ruptures in Chinese society in modern times have been so profound that many of the most salient features of the Chinese tradition, including the kind of Confucian humanism we were disposed to study, seem little more than distant echoes.

Despite my fears that a sympathetic reading of the *Confucian Analects, Mencius, Hsün Tzu, Reflections on Things at Hand,* and *Instructions for Practical Living* might seem like outmoded feudal ideology, the response to the material and the communication among us in lectures, seminars, small group discussions, and informal conversations was extraordinary. No one seemed in the least offended when I remarked, jokingly, that I was introducing a "foreign culture" subject. They even tolerated my paraphrasing of Clifford Geertz's idea, the liberating experience of confronting radical otherness, and my suggestion that the reintroduction of Confucianism – a form of inclusive humanism, as I interpreted it[22] – could serve for comparative purposes as a "radical otherness" to the Marxist mode of analysis with which they were so familiar. In being confronted with this "foreign culture" subject, they were, in theory, being offered the possibility of a liberating experience.

Before long, however, I came to realise that Confucianism, far from being foreign, is an integral part of what a leading contemporary thinker in China, Li Tze-hou 李澤厚, persuasively argues is the "psychocultural construct" of the contemporary Chinese intellectual, no less than of the Chinese peasant. The problem, indeed, is that they have been for so long, so thoroughly, and often so unreflectively immersed in this tradition that its very familiarity has bred contempt for it. Few could see much potential for creative transformation in a feudal ideology that has so repeatedly frustrated China's quest for modernity. Indeed, their lived experience in a society shaped by traditional habits of the heart has definitively, if not

---

[22] Tu Wei-ming 杜維明, "Toward a Third Epoch of Confucian Humanism: A Background Understanding", in *Confucianism: The Dynamics of Tradition*, Irene Eber, ed. (New York: Macmillan, 1986), pp. 3–21.

conclusively, persuaded them that the Confucian heritage – the embodiment of authoritarianism, bureaucratism, nepotism, conservatism, and male chauvinism – must be thoroughly critiqued again. As iconoclasts, they are indeed children of the May Fourth movement.

My attempts to show that the Confucian tradition, as an inclusive humanism, needs to be studied for its own sake as a necessary precondition to any critical reappraisal of its modern significance struck a number of sympathetic chords in my audience, which grew substantially when I gave later presentations at other universities and at scholarly conferences in other cities. Still, on several occasions, while I was speaking, the image of Rabbi Israel of Rishin – seated in his golden chair and telling the story of how it was done – did come to mind.

Certain colleagues and students who became my friends (and, on occasion, my fellow travellers) helped, by their persistent questioning, to make me acutely aware of my own boundaries: Would I have discovered the symbolic and spiritual resources overflowing from the Confucian tradition had I myself been raised in China? Educated in Taiwan from fifth grade through college, how could I possibly appreciate the dynamic iconoclastic spirit of the May Fourth movement? My experience as both a graduate student and a college teacher in the United States since 1962 must in important ways have conditioned my sense of the Chinese reality, both past and present. How can I be thoroughly critical of China's past, when I present it to American students as a subject worth studying?

Since 1966, when I first taught a course on cultural values and social change in contemporary China at my alma mater, Tunghai University (Taiwan), I have been greatly interested in the revival of Confucian studies in industrial East Asia. The interest was enhanced in 1982 when I accepted the challenging task of trying to introduce Confucian ethics to interested secondary school students in Singapore. To be sure, the narrowly defined Weberian question of identifying the functional equivalent of the Protestant ethic in the so-called post-Confucian states (Japan, South Korea, Taiwan, Hong Kong, and Singapore) did not greatly excite my intellectual passion, though I became fascinated by the profound implications that the Weberian mode of analysis has for both comparative cultural and religious studies. Today, examining the contribution that the Confucian tradition can make to human self-understanding in an increasingly secularised and pluralistic world, together with exploring the authentic possibility of thinking both philosophically and religiously about perennial human concerns from Confucian roots, are projects that delight me. While motivated by a strong desire to give a sympathetic and fair reading of the Confucian message to students at Peking University when the opportunity presented itself, might

I have given more emphasis to the tragic fact that the great Confucian ideas, as they became crystallised in the power relationships of an oppressive polity, must inevitably enslave the mind, had I been exposed firsthand to its contemporary manifestation?

China is today at an ideological crossroads. The inner strength of the Chinese intelligentsia has been sapped by the collusion of feudal Chinese traditionalism (the remnants of a politicised Confucian moralism) and modern Western collectivism (the outmoded practices of Leninist dictatorship). To release and cultivate the vital energy for self-transformation, the Chinese intellectuals need to tap the resources of both their own tradition and that of the West. That is possible if they are able to identify the two narrow ridges between traditional feudalism and Confucian humanism, between bourgeois capitalism and democratic liberalism. If they are willing to attain the new by reanimating the old, to revitalise the self by embodying the other, a fruitful path could be the creative interaction between Confucian humanism and democratic liberalism in a socialist context. That, in Edward Shils's wise counsel, is "a task for patient watchfulness and tact of the utmost delicacy".[23]

---

[23] Edward Shils, *Tradition* (Chicago: The University of Chicago Press, 1981), p. 330.

Bibliography of
Tu Wei-ming

1968

"The Creative Tension between *Jen* and *Li*", *Philosophy East and West*, XVIII: 1–2 (January–April 1968), 29–39.

The Quest for Self-Realization – A Study of Wang Yang-ming's Formative Years (1472–1509), thesis presented to the Committee on the Degree of Doctor of Philosophy in History and Far Eastern Languages (Harvard University, 1968), 271 pp.

"Towards an Integrated Study on Confucianism", paper presented to the 14th International Congress of Philosophy (Wien: Akten des XIV Kongresses für Philosophie, 2–9 September, 1968), V:532–537.

1970

Traditional China, coedited with James T. C. Liu (Prentice-Hall, 1970), 179 pp.

San-nien ti hsü-ai 三年的畜艾 (Three years of cultivating the moxa; Taipei: Chih-wen 志文 Book Co., 1970), 191 pp.

"The Unity of Knowing and Acting – From a Neo-Confucian Perspective", in *Philosophy: Theory and Practice*, ed., T. M. P. Mahadevan (Madras: Proceedings of the International Seminar on World Philosophy, December 7–17, 1970), pp. 190–205.

1971

"The Neo-Confucian Concept of Man", *Philosophy East and West* XXI:1 (January 1971), 79–87.

"Mind and Human Nature", review article, *The Journal of Asian Studies*, XXX:3 (May 1971), 642–647.

1972

"*Li* as Process of Humanization", *Philosophy East and West*, XXII:2 (April 1972), 187–201.

1973

"Jih-pen T'ien-li ta-hsüeh ts'ang 'Wang Yang-ming chiang-hsüeh ta-wen ping ch'ih-tu' chüan ch'u-t'an 日本天理大學藏王陽明講學答問並尺牘卷初探 (A preliminary examination of Wang Yang-ming's unpublished letters from the T'ien-li University collection in Japan), *Ta-lu tsa-chih* 大陸雜誌, XLVI:3 (March 1973).

"Subjectivity and Ontological Reality – An Interpretation of Wang Yang-ming's Mode of Thinking", *Philosophy East and West*, XXIII: 1–2 (January–April 1973), 187–205.

"Wang Yang-ming ta Chou Tao-t'ung shu wu-feng" 王陽明答周道通書五封 (Wang Yang-ming's five unpublished letters to Chou Tao-t'ung), *Ta-lu tsa-chih*, XLVII:2 (August 1973).

"On the Spiritual Development of Confucius' Personality", paper read at the XXVII International Congress of Orientalists in Ann Arbor, Michigan (August 7, 1967), *Ssu-yü yen* 思與言 (Thought and Word), XI:3 (September 1973), 29–37.

1974

"An Introductory Note on Time and Temporality", *Philosophy East and West*, XXIV:2 (April 1974), 119–122.

"Reconstituting the Confucian Tradition", review article, *The Journal of Asian Studies*, XXXIII:3 (May 1974), 441–454.

"An Inquiry into Wang Yang-ming's Four-Sentence Teaching", *The Eastern Buddhist*, new series VII:2 (October 1974), 32–48.

1975

"Yen Yüan: From Inner Experience to Lived Concreteness", in *The Unfolding of Neo-Confucianism*, ed., Wm. T. de Bary (New York: Columbia University Press, 1975), pp. 511–541.

1976

"Ou-yang Te", in *Dictionary of Ming Biography*, eds., L. Carrington Goodrich and Chaoying Fang (New York: Columbia University Press, 1976), pp. 1102–1104.

"The Confucian Perception of Adulthood", *Daedalus*, 105:2 (April 1976), 109–123.

Centrality and Commonality: An Essay on Chung-yung, monograph no. 3 of the Society for Asian and Comparative Philosophy (Honolulu: The University Press of Hawaii, 1976), 181 pp.

"Hsiung Shih-li's Quest for Authentic Existence", in *The Limits of Change*, ed., Charlotte Furth (Cambridge: Harvard University Press, 1976), pp. 424–275; 396–400.

"Transformational Thinking as Philosophy", review article, *Philosophy East and West*, XXVI (January–April 1976), 75–80.

"Confucianism: Symbol and Substance in Recent Times", *Asian Thought and Society: an International Review*, I:1 (April 1976), 42–66.

Jen-wen hsin-ling te chen-tang 人文心靈的震盪 (The resonance of the humanist mind; Taipei: China Times Publication Co., 1976), 197 pp.

Neo-Confucian Thought in Action: Wang Yang-ming's Youth (1472–1509) (Berkeley: University of California Press, 1976), 218 pp.

"Wang Yang-ming's Youth: A Personal Reflection on the Method of My Research", *Ming Studies*, no. 3 (1976), 11–17.

1977

"Inner Experience: The Basis of Creativity in Neo-Confucian Thinking", in *Artists and Tradition, Uses of the Past in Chinese Culture*, ed., Christian Murck (Princeton: The Art Museum, Princeton University, 1977), pp. 9–15.

"Chinese Perceptions of America", in *Dragon and Eagle: United States-China Relations, Past and Future*, eds., Michel Oksenberg and Robert B. Oxnam (New York: Basic Books, 1977), pp. 87–106.

1978

"On the Mencian Perception of Moral Self-Development", *The Monist*, 61.1 (January 1978), 72–81.

"The *Problematik* of Kant and the Issue of Transcendence: A Reflection on 'Sinological Torgue'", *Philosophy East and West*, XXVIII:2 (April 1978), 215–221.

"The 'Moral Universal' from the Perspective of East Asian Thought", in *Morality as a Biological Phenomenon*, ed., Gunther S. Stent (Berlin: Dahlem Konferenzen, 1978), pp. 187–207.

"Yi Hwang's Perception of the Mind", *T'oegye Hakpo*, No. 19 (October 1978), 76–88. [Also available in Korean translation].

"T'oegye hsin-hsing lun shu-hou" 退溪心性論書後 (Further thoughts on Yi Hwang's perception of the mind), *T'oegye Hakpo*, No. 20 (December 1978), 18–21 [Available in Korean translation only].

1979

Humanity and Self-Cultivation: Essays in Confucian Thought (Berkeley: Asian Humanities Press, 1979), 364 pp.

"Shifting Perspectives on Text and History: A Reflection on Shelly Errington's Paper", *Journal of Asian Studies*, XXXVIII:2 (February 1979), 245–251.

"The Value of the Human in Classical Confucian Thought", *Humanitas*, XV:2 (May 1979), 161–176.

"Ultimate Self-Transformation as a Communal Act: Comments on Modes of Self-Cultivation in Traditional China", *Journal of Chinese Philosophy*, 6 (1969), 237–246.

"*Hsi-yu Chi* as an Allegorical Pilgrimage in Self-Cultivation", review, *History of Religions*, 19.2 (November, 1979), 177–184.

"The 'Thought of Huang-Lao': A Reflection on the Lao Tzu and Huang Ti Texts in the Silk Manuscripts of Ma-wang-tui", *The Journal of Asian Studies*, XXXIX:1 (November 1979), 95–110.

"A Note on Wittfogel's Science of Society", *Bulletin of Concerned Asian Scholars*, 11.4 (October–December 1979), 38–39.

1980

"Neo-Confucian Ontology: A Preliminary Questioning", *Journal of Chinese Philosophy* 7 (1980), 93–114.

"A Religiophilosophical Perspective on Pain", in *Pain and Society*, eds. H.W. Kosterlitz and L.Y. Terenius (Berlin: Dahlem Konferenzen, 1980), pp. 63–78.

1981

"*Jen* as a Living Metaphor in the Confucian *Analects*", *Philosophy East and West*, 31.1 (January 1981), 45–54.

"Ts'ung i tao yen" 從意到言 (From intention to word), *Chung-hua wen-shih lun-ts'ung* 中華文史論叢 (Shang-hai: January, 1981), 225–261.

"Shih-t'an Chung-kuo che-hsüeh chung ti san-ko chi-tiao" 試談中國哲學中的三個基調 (A preliminary discussion on the three basic motifs in Chinese philosophy), *Chung-kuo che-hsüeh shih yen-chiu* 中國哲學史研究 (Beijing, March 1981), 19–25.

"Kung Tzu jen-hsüeh chung ti tao hsüeh cheng" 孔子仁學中的道學政 (The Way, Learning and Politics in Confucius' Learning of Humanity), *Chung-kuo che-hsüeh* 中國哲學 (Beijing, 1981), 17–32.

1982

"T'oegye's Creative Interpretation of Chu Hsi's Philosophy of Principle", *Korean Journal*, XXII:2 (February 1982), 4–15.

"Towards an Understanding of Liu Yin's Confucian Eremitism", in Hoklam Chan and Wm. T. de Bary, eds., *Yüan Thought: Chinese Thought and Religion under the Mongols* (New York: Columbia University Press, 1982), pp. 233–277.

1983

"Perceptions of Learning (*hsüeh*) in Early Ch'ing Thought", in *Symposium in Commemoration of Professor T'ang Chün-i* (Taipei: Student Book Co., 1983), pp. 27–61.

"Die neokonfuzianische Ontologie", in Wolfgang Schluchter ed., *Max Webers Studie über Konfuzianismus und Taoismus* (Frankfurt: Suhrkam, 1983), pp 271–297. A German translation of "Neo-Confucian Ontology: A Preliminary Questioning" published in 1980.

1984

"The Idea of the Human in Mencian Thought: An Approach to Chinese Aesthetics", in Susan Bush and Christian Murck, eds., *Theories of the Arts in China* (Princeton: Princeton University Press, 1984), pp. 57–73.

"A Confucian Perspective on Learning to be Human", in *The World's Religious Traditions*, ed., Frank Whaling (Edinburgh: T. & T. Clark, 1984), pp. 55–71.

"On Neo-Confucianism and Human-Relatedness", in *Religion and Family in East Asia*, eds., George De Vos and T. Sofue (Osaka: The National Museum of Ethnology, 1984), pp. 111–125.

"The Continuity of Being: Chinese Visions of Nature", in *On Nature*, Vol. 6 of *Boston University Studies in Philosophy and Religion*, ed., Leroy S. Rouner (Notre Dame, Ind.: University of Notre Dame Press, 1984), pp. 113–129.

"Wei-Chin Hsüan-hsüeh chung ti t'i-yen ssu-hsiang – shih-lun Wang Pi 'sheng-jen t'i-wu' kuan-nien ti che-hsüeh i-i" 魏晉玄學中的體驗思想－試論王弼'聖人體無'觀念的哲學意義 (Personal experiential thought in the Wei-Chin period – a preliminary discussion on the philosophical meaning of Wang Pi's concept, "the sage embodies nothingness"), *Yen-yüan lun-hsüeh chi* 燕園論學集 (Essays in memory of T'ang Yung-t'ung's ninetieth birthday; Beijing: Peking University Press, 1984), pp. 197–213.

"Ts'ung shen-hsin-ling-shen ssu ch'en-ts'i k'an Ju-chia ti jen-hsüeh" 從身心靈神四層次看儒家的人學 (Confucian humanist learning in the four related perspectives of body, mind, soul and spirit; Hong Kong: *Ming-pao yüeh-kan* 明報月刊, December 1984), 41–44.

1985

"Sung-Ju chiao-yü kuan-nien ti pei-ching" 宋儒教育觀念的背景 ("A Background for Understanding the Idea of Education in the Sung"), trans., Lin Cheng-chen 林正珍, *Historical Review* (Taiwan University), no. 9 (January 1985), pp. 43–57.

Confucian Thought: Selfhood as Creative Transformation (Albany, New York: State University of New York Press, 1985), 203 p.

"Subjectivity in Liu Tsung-chou's Philosophical Anthropology", in *Individualism and Holism: The Confucian and Taoist Perspectives*, ed. Donald J. Munro (Ann Arbor: University of Michigan Press, 1985), pp. 215–235.

"Yi T'oegye's Perception of Human Nature: A Preliminary Inquiry into the Four-Seven Debate in Korean Confucianism", in *The Rise of Neo-Confucianism in Korea*, eds., Wm. T. de Bary and Jahyun Haboush (New York: Columbia University Press, 1985), pp. 261–281.

1986

"Ju-hsüeh ti-san-ch'i fa-chan ti ch'ien-ching wen-ti" 儒學第三期發展的前景問題 ("On the so-called 'Third Epoch of Confucian Humanism'"), *Ming-pao Monthly* 明報月刊 (Hong Kong), no. 21.1 (January 1986), pp. 27–32; no. 21.2 (February 1986), pp. 36–38; no. 21.3 (March 1986), pp. 65–68.

"An Inquiry on the Five Relationships in Confucian Humanism", in *The Psycho-Cultural Dynamics of the Confucian Family*, edited by Walter H. Slote (Seoul: International Cultural Society of Korea, 1986), pp. 175–190.

"Ts'ung shih-chieh ssu-ch'ao k'an Ju-hsüeh yen-chiu de hsin fa-chan" 從世界思潮看儒學研究的新發展 ("New Directions in Confucian Studies in the Perspective of World Thoughts"), *Chiu-chou hsüeh-k'an* 九州學刊 (Chinese Cultural Quarterly; Hong Kong: The Hong Kong Institute for Promotion of Chinese Culture, 1986), vol. 1, no. 1.

"Toward a Third Epoch of Confucian Humanism: A Background Understanding", in *Confucianism: The Dynamics of Tradition*, ed. Irene Eber (New York: Macmillan, 1986), pp. 3–21.

"The Structure and Function of the Confucian Intellectual in Ancient China", in *The Origins and Diversity of Axial Age Civilizations*, ed., S.N. Eisenstadt (Albany, New York: State University of New York Press), pp. 360–373.

"Lun Ju-chia de t'i-chih – te-hsing chih chih de han-i" 論儒家的體知－德性之知的涵義 ("On the 'Experiential Knowing' in Confucian Thought – The Implications of Moral Knowledge"), in *Ju-chia lun-li yen-t'ao-hui lun-wen chi* 儒家倫理研討會論文集 (*Collection of Essays on Confucian Ethics*), ed. Liu Shu-hsien 劉述先 (Singapore: Institute of East Asian Philosophies, 1987), pp. 98–111.

"Profound Learning, Personal Knowledge, and Poetic Vision", *The Vitality of the Lyric Voice*, eds., Shuen-fu Lin and Stephen Owen (Princeton: Princeton University Press, 1986), pp. 3–31.

1987

"The Chinese Intellectual's Way of Being Religious", *Faith*, May 1987, vol. 1, issue 1, 25–28.

"Iconoclasm, Holistic Vision, and Patient Watchfulness: A Personal Reflection on the Modern Chinese Intellectual Quest", *Daedalus*, vol. 116, no. 2 (spring 1987), 75–94.

"The Religious Situation in the People's Republic of China Today", in *Religion in Today's World*, ed. Frank Whaling (Edinburgh: T & T Clark 1987), pp. 279–291.

"A Chinese Perspective on Pain", *Acta Neurochirurgica*, Suppl. 38, 147–151 (1987).

"Confucian Studies in the People's Republic", *Humanities*, VIII: 5 (September/October 1987), 14–16, 34–35.

1988

"Confucius and Confucianism", *Encyclopaedia Britannica*, Macropaedia (15th edition, 1988), vol. 16, pp. 653–662.

"Nature in Confucian Humanism", *Essays on Perceiving Nature*, ed. Diana Macintyre Deluca (Honolulu: The Perceiving Nature Conference Committee, 1988), pp. 99–110.

"A Confucian Perspective on the Rise of Industrial East Asia", 1687th State Meeting Report, *Bulletin of the American Academy of Arts and Sciences*, vol. XLII, no. 1 (October 1988), 32–50.

"Lun Lu Hsiang-shan ti shih-hsüeh" 論陸象山的實學 (On the real learning of Lu Hsiang-shan), *Chung-kuo che-hsüeh-shih yen-chiu*, no. 32 (July 1988), 56–69.

1989

Way, Learning and Politics: Essays on the Confucian Intellectual (Singapore: The Institute of East Asian Philosophies, 1989)

Ju-hsüeh ti-san ch'i fa-chan ti ch'ien-ching wen-t'i 儒學第三期發展的前景問題(The *Problematik* of the development of the "third epoch" of Confucian learning; Taipei: Lien-ching 聯經, 1989).

Centrality and Commonality: An Essay on Confucian Religiousness, a revised and enlarged edition of *Centrality and Commonality: An Essay on Chung-yung* (Albany, New York: State University of New York Press, 1989).

Hsin-chia-p'o ti t'iao-chan: hsin Ju-chia lun-li yü ch'i-yeh ching-shen 新加坡的挑戰:新儒家倫理與企業精神 (The Singapore challenge: new Confucian ethics and the entrepreneurial spirit; Chinese translation of

Confucian Ethics Today: The Singapore Challenge; Beijing: Sanlian 三聯, 1989).

1990

Ju-chia chih-wo i-shih ti fan-ssu 儒家自我意識的反思 (Reflection on the Confucian Self-Consciousness; Taipei: Lien-ching 聯經, 1990).

1991

"Konfuzianischer Humanismus und Demokratie," in *Europa und die Civil Society*, ed. Krzysztof Michalski (Stuttgart, Germany: Klett-Cotta, 1991), pp. 222–244.

"Cultural China: The Periphery as the Center," *Daedalus*, Spring 1991, 1-32.

"The Search for Roots in East Asia: The Case of the Confucian Revival," in Martin E. Marty and R. Scott Appleby, eds., *Fundamentalisms Observed* (Chicago: University of Chicago Press).

Ju-chia ssu-hsiang hsin-lun 儒家思期新論 (A new discourse on Confucian thought, a Chinese translation of *Confucian Thought: Selfhood as Creative Self-Transformation;* Chekiang People's Publishers, 1991).

Editor, *The Triadic Accord: Confucian Ethics, Industrial East Asia, and Max Weber* (Singapore: Institute of East Asian Philosophies, 1991).

1992

"The Enlightenment Mentality and the Chinese Intellectual Dilemma," in *Perspectives on Modern China: Four Anniversaries*, eds., Kenneth Lieberthal, et al (Armonk, N.Y.: M. E. Sharpe), pp. 103–118.

"Intellectual Effervescence in China," in *Exit from Communism, Daedalus,* Spring 1992, 251-292.

Co-editor, *The Confucian World Observed: A Contemporary Discussion of Confucian Humanism in East Asia* (Honolulu: East-West Center/ University of Hawaii Press, 1992).

Jen-hsing yü chih-wo hsiu-yang 人性與自我修養 (human nature and self-cultivation, second Chinese translation of *Humanity and Self-Cultivation*; Taipei: Lien-ching 聯經, 1992).

"Core Values and the Possibility of a Fiduciary Community," in *Re-structuring for World Peace on the Threshold of the Twentieth-First Century*," eds., Katherine Tehranian and Majid Tehranian (Cresskill, New Jersey: Hampton Press, 1992), pp. 333–345.

Ju-chia ch'uan-t'ung ti hsien-tai chuan-hua: Tu Wei-ming hsin-Ju-hsüeh lun-wen chi-yao 儒家傳統的現代轉化：杜維明新儒學論文輯要 (the modern transformation of the Confucian tradition: an anthology of Tu Wei-ming's New Confucian writings), comps., Yue Hua 岳華 and Guan Tong 關東 (Beijing: Chinese Radio and Television Publishers, 1992).

Index

Index prepared by Thomas Selover